AF795352

VOLUME EIGHTY FOUR

ADVANCES IN PHARMACOLOGY

VOLUME EIGHTY FOUR

ADVANCES IN PHARMACOLOGY

Pharmacology of Restless Legs Syndrome (RLS)

Edited by

STEFAN CLEMENS

Brody School of Medicine, Department of Physiology, East Carolina University, Greenville, NC, United States

IMAD GHORAYEB

Aquitaine Institute for Cognitive and Integrative Neuroscience, Bordeaux University, CNRS-UMR 5287, Bordeaux, France

Serial Editor

S.J. ENNA

University of Kansas Medical Center, Kansas City, KS, United States

Managing Editor

LYNN LECOUNT

University of Kansas Medical Center, School of Medicine, Kansas City, KS, United States

ELSEVIER

ACADEMIC PRESS

An imprint of Elsevier

Academic Press is an imprint of Elsevier
50 Hampshire Street, 5th Floor, Cambridge, MA 02139, United States
525 B Street, Suite 1650, San Diego, CA 92101, United States
The Boulevard, Langford Lane, Kidlington, Oxford OX5 1GB, United Kingdom
125 London Wall, London, EC2Y 5AS, United Kingdom

First edition 2019

Copyright © 2019 Elsevier Inc. All rights reserved.

No part of this publication may be reproduced or transmitted in any form or by any means, electronic or mechanical, including photocopying, recording, or any information storage and retrieval system, without permission in writing from the publisher. Details on how to seek permission, further information about the Publisher's permissions policies and our arrangements with organizations such as the Copyright Clearance Center and the Copyright Licensing Agency, can be found at our website: www.elsevier.com/permissions.

This book and the individual contributions contained in it are protected under copyright by the Publisher (other than as may be noted herein).

Notices
Knowledge and best practice in this field are constantly changing. As new research and experience broaden our understanding, changes in research methods, professional practices, or medical treatment may become necessary.

Practitioners and researchers must always rely on their own experience and knowledge in evaluating and using any information, methods, compounds, or experiments described herein. In using such information or methods they should be mindful of their own safety and the safety of others, including parties for whom they have a professional responsibility.

To the fullest extent of the law, neither the Publisher nor the authors, contributors, or editors, assume any liability for any injury and/or damage to persons or property as a matter of products liability, negligence or otherwise, or from any use or operation of any methods, products, instructions, or ideas contained in the material herein.

ISBN: 978-0-12-816758-8
ISSN: 1054-3589

For information on all Academic Press publications
visit our website at https://www.elsevier.com/books-and-journals

Publisher: Zoe Kruze
Acquisition Editor: Fiona Pattison
Editorial Project Manager: Shellie Bryant
Production Project Manager: Vignesh Tamil
Cover Designer: Alan Studholme

Typeset by SPi Global, India

ELSEVIER Book Aid International
Working together
to grow libraries in
developing countries
www.elsevier.com • www.bookaid.org

Contents

Section II
Disease models/genetics

Section III
Treatments and treatment complications

Contributors

Michael Aschner
Department of Molecular Pharmacology, Albert Einstein College of Medicine, Bronx, NY, United States

Oliviero Bruni
Pediatric Sleep Center, Department of Developmental and Social Psychology, Sapienza University, Rome, Italy

Irene Cano-Pumarega
Sleep Research Institute, Madrid, Spain

Vicent Casadó
Centro de Investigación Biomédica en Red sobre Enfermedades Neurodegenerativas (CIBERNED), Madrid; Institute of Biomedicine of the University of Barcelona (IBUB); Department of Biochemistry and Molecular Biomedicine, Faculty of Biology, University of Barcelona, Barcelona, Spain

Verònica Casadó-Anguera
Centro de Investigación Biomédica en Red sobre Enfermedades Neurodegenerativas (CIBERNED), Madrid; Institute of Biomedicine of the University of Barcelona (IBUB); Department of Biochemistry and Molecular Biomedicine, Faculty of Biology, University of Barcelona, Barcelona, Spain

Francesca Casoni
Department of Clinical Neurosciences, IRCCS San Raffaele Scientific Institute, Neurology—Sleep Disorders Center, Milan, Italy

Pan Chen
Department of Molecular Pharmacology, Albert Einstein College of Medicine, Bronx, NY, United States

Brian Chiou
Department of Neurosurgery, Penn State College of Medicine, Hershey, PA, United States

Stefan Clemens
Brody School of Medicine, Department of Physiology, East Carolina University, Greenville, NC, United States

James R. Connor
Department of Neurosurgery, Penn State College of Medicine, Hershey, PA, United States

Antoni Cortés
Centro de Investigación Biomédica en Red sobre Enfermedades Neurodegenerativas (CIBERNED), Madrid; Institute of Biomedicine of the University of Barcelona (IBUB); Department of Biochemistry and Molecular Biomedicine, Faculty of Biology, University of Barcelona, Barcelona, Spain

Lourdes DelRosso
University of Washington and Seattle Children's Hospital, Seattle, WA, United States

Luigi Ferini-Strambi
Department of Clinical Neurosciences, IRCCS San Raffaele Scientific Institute, Neurology—Sleep Disorders Center; Faculty of Psychology, "Vita-Salute" San Raffaele University, Milan, Italy

Sergi Ferré
Integrative Neurobiology Section, National Institute on Drug Abuse, Intramural Research Program, National Institutes of Health, Baltimore, MD, United States

Raffale Ferri
Oasi Research Institute—IRCCS, Troina, Italy

Andrea Galbiati
Department of Clinical Neurosciences, IRCCS San Raffaele Scientific Institute, Neurology—Sleep Disorders Center; Faculty of Psychology, "Vita-Salute" San Raffaele University, Milan, Italy

Diego García-Borreguero
Sleep Research Institute, Madrid, Spain

Imad Ghorayeb
Clinical Neurophysiology Department, Clinical Neurosciences Pole, Bordeaux Teaching Hospital; Aquitaine Institute for Cognitive and Integrative Neuroscience, Bordeaux University, CNRS-UMR 5287, Bordeaux, France

Xavier Guitart
Integrative Neurobiology Section, National Institute on Drug Abuse, Intramural Research Program, National Institutes of Health, Baltimore, MD, United States

Omamuyovwi Meashack Ijomone
Department of Molecular Pharmacology, Albert Einstein College of Medicine, Bronx, NY, United States; Department of Human Anatomy, Federal University of Technology, Akure, Nigeria

Daniel D. Lam
Institute of Neurogenomics, Helmholtz Zentrum München, Neuherberg; Lehrstuhl für Neurogenetik und Institut für Humangenetik, School of Medicine, Klinikum Rechts der Isar, Technische Universität München, Munich, Germany

Giuseppe Lanza
Oasi Research Institute—IRCCS, Troina, Italy

Kun He Lee
Department of Molecular Pharmacology, Albert Einstein College of Medicine, Bronx, NY, United States

Celia Garcia Malo
Sleep Research Institute, Madrid, Spain

Estefanía Moreno
Centro de Investigación Biomédica en Red sobre Enfermedades Neurodegenerativas (CIBERNED), Madrid; Institute of Biomedicine of the University of Barcelona (IBUB); Department of Biochemistry and Molecular Biomedicine, Faculty of Biology, University of Barcelona, Barcelona, Spain

Walter Paulus
Department of Clinical Neurophysiology, University Medical Center Göttingen, Georg August University, Göttingen, Germany

César Quiroz
Integrative Neurobiology Section, National Institute on Drug Abuse, Intramural Research Program, National Institutes of Health, Baltimore, MD, United States

William Rea
Integrative Neurobiology Section, National Institute on Drug Abuse, Intramural Research Program, National Institutes of Health, Baltimore, MD, United States

Sofía Romero
Sleep Research Institute, Madrid, Spain

Aaro V. Salminen
Institute of Neurogenomics, Helmholtz Zentrum München, Neuherberg; Department of Neurology, Klinikum Rechts der Isar, Technische Universität München, Munich, Germany

Claudia Trenkwalder
Department of Neurosurgery, University Medical Center, Göttingen; Paracelsus-Elena Hospital, Center of Parkinsonism and Movement Disorders, Kassel, Germany

Quinn W. Wade
Department of Neurosurgery, Penn State College of Medicine, Hershey, PA, United States

Vivian Wanner
Instituto Europeo del Sueño, Santiago, Chile

Juliane Winkelmann
Institute of Neurogenomics, Helmholtz Zentrum München, Neuherberg; Lehrstuhl für Neurogenetik und Institut für Humangenetik, School of Medicine, Klinikum Rechts der Isar, Technische Universität München; Munich Cluster for Systems Neurology (SyNergy), Munich, Germany

Preface

Restless Legs Syndrome (RLS) is a chronic ailment of the nervous system that has only in recent years become more widely accepted as a clinical disorder with its own distinct features. Yet in the literature, evidence of this sometimes debilitating condition goes back to 1685 when the English physician Thomas Willis first described the symptoms, and it was none other than Mark Twain who let Huckleberry Finn talk in 1885 about "There was a place on my ankle that got to itching; but I dasn't scratch it .... Seemed like I'd die if I couldn't scratch. Well, I've noticed that thing plenty of times since. If you are with the quality, or at a funeral, or trying to go to sleep ... you will itch all over in upwards of a thousand places."

The Swedish neurologist Karl Ekbom first defined and used in the mid-1940s the term Restless Legs Syndrome for a "hitherto overlooked disease in the legs," but, despite a gradual and substantial increase in scientific studies since, as of 2014 "the pathophysiological features of RLS remain undetermined" (Chokroverty, N Engl J Med).

One of the key diagnostic criteria of RLS is its circadian feature, with the symptoms, which mostly or predominantly or exclusively affect the legs, occurring late in the day or in the night, but always at rest. With an overall prevalence of 3%–8% in the general population, independent of the severity, it is one of the most common and costly neurological disorders.

After a first serendipitous observation that RLS is responsive to dopaminergics subsequent studies focused on this monoamine and RLS was considered a possible dopamine-related disorder. However, more recent studies have found a lack of evidence of a dopamine dysfunction in RLS patients and highlighted the influence of familial components (genetics), iron metabolism, and underlined the role of the basal ganglia and the spinal cord as putative key areas in the CNS that mediate the symptomatology. While the pathophysiology of this disorder is extremely stereotypical in the clinic, a number of additional factors or comorbidities have been identified (gender, pregnancy, late-stage renal disease) that are associated with RLS symptoms but causality has not yet been confirmed. Pediatric cases of RLS do exist; however, the disorder usually emerges later in life, and the lack of a single clear identified trigger or cause suggests that RLS is a disorder of multifactorial origin. Mounting evidence indicates that altered genetic characteristics of select genes during early development may provide the pathophysiological environment for RLS to emerge later in life.

Dopaminergic treatments, while initially very successful when focused on inhibitory D2 and D3 receptors, have been hampered in their long-term success by the gradual emergence of adverse effects that cause a worsening of the symptoms (augmentation), tolerance, and impulse control disorder. Alternative nonspecific treatment options, originally developed to combat other diseases including neurological pain conditions, are being used to alleviate the symptomatology and target Ca^{2+} channels, glutamate and GABA pathways, as well as adenosine, opioid receptors, and the cannabinoid system. Other avenues, including iron supplementation therapies, are explored to mitigate some of the contributing factors with however unpredictable results.

Over the past decade, new developments have deepened our understanding of RLS, its possible genetic and other causes, its symptomatology, and its responsiveness to the different drug classes. New pharmacological tools and approaches, both basic science and in the clinic, are being used to address many of the unmet needs for RLS patients. Yet, and surprisingly, despite these efforts, the corresponding dysfunctions in the underlying sensorimotor presentation are still not fully understood. This volume provides a summary of these recent advances in the field, whether dissecting the roles and interactions of genes as obtained from human GWAS studies, the cooperation of different dopamine receptors with each other or with other receptor families in animal models of RLS, or the impact of the different treatment options in the clinic.

We are sincerely grateful to our colleagues and friends who are contributing to this volume, and we hope that the selected cross sections of these latest developments will provide a useful reference for researchers of the RLS community, and hopefully/possibly even beyond.

Stefan Clemens
Brody School of Medicine,
Department of Physiology,
East Carolina University,
Greenville, NC, United States

Imad Ghorayeb
Aquitaine Institute for Cognitive and Integrative Neuroscience,
Bordeaux University, CNRS-UMR 5287,
Bordeaux, France

SECTION I

Pathophysiology

CHAPTER ONE

Adenosine mechanisms and hypersensitive corticostriatal terminals in restless legs syndrome. Rationale for the use of inhibitors of adenosine transport

Sergi Ferré[a,*], César Quiroz[a], William Rea[a], Xavier Guitart[a], Diego García-Borreguero[b]

[a]Integrative Neurobiology Section, National Institute on Drug Abuse, Intramural Research Program, National Institutes of Health, Baltimore, MD, United States
[b]Sleep Research Institute, Madrid, Spain
*Corresponding author: e-mail address: sferre@intra.nida.nih.gov

Contents

Abstract

Our working hypothesis is that a hypoadenosinergic state is a main pathogenetic factor that determines the sensory-motor symptoms and hyperarousal of restless legs syndrome (RLS). We have recently demonstrated that brain iron deficiency (BID) in rodents, a well-accepted animal model of RLS, is associated with a generalized downregulation of adenosine A_1 receptors (A1R) in the brain and with hypersensitivity of corticostriatal glutamatergic terminals. Here, we first review the experimental evidence for a pivotal role of adenosine and A1R in the control of striatal glutamatergic transmission and the rationale for targeting putative downregulated striatal A1R in RLS patients, which is supported by recent clinical results obtained with dipyridamole, an inhibitor of the

ISSN 1054-3589
https://doi.org/10.1016/bs.apha.2018.12.005

nucleoside transporters ENT1 and ENT2. Second, we perform optogenetic-microdialysis experiments in rats to demonstrate that A1R determine the sensitivity of corticostriatal glutamatergic terminals and the ability of dipyridamole to counteract optogenetically-induced corticostriatal glutamate release in both animals with BID and controls. Thus, a frequency of optogenetic stimulation that was ineffective at inducing cortico-striatal glutamate release in control rats became effective with the local perfusion of a selective A1R antagonist. Furthermore, in animals with and without BID, the striatal application of dipyridamole blocked the optogenetic-induced glutamate release and decreased basal levels of glutamate, which was counteracted by the A1R antagonist. The results support the clinical application of ENT1 inhibitors in RLS.

Abbreviations

A1R	adenosine A_1 receptor
A2AR	adenosine A_{2A} receptor
AAV	adeno-associated virus
BID	brain iron deficiency
BP	binding potential
CAMKII	Ca^{2+}/calmodulin-dependent protein kinase II
ChR2	channelrhodopsin 2
CPT	cyclopentyltheophylline
CSF	cerebrospinal fluid
D2R	dopamine D_2 receptor
EYFP	enhanced yellow fluorescence protein
ENT	equilibrative nucleoside transported
PLMS	periodic limb movements during sleep
RLS	restless legs syndrome
TfR	transferrin receptor
TH	tyrosine hydroxylase
VDCC	voltage-dependent calcium channels

1. Introduction

Restless legs syndrome (RLS) can be pathophysiologically separated into two clinical phenomena: Deficits of sensorimotor integration that produce akathisia and periodic limb movements during sleep (PLMS) and an enhanced arousal state (hyperarousal) (Ferré, García-Borreguero, Allen, & Earley, 2018). Akathisia is described as a feeling of restlessness and an urgent need to move. PLMS have very specific characteristics: they consist on repetitive episodes of leg movement activity (at least 4 in a row) with a duration of up to 10s and an inter-movement interval of 5–90s (Ferri, 2012). Hyperarousal manifests, first, as a short sleep time with episodes of arousals during sleep, related but not caused by PLMS; thus, in about half of all cases, the onset of the episodes of arousal precedes the onset of the leg movements (Ferri et al., 2015). Second, hyperarousal manifests as a lack of profound sleepiness during the day, which would be expected given the significant sleep loss at night (Allen, Stillman, & Myers, 2010).

Altered dopaminergic function plays an important role in PLMS and akathisia in RLS, which is supported by the remarkable initial therapeutic response with L-dopa and dopamine D_2-like receptor agonists, such as pramipexole and ropinirole (Earley et al., 2014). But there is also evidence for biochemical alterations in the dopaminergic system. The dopaminergic profile in postmortem tissue from RLS patients includes an increased tyrosine hydroxylase (TH) activity in the substantia nigra and in the striatum and a decreased density of striatal dopamine D_2 receptors (D2R), compatible with a presynaptic hyperdopaminergic state, where downregulation of D2R would represent an adaptive postsynaptic effect of an increased dopamine synthesis and release (Earley et al., 2014). In fact, the clinical dopaminergic profile in RLS patients includes abnormally high CSF levels of the dopamine metabolite 3-ortho-methyldopa (3-OMD), interpreted to indicate increased TH activity (Allen, Connor, Hyland, & Earley, 2009).

On the other hand, dopamine receptor agonists are little effective for the hyperarousal component of RLS, where glutamatergic mechanisms seem to be involved. A study by Allen, Barker, Horská, and Earley (2013), using magnetic resonance spectroscopy (MRS) in subjects with RLS compared to controls, showed an increased thalamic concentration of glutamate, which correlated with the time spent awake during the sleep period. These findings therefore suggested a presynaptic hyperglutamatergic state in RLS that could be involved with the hyperarousal state, but also with the sensory-motor symptoms of RLS. In fact, glutamatergic mechanisms play a central role in the therapeutic effects of $\alpha_2\delta$-ligands, such as gabapentin, which are effective for both the sensory-motor symptoms and the hyperarousal (Garcia-Borreguero et al., 2014). Thus, $\alpha_2\delta$-ligands target the $\alpha_2\delta$-subunits of calcium channels localized in glutamatergic terminals, inhibiting glutamate release (Dooley, Taylor, Donevan, & Feltner, 2007).

Brain iron deficiency (BID) is now well recognized as a main initial pathophysiological mechanism in the development of RLS, which is supported by results obtained from cerebrospinal fluid (CSF) analysis and from brain imaging and postmortem studies (Earley et al., 2014). BID in RLS seems to result from alterations of iron acquisition by the brain, a dysregulation of iron transportation by the blood-brain barrier (Earley et al., 2014). The involvement of BID in RLS is promoting the use of iron therapy in refractory RLS, as shown in the Mayo Clinic recommendations (Silber et al., 2013). BID in rodents during the postweaning period represents a valid pathogenetic model of RLS, since it recapitulates, not only similar behavioral changes of RLS (Dean, Allen, O'Donnell, & Earley, 2006; Lai et al., 2017), but also the main observed biochemical changes, such as the presynaptic hyperdopaminergic state, with the increase in striatal and nigral TH activity and the reduced striatal density of D2R (Connor et al., 2009). It has been suggested that the chain of events that connect BID to an increase in TH expression involves a BID-induced increase in the expression of the hypoxia inducible factor 1α (HIF-1 α) (Earley et al., 2014). However, increased striatal TH activity could also be secondary to increased striatal glutamatergic transmission (see below).

We recently obtained the first clear experimental evidence for a BID-dependent increase in presynaptic glutamatergic transmission in the BID rat model of RLS, using a new *in vivo* optogenetic-microdialysis method (Yepes et al., 2017). In this method, a virus expressing the light-sensitive ion channel channelrhodopsin and a green fluorescent protein is injected in the cortex and, after some weeks, channelrhodopsin is selectively expressed by striatal glutamatergic terminals. Then, a microdialysis probe with an embedded optical fiber is implanted in the striatum, which allows the measurement of light-induced stimulation of glutamate release by corticostriatal glutamatergic terminals (Quiroz, Orrú, et al., 2016). The method also allows the analysis of the effect of the local perfusion of different drugs directly within the same area being sampled for glutamate (Quiroz, Orrú, et al., 2016). The study showed that BID in rats produces hypersensitivity of corticostriatal glutamatergic terminals, which released glutamate with lower frequency of optogenetic stimulation than controls (60 Hz versus 100 Hz) (Yepes et al., 2017). We hypothesized that BID-induced hypersensitivity of corticostriatal glutamatergic terminals represents a main pathogenetic mechanism involved in the sensory-motor symptoms of RLS (Yepes et al., 2017). Since we previously demonstrated that optogenetically-induced glutamate release from corticostriatal terminals locally induces striatal dopamine release, we also hypothesized that hypersensitivity of corticostriatal glutamatergic terminals could also be involved in the BID-induced hyperdopaminergic state of RLS (Ferré, García-Borreguero, et al., 2018; Ferré, Quiroz, et al., 2018). Significantly, local application of either the $\alpha_2\delta$ ligand gabapentin or the dopamine receptor agonists pramipexole or ropinirole blocked completely glutamate release induced by optogenetic stimulation, both in controls (at 100 Hz) and in animals with BID (at 60 Hz) (Yepes et al., 2017). This implied that dopamine receptors and voltage-dependent calcium channels (VDCC) expressing $\alpha_2\delta$ units localized in striatal glutamatergic terminals might represent key targets for the therapeutic effects of both dopamine receptor agonists and $\alpha_2\delta$ ligands in RLS. The apparently inexplicable efficacy of dopamine receptor agonists in the frame of a hyperdopaminergic state could then be explained by their action on presynaptic, and not postsynaptic, striatal dopamine receptors. Activation of presynaptic dopamine receptors localized in glutamatergic terminals would locally inhibit glutamate-dependent dopamine release. An additional implication is that the use of the optogenetic-microdialysis method in BID rats provides an animal model to screen new putative therapeutically effective treatments for RLS (Yepes et al., 2017).

Adenosine plays an important modulatory role of the function of corticostriatal terminals. This control is mediated by adenosine A_1 and A_{2A} receptors (A1R and A2AR), which establish intermolecular interactions forming A1R-A2AR heteromers (Ciruela et al., 2006; Navarro, Cordomí, Brugarolas, et al., 2018). These heteromers work as an adenosine concentration-dependent switch, which determines opposite effects of adenosine on glutamate release depending on a predominant A1R or A2AR activation in the heteromer. Adenosine has more affinity for A1R than for A2AR and, therefore, low concentrations of adenosine activate A1R, which induces an inhibition of glutamate release. On the other hand, with high concentrations of adenosine (obtained upon conditions of strong glutamatergic input, with the consequent neuronal and glial ATP release and conversion of ATP on adenosine), simultaneous activation of the A2AR leads to allosteric interactions that lead to a decrease in the affinity and efficacy of adenosine for the A1R (Ciruela et al., 2006; Navarro, Cordomí, Brugarolas, et al., 2018). The molecular mechanisms of these allosteric interactions are beginning to be understood and they are related to the specific tetrameric quaternary structure of the A1R-A2AR heteromer (Navarro, Cordomí, Brugarolas, et al., 2018).

We have recently shown that BID in rodents causes a generalized downregulation of A1R in the brain (Quiroz, Gulyani, et al., 2016). Based on these results, we have hypothesized that a hypoadenosinergic state, secondary to A1R downregulation, could be mostly responsible for the hyperglutamatergic and hyperdopaminergic states of RLS that determine the sensory-motor symptoms of RLS as well as the hyperarousal component

(Ferré, García-Borreguero, et al., 2018; Ferré, Quiroz, et al., 2018). More specifically, in view of the key inhibitory role of A1R on striatal glutamate release, A1R downregulation should be mostly responsible for the BID-induced hypersensitivity of corticostriatal glutamatergic terminals (Ferré, García-Borreguero, et al., 2018; Ferré, Quiroz, et al., 2018). We therefore predicted that equilibrative nucleoside transporter inhibitors, by increasing the striatal extracellular levels of adenosine (which would facilitate the binding probability of adenosine to the lower expressed A1R; see Section 4), could provide a new therapeutic approach for RLS. In fact, we have recently reported encouraging results with the non-selective ENT1/ENT2 dipyridamole in an open trial with RLS patients (García-Borreguero et al., 2018). The goal of the present study was to further support the A1R-dependent hypoadenosinergic-state hypothesis and its involvement in the BID-induced hypersensitivity of corticostriatal terminals, as well as its possible therapeutic implications. Our preclinical and clinical studies would predict that striatal application of an A1R blocker should produce hypersensitivity of corticostriatal terminals. We would then expect that, the same way as in rats with BID, in naïve rats, an A1R antagonist should reduce the frequency of optogenetic stimulation necessary to induce corticostriatal glutamate release. Furthermore, dipyridamole, by increasing the striatal extracellular concentration of adenosine and the activation of presynaptic A1R, should be able to counteract optogenetic-induced glutamate release in both naïve rats and in rats with BID. Finally, we would also expect that this putative effect of dipyridamole should be counteracted by an A1R blocker.

2. Materials and methods

2.1 Animals

Male Sprague-Dawley albino rats (Charles River Laboratories, Wilmington, MA), weighing 100–150 g and 280–360 g at the time of the first and second surgeries, respectively, were used in the experiments. Animals were housed 2 per cage and kept on a 12/12-h dark/light cycle with food and water available ad libitum. All animals used in the study were maintained in accordance with the guidelines of the National Institutes of Health Animal Care and the animal research conducted to perform this study was approved by the NIDA IRP Animal Care and Use Committee (protocol #: 15-BNRB-73). The rats were divided into two groups: the control group was fed with a diet containing an essential amount of iron (48 ppm iron, Catalog TD 80394,

Harlan-Teklad, Madison, WI) and the BID group was fed with a diet containing a low iron concentration (4 ppm iron, Catalog TD 80396, Harlan-Teklad). The other contents of the diet were the same. Diets were started immediately after weaning, at 21 days of age, and continued for 4 weeks, when microdialysis experiments were performed.

2.2 Assessment of iron deficiency

Systemic iron deficiency was assessed by measuring the hematocrit content from blood collected before perfusion at the end of the microdialysis experiments to control for the efficiency of the iron-deficient diet. A hematocrit below 20% indicated a successful diet, as we previously showed in our previous studies that it is associated with significant BID (Quiroz et al., 2010; Yepes et al., 2017).

2.3 Surgical procedures

Four weeks before the microdialysis experiments, the animals, weighing between 100 and 150 g, were anesthetized with 3 mL/kg of Equithesin (4.44 g of chloral hydrate, 0.972 g of Na pentobarbital, 2.124 g of $MgSO_4$, 44.4 mL of propylene glycol, 12 mL of ethanol and distilled H_2O up to 100 mL of final solution, NIDA Pharmacy, Baltimore, MD). A unilateral injection of an adeno-associated virus (AAV) encoding channelrhodopsin 2 (ChR2) fused to enhanced yellow fluorescence protein (EYFP) under control of the Ca^{2+}/calmodulin-dependent protein kinase II (CaMKII) neuronal promoter (AAV-CaMKIIa-hChR2(H134R)-EYFP; University of North Carolina core vector facility) was delivered in the agranular motor cortex; coordinates of injection were 2.5 mm anterior, 3 mm lateral and −5 mm ventral with respect to bregma. Virus (0.5 μL of purified and concentrated AAV, 1×10^{12} infectious units/mL) was injected using a 105 μm-thick silica tubing injector coupled directly to a 1 μL-syringe driven by an infusion pump. Virus suspension was injected over a 10-min period at a rate of 50 nL/min and the injector was left in place for an additional 10 min to allow diffusion of the suspension. Four weeks after virus injection, with the rats weighing 280–360 g, a modified microdialysis probe (optogenetic-microdialysis probe) with an embedded light-guiding optic fiber (see below) was implanted into the lateral striatum under Equithesin anesthesia (3 mL/kg); coordinates were 0 mm anterior, 4.5 lateral and −7 mm ventral with respect to bregma. The probes were fixed to the skull with stainless steel screws and dental glass ionomer cement.

2.4 Intracranial optogenetic stimulation

An optogenetic-microdialysis probe with a 125 µm-diameter optic fiber (0.22 numerical aperture) embedded in a microdialysis probe was used for optogenetic stimulation of glutamate release by cortico-striatal terminals (Quiroz, Orrú, et al., 2016; Yepes et al., 2017). The tip of the optic fiber was given a conical shape to allow a local light dispersion through and around the working portion of the dialyzable membrane. The conical sculpted tip with the cladding fused to the core was obtained by pulling the fiber with a Flamming-Brown pipette puller (Sutter Instruments, Novato, CA), fitted with a custom platinum heating filament of circular cross-section (1 mm in diameter) and a holder specifically designed for the diameter of the optic fiber. Optical stimulation was delivered coupling the light guiding port of the implanted optogenetic-microdialysis probe to a 473-nm solid-state laser module driven by an electrical stimulator (Grass S88 stimulator). Light pulses were applied over a 20-min period in 160-ms trains of 1-ms pulses at a frequency of 60 or 100 Hz and intensity of 5–8 mW at the probe tip (one train/s). Light intensity at the probe tip was measured before implantation using an integrating sphere silicon photodiode power sensor designed for optical power measurements independent of beam shape and divergence (model S144C, Thor Labs, Newton, NJ).

2.5 *In vivo* microdialysis

Microdialysis sampling was performed to analyze the extracellular concentrations of striatal glutamate of freely moving rats 24 h after probe implantation. An artificial cerebrospinal solution (aCSF; 144 NaCl, 4.8 KCl, 1.7 $CaCl_2$, and 1.2 $MgCl_2$, in mM) with or without the A1R antagonist cyclopentyltheophylline (CPT; 300 µM, Millipore-Sigma, Saint Louis, MO) or the ENT1/ENT2 inhibitor dipyridamole (1 µM, Tocris-Bio-Techne, Minneapolis, MN), was pumped through the optogenetic-microdialysis probe at a constant rate of 1 µL/min. After a washout period of 90 min, dialysate samples were collected for 60 min of baseline sampling at 20-min intervals. After baseline sampling, optogenetic stimulation was applied for 20 min and 20-min samples were taken for 80 additional min after the beginning of the stimulation. Glutamate content was measured by HPLC coupled to a glutamate oxidase enzyme reactor and electrochemical detector (Eicom, San Diego, CA). At the end of the microdialysis experiment, animals were deeply anesthetized with Equithesin and perfused transcardially with 0.1 M phosphate buffered saline (PBS), followed by

4% formaldehyde in 0.1M PBS, pH 7.4. Brains were stored in the same fixative and then transferred into a solution of 20% sucrose/0.1M sodium phosphate, pH 7.4, solution for 48h at 4°C. Forty micrometer coronal sections were cut in a Leica (Nussloch, Germany) CM3050S cryostat at −20°C, collected in PBS, and stored in antifreeze-buffered solution (20% ethylene glycol, 10% glycerol, and 10% sucrose in PBS) at −80°C until processing. Sections were then evaluated for probe localization and ChR2-EYFP expression using a Typhoon multimode laser scanner (GE life Sciences, Piscataway, NJ). Confocal fluorescence microscopy images were acquired with a Zeiss microscope (Examiner Z1, Zeiss, Gottingen, Germany) fitted with a confocal laser module (LSM-710, Zeiss).

3. Results

As shown in a previous study (Yepes et al., 2017), in animals with a control diet, a frequency of optogenetic stimulation of 60Hz did not produce striatal glutamate release (circles in Fig. 1), while 100Hz produced a

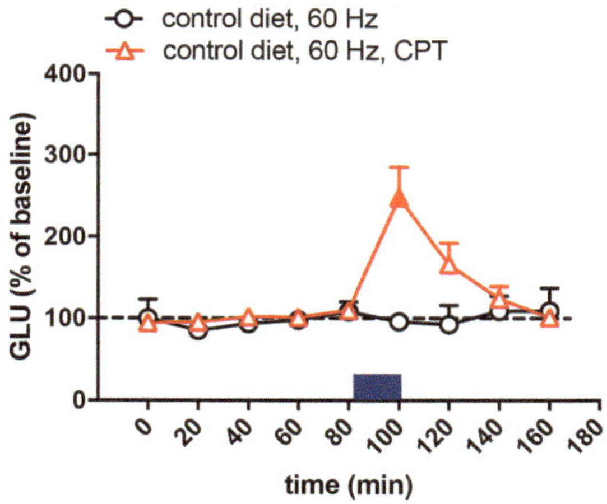

Fig. 1 Glutamate release induced by low-frequency (60Hz) of optogenetic stimulation of the corticostriatal terminals in the lateral striatum of rats with control diet with (triangles) and without (circles) perfusion of the A1R antagonist CPT (300 μM). CPT is constantly perfused since the beginning of glutamate sampling and the period of optogenetic stimulation (20min) is represented by a blue rectangle. Results are expressed as means + S.E.M. of percentage of the average of the first three basal values (n = 9 and 7 per group). Filled symbols represent significantly different means as compared to the mean of the first three basal values ($P < 0.05$; repeated measures ANOVA, followed by Dunnett's multiple comparisons test).

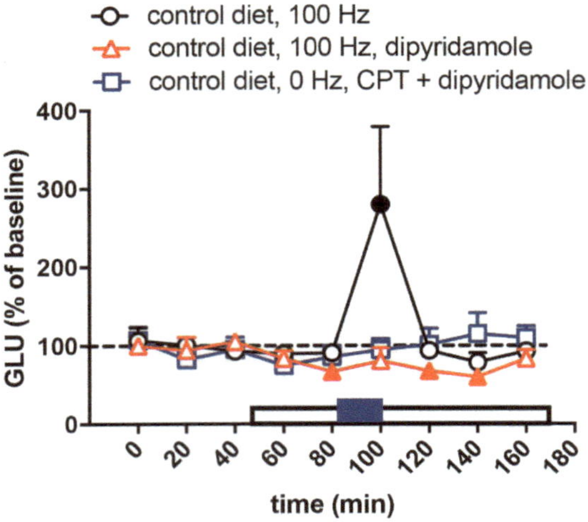

Fig. 2 Glutamate release induced by high-frequency (100 Hz) of optogenetic stimulation of the corticostriatal terminals in the lateral striatum of rats with control diet with (triangles) and without (circles) perfusion of the ENT1/ENT2 inhibitor dipyridamole (1 μM). The plot with squares represents the effect of co-perfusion of the A1R antagonist CPT (300 μM) and dipyridamole (1 μM), without optogenetic stimulation. CPT is constantly perfused since the beginning of glutamate sampling. The period of dipyridamole perfusion is represented by an empty rectangle and the period of optogenetic stimulation (20 min) is represented by a blue rectangle. Results are expressed as means + S.E.M. of percentage of the average of the first three basal values ($n = 7$–8 per group). Filled symbols represent significantly different means as compared to the mean of the first three basal values ($P < 0.05$; repeated measures ANOVA, followed by Dunnett's multiple comparisons test).

significant effect (circles in Fig. 2). Also, as previously shown (Yepes et al., 2017), the corticostriatal terminals of animals with BID were more sensitive to the optogenetic stimulation and glutamate release was obtained with the lower frequency, at 60 Hz (circles in Fig. 3). Nevertheless, 60 Hz also produced glutamate release in animals with control diet with perfusion of the A1R antagonist CPT (triangles in Fig. 1), indicating that A1R blockade increases the sensitivity of the corticostriatal terminals to release glutamate. The concentration of CPT perfused through the microdialysis probe (300 μM) was previously shown to be effective at modulating striatal glutamate release by selectively acting on presynaptic A1R (Borycz et al., 2007; Quarta et al., 2004). In rats with a control diet, perfusion of the ENT1/ENT2 inhibitor dipyridamole (1 μM) produced a small but significant decrease in the basal striatal extracellular concentration of glutamate before and after the optogenetic stimulation (80-min, 120-min and 140-min samples in Fig. 2; triangles). In addition, dipyridamole completely blocked

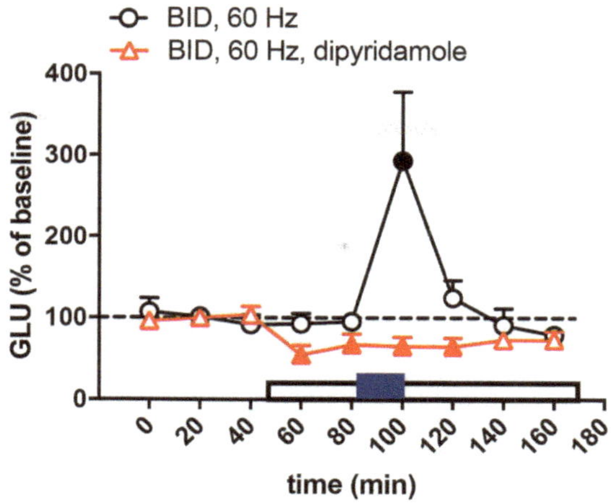

Fig. 3 Glutamate release induced by low-frequency (60 Hz) of optogenetic stimulation of the corticostriatal terminals in the lateral striatum of rats with BID with (triangles) and without (circles) perfusion of the ENT1/ENT2 inhibitor dipyridamole (1 μM). The period of dipyridamole perfusion is represented by an empty rectangle and the period of optogenetic stimulation (20 min) is represented by a blue rectangle. Results are expressed as means + S.E.M. of percentage of the average of the first three basal values ($n = 7$–8 per group). Filled symbols represent significantly different means as compared to the mean of the first three basal values ($P < 0.05$; repeated measures ANOVA, followed by Dunnett's multiple comparisons test).

glutamate release induced by optogenetic stimulation (100-min sample in Fig. 2; triangles). The specific involvement of A1R on the effects of dipyridamole could be confirmed by the ability of CPT (300 μM) to counteract the dipyridamole-induced decrease in the basal extracellular levels of glutamate (80-min, 120-min and 140-min samples in Fig. 2; squares). These results, therefore confirm the A1R-mediated effects of dipyridamole. Importantly, in rats with BID, dipyridamole also decreased basal levels of glutamate (60-min, 80-min and 120-min samples in Fig. 3; triangles) and optogenetic-induced increase in extracellular concentration of glutamate (100-min sample in Fig. 3; triangles). These results validate once more the use of the optogenetic-microdialysis method in BID rats as a model to identify new pharmacological treatments for RLS (see Section 4).

4. Discussion

The results of the present experiments support our hypothesis of a key role of adenosine and A1R in the modulation of corticostriatal glutamatergic transmission and their possible use as targets for drug development in RLS.

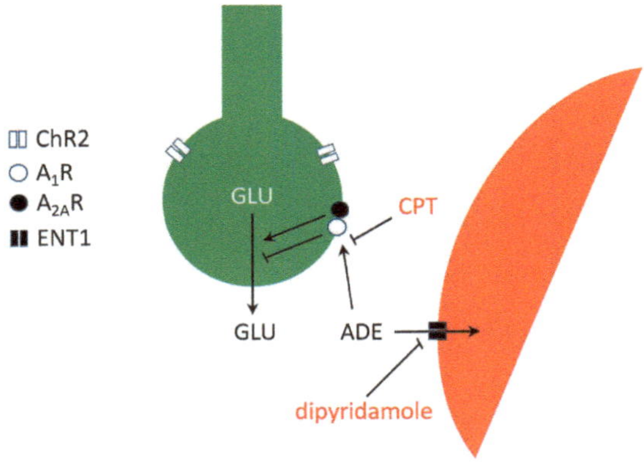

Fig. 4 Scheme representing the A1R-mediated modulation glutamate release by corticostriatal terminals (in green). The ability of endogenous adenosine (ADE) to inhibit glutamate release under basal conditions or upon optogenetic stimulation of channelrhodopsin 2 (ChR2)-expressing terminals is increased by blocking its transport to astrocytes (in red) with the ENT1/ENT2 inhibitor dipyridamole or by blocking its binding to A1R with the A1R antagonist CPT.

In addition, they confirm the preclinical efficacy of the ENT1/ENT2 inhibitor dipyridamole in the BID rodent. As previously predicted (Ferré, Quiroz, et al., 2018), dipyridamole counteracted optogenetically-induced glutamate release by corticostriatal terminals in naïve and BID rats. The results of the present experiments are schematically summarized in Fig. 4, which implies that manipulations of the endogenous levels of adenosine or its binding potential (BP) to the A1R significantly determine the sensitivity of corticostriatal nerve terminals to release glutamate.

BP is an operational measure of receptor occupancy by an endogenous or exogenous ligand, which determines the instantaneous functional receptor response, and is denoted as the product of maximum density of the receptor (B_{max}) and the affinity of the specific ligand to its receptor (i.e., $\text{BP} = B_{\text{max}} \times 1/K_{\text{D}}$) (Mintun, Raichle, Kilbourn, Wooten, & Welch, 1984). According to the Law of Mass Action, the rate of any reaction is proportional to the concentrations of the reactants. Applied to ligand-receptor interactions, the concentration of ligand-receptor complex (receptor occupancy and, therefore, receptor activation when the ligand is an agonist) depends on the concentration of ligand and receptor (receptor density) and to the affinity of the ligand for the receptor. This is, nevertheless, an oversimplification and there are additional factors that determine the ligand-receptor encounter probability, such as receptor clustering, which increases rebinding probability. Recent studies are providing strong evidence for pre-coupling of specific receptors and their specific associated signaling proteins and effectors (Navarro, Cordomí, Casadó-Anguera, et al., 2018). These macromolecular complexes can form high-order oligomers that include the same and different receptors (receptor heteromers), allowing, not only the very efficient receptor response upon very low concentrations of the ligands (Civciristov et al., 2018), but also very specific interactions between different ligands at specific effectors (Navarro, Cordomí, Casadó-Anguera, et al., 2018). In any case, here we use the concepts of BP and ligand-receptor encounter probability to provide the rationale for increasing the concentration of the endogenous ligand (adenosine) to compensate the decrease in the density of its receptor (A1R).

Our pathogenetic working hypothesis in RLS, a BID-induced A1R downregulation that leads to hypersensitive corticostriatal glutamatergic terminals (Ferré, García-Borreguero, et al., 2018; Ferré, Quiroz, et al., 2018), would imply a decrease in the BP of endogenous adenosine and would predict that dipyridamole should lead to an increase in the occupancy of A1R by increasing the concentration of endogenous adenosine. The BID-induced decrease in adenosine BP to A1R was mimicked by the A1R antagonist CPT, which expectedly produced hypersensitivity of corticostriatal terminals. In addition, dipyridamole significantly reduced, through an A1R-dependent mechanism (blocked by CPT), optogenetically-induced cortico-striatal glutamate release in naïve and BID rats.

An interesting result of the present study is the complete blockade of optogenetically-induced glutamate release produced by the A1R-mediated effect of dipyridamole, which is in contrast with the previously reported partial inhibitory effect of A1R agonists (at most, 50%) observed in synaptosomal preparations of not only striatal, but also hippocampal, cortical and spinal tissue (Ambrósio, Malva, Carvalho, & Carvalho, 1997; Ciruela et al., 2006; Li & Eisenach, 2005; Marchi et al., 2002). One plausible explanation is the presence of additional A1R-modulated cellular components in the *in vivo* microdialysis preparation, such as the cholinergic interneurons. Thus, corticostriatal inputs directly activate cholinergic interneurons (Kosillo, Zhang, Threlfell, & Cragg, 2016) and striatal acetylcholine release promotes glutamate release by activation of α_7-nicotinic receptors localized in the corticostriatal terminals (Kaiser & Wonnacott, 2000; Quarta et al., 2004). The cholinergic component of glutamate release can then be modulated by adenosine, which exerts a significant inhibitory control of the excitability of the striatal cholinergic interneurons by acting on A1R, their predominantly expressed adenosine receptor subtype (Song, Tkatch, & Surmeier, 2000).

Astrocytes could also constitute an additional significant player, since they are believed to amplify neuronal glutamate release and they also express A1R (Daré, Schulte, Karovic, Hammarberg, & Fredholm, 2007; Ferré et al., 2007).

In the brain, adenosine uptake occurs primarily by facilitated diffusion via equilibrative transporters, which inhibition leads to an increase in the extracellular concentration of adenosine (Cunha, 2016; Dulla & Masino, 2013; Parkinson et al., 2011). There are four different subtypes of equilibrative transporters, ENT1-ENT4, from which ENT1 and ENT2 are the most expressed in the brain, predominantly in astrocytes, but also in neurons (Parkinson et al., 2011). In fact, astrocytes are also the main source of extracellular adenosine, released as ATP and rapidly converted in adenosine by means of ecto-nucleotidases (Cunha, 2016; Dulla & Masino, 2013), and it has been demonstrated that astrocytic ATP release plays a major in the A1R-mediated regulation of adenosine on presynaptic glutamate transmission (Hines & Haydon, 2013). Some studies indicate that ENT1 plays a more salient role than ENT2 in determining the extracellular concentration of adenosine in the brain (Alanko, Porkka-Heiskanen, & Soinila, 2006), and ENT1 (but not ENT2) is often regionally co-localized with A1R, supporting a more significant role of ENT1 in the transport of adenosine that controls A1R function (Jennings et al., 2001). Therefore, it would be desirable to develop still non-available selective ENT1 inhibitors.

Meanwhile, apart from the present preclinical results, there are two additional reasons that support the clinical use of the ENT1/ENT2 inhibitor dipyridamole in RLS patients, instead of selective A1R agonists. First, selective A1R agonists cannot be used clinically because of their strong cardiovascular side effects, bradycardia and hypotension (Schindler et al., 2005). Second, dipyridamole is already extensively used clinically as antiplatelet, to prevent stroke and heart attack, with relatively infrequent side effects (Kim & Liao, 2008). However, the possible use of dipyridamole (and other ENT1/ENT2 inhibitors) for RLS could be questioned in view of its previously reported low brain penetrability (Parkinson et al., 2011; Sollevi, 1986). Nevertheless, we recently demonstrated its ability to modulate postsynaptic striatal A1R and A2AR with systemic administration of dipyridamole in reserpinized mice (Ferré, Quiroz, et al., 2018). Furthermore, as predicted from the "hypoadenosinergic state" hypothesis of RLS pathophysiology, an open trial of dipyridamole with 15 untreated idiopathic RLS patients provided very encouraging results (García-Borreguero et al., 2018). These preliminary clinical results suggest that dipyridamole has significant therapeutic effects, not only on the sensory-motor symptoms, but also for the hyperarousal. In fact, as recently reviewed (Ferré, García-Borreguero, et al., 2018), A1R downregulation in areas that control the ascending arousal systems might be also a main pathogenetic mechanism involved in the hyperarousal and sleep disruption in RLS. These clinical results, nevertheless, need now to be consolidated with a placebo-controlled study.

Acknowledgments

Work supported by the intramural funds of the National Institute on Drug Abuse.

Conflict of interest

The authors have no conflicts of interest to declare.

References

Alanko, L., Porkka-Heiskanen, T., & Soinila, S. (2006). Localization of equilibrative nucleoside transporters in the rat brain. *Journal of Chemical Neuroanatomy*, *31*, 162–168.

Allen, R. P., Barker, P. B., Horská, A., & Earley, C. J. (2013). Thalamic glutamate/glutamine in restless legs syndrome: Increased and related to disturbed sleep. *Neurology*, *80*, 2028–2034.

Allen, R. P., Connor, J. R., Hyland, K., & Earley, C. J. (2009). Abnormally increased CSF 3-ortho-methyldopa (3-OMD) in untreated restless legs syndrome (RLS) patients indicates more severe disease and possibly abnormally increased dopamine synthesis. *Sleep Medicine*, *10*, 123–128.

Allen, R. P., Stillman, P., & Myers, A. J. (2010). Physician-diagnosed restless legs syndrome in a large sample of primary medical care patients in western Europe: Prevalence and characteristics. *Sleep Medicine*, *11*, 31–37.

Ambrósio, A. F., Malva, J. O., Carvalho, A. P., & Carvalho, C. M. (1997). Inhibition of N-,P/Q- and other types of Ca^{2+} channels in rat hippocampal nerve terminals by the adenosine A1 receptor. *European Journal of Pharmacology*, *340*, 301–310.

Borycz, J., Pereira, M. F., Melani, A., Rodrigues, R. J., Köfalvi, A., Panlilio, L., et al. (2007). Differential glutamate-dependent and glutamate-independent adenosine A1 receptor-mediated modulation of dopamine release in different striatal compartments. *Journal of Neurochemistry*, *101*, 355–363.

Ciruela, F., Casadó, V., Rodrigues, R. J., Luján, R., Burgueño, J., Canals, M., et al. (2006). Presynaptic control of striatal glutamatergic neurotransmission by adenosine A1-A2A receptor heteromers. *Journal of Neuroscience*, *26*, 2080–2087.

Civciristov, S., Ellisdon, A. M., Suderman, R., Pon, C. K., Evans, B. A., Kleifeld, O., et al. (2018). Preassembled GPCR signaling complexes mediate distinct cellular responses to ultralow ligand concentrations. *Science Signaling*, *11*(551). eaan1188.

Connor, J. R., Wang, X. S., Allen, R. P., Beard, J. L., Wiesinger, J. A., Felt, B. T., et al. (2009). Altered dopaminergic profile in the putamen and substantia nigra in restless leg syndrome. *Brain*, *132*, 2403–2412.

Cunha, R. A. (2016). How does adenosine control neuronal dysfunction and neurodegeneration? *Journal of Neurochemistry*, *139*, 1019–1055.

Daré, E., Schulte, G., Karovic, O., Hammarberg, C., & Fredholm, B. B. (2007). Modulation of glial cell functions by adenosine receptors. *Physiology and Behavior*, *92*, 15–20.

Dean, T., Jr., Allen, R. P., O'Donnell, C. P., & Earley, C. J. (2006). The effects of dietary iron deprivation on murine circadian sleep architecture. *Sleep Medicine*, 7, 634–640.

Dooley, D. J., Taylor, C. P., Donevan, S., & Feltner, D. (2007). Ca^{2+} channel α2δ ligands: Novel modulators of neurotransmission. *Trends in Pharmacological Sciences*, *28*, 75–82.

Dulla, C. G., & Masino, S. A. (2013). Physiology and metabolic regulation of adenosine: Mechanisms. In S. Masino & D. Boison (Eds.), *Adenosine. A key link between metabolism and brain activity* (pp. 87–107). New York: Springer.

Earley, C. J., Connor, J., Garcia-Borreguero, D., Jenner, P., Winkelman, J., Zee, P. C., et al. (2014). Altered brain iron homeostasis and dopaminergic function in restless legs syndrome (Willis-Ekbom disease). *Sleep Medicine*, *15*, 1288–1301.

Ferré, S., Agnati, L. F., Ciruela, F., Lluis, C., Woods, A. S., Fuxe, K., et al. (2007). Neurotransmitter receptor heteromers and their integrative role in 'local modules': The striatal spine module. *Brain Research Reviews*, *55*, 55–67.

Ferré, S., García-Borreguero, D., Allen, R. P., & Earley, C. J. (2018). New insights into the neurobiology of restless legs syndrome. *The Neuroscientist*. https://doi.org/10.1177/1073858418791763.

Ferré, S., Quiroz, C., Guitart, X., Rea, W., Seyedian, A., Moreno, E., et al. (2018). Pivotal role of adenosine neurotransmission in restless legs syndrome. *Frontiers in Neuroscience*, *11*, 722.

Ferri, R. (2012). The time structure of leg movement activity during sleep: The theory behind the practice. *Sleep Medicine*, *13*, 433–441.

Ferri, R., Rundo, F., Zucconi, M., Manconi, M., Bruni, O., Ferini-Strambi, L., et al. (2015). An evidence-based analysis of the association between periodic leg movements during sleep and arousals in restless legs syndrome. *Sleep*, *38*, 919–924.

García-Borreguero, D., Guitart, X., Garcia Malo, C., Cano-Pumarega, I., Granizo, J. J., & Ferré, S. (2018). Treatment of restless legs syndrome/Willis-Ekbom disease with the nonselective ENT1/ENT2 inhibitor dipyridamole: Testing the adenosine hypothesis. *Sleep Medicine*, *45*, 94–97.

Garcia-Borreguero, D., Patrick, J., DuBrava, S., Becker, P. M., Lankford, A., Chen, C., et al. (2014). Pregabalin versus pramipexole: Effects on sleep disturbance in restless legs syndrome. *Sleep*, *37*, 635–643.

Hines, D. J., & Haydon, P. J. (2013). Physiology and metabolic regulation of adenosine: Mechanisms. In S. Masino & D. Boison (Eds.), *Adenosine. A key link between metabolism and brain activity* (pp. 157–177). New York: Springer.

Jennings, L. L., Hao, C., Cabrita, M. A., Vickers, M. F., Baldwin, S. A., Young, J. D., et al. (2001). Distinct regional distribution of human equilibrative nucleoside transporter proteins 1 and 2 (hENT1 and hENT2) in the central nervous system. *Neuropharmacology*, *40*, 722–731.

Kaiser, S., & Wonnacott, S. (2000). Alpha-bungarotoxin-sensitive nicotinic receptors indirectly modulate [(3)H]dopamine release in rat striatal slices via glutamate release. *Molecular Pharmacology*, *58*, 312–318.

Kim, H. H., & Liao, J. K. (2008). Translational therapeutics of dipyridamole. *Arteriosclerosis, Thrombosis, and Vascular Biology*, *28*, s39–s42.

Kosillo, P., Zhang, Y. F., Threlfell, S., & Cragg, S. J. (2016). Cortical control of striatal dopamine transmission via striatal cholinergic interneurons. *Cerebral Cortex*, *26*, 4160–4169.

Lai, Y. Y., Cheng, Y. H., Hsieh, K. C., Nguyen, D., Chew, K. T., Ramanathan, L., et al. (2017). Motor hyperactivity of the iron-deficient rat—an animal model of restless legs syndrome. *Movement Disorders*, *32*, 1687–1693.

Li, X., & Eisenach, J. C. (2005). Adenosine reduces glutamate release in rat spinal synaptosomes. *Anesthesiology*, *103*, 1060–1065.

Marchi, M., Raiteri, L., Risso, F., Vallarino, A., Bonfanti, A., Monopoli, A., et al. (2002). Effects of adenosine A1 and A2A receptor activation on the evoked release of glutamate from rat cerebrocortical synaptosomes. *British Journal of Pharmacology*, *136*, 434–440.

Mintun, M. A., Raichle, M. E., Kilbourn, M. R., Wooten, G. F., & Welch, M. J. (1984). A quantitative model for the in vivo assessment of drug binding sites with positron emission tomography. *Annals of Neurology, 15*, 217–227.
Navarro, G., Cordomí, A., Brugarolas, M., Moreno, E., Aguinaga, D., Pérez-Benito, L., et al. (2018). Cross-communication between G(i) and G(s) in a G-protein-coupled receptor heterotetramer guided by a receptor C-terminal domain. *BMC Biology, 16*, 24.
Navarro, G., Cordomí, A., Casadó-Anguera, V., Moreno, E., Cai, N.-S., Cortés, A., et al. (2018). Evidence for functional pre-coupled complexes of receptor heteromers and adenylyl cyclase. *Nature Communications, 9*, 1242.
Parkinson, F. E., Damaraju, V. L., Graham, K., Yao, S. Y., Baldwin, S. A., Cass, C. E., et al. (2011). Molecular biology of nucleoside transporters and their distributions and functions in the brain. *Current Topics in Medicinal Chemistry, 11*, 948–972.
Quarta, D., Borycz, J., Solinas, M., Patkar, K., Hockemeyer, J., Ciruela, F., et al. (2004). Adenosine receptor-mediated modulation of dopamine release in the nucleus accumbens depends on glutamate neurotransmission and N-methyl-D-aspartate receptor stimulation. *Journal of Neurochemistry, 91*, 873–880.
Quiroz, C., Gulyani, S., Ruiqian, W., Bonaventura, J., Cutler, R., Pearson, V., et al. (2016). Adenosine receptors as markers of brain iron deficiency: Implications for restless legs syndrome. *Neuropharmacology, 111*, 160–168.
Quiroz, C., Orrú, M., Rea, W., Ciudad-Roberts, A., Yepes, G., Britt, J. P., et al. (2016). Local control of extracellular dopamine levels in the medial nucleus accumbens by a glutamatergic projection from the infralimbic cortex. *Journal of Neuroscience, 36*, 851–859.
Quiroz, C., Pearson, V., Gulyani, S., Allen, R., Earley, C., & Ferré, S. (2010). Up-regulation of striatal adenosine A(2A) receptors with iron deficiency in rats: Effects on locomotion and cortico-striatal neurotransmission. *Experimental Neurology, 224*, 292–298.
Schindler, C. W., Karcz-Kubicha, M., Thorndike, E. B., Müller, C. E., Tella, S. R., Ferré, S., et al. (2005). Role of central and peripheral adenosine receptors in the cardiovascular responses to intraperitoneal injections of adenosine A1 and A2A subtype receptor agonists. *British Journal of Pharmacology, 144*, 642–650.
Silber, M. H., Becker, P. M., Earley, C., Garcia-Borreguero, D., Ondo, W. G., & Medical Advisory Board of the Willis-Ekbom Disease Foundation. (2013). Willis-Ekbom disease foundation revised consensus statement on the management of restless legs syndrome. *Mayo Clinic Proceedings, 88*, 977–986.
Sollevi, A. (1986). Cardiovascular effects of adenosine in man; possible clinical implications. *Progress in Neurobiology, 27*, 319–349.
Song, W. J., Tkatch, T., & Surmeier, D. J. (2000). Adenosine receptor expression and modulation of Ca(2+) channels in rat striatal cholinergic interneurons. *Journal of Neurophysiology, 83*, 322–332.
Yepes, G., Guitart, X., Rea, W., Newman, A. H., Allen, R. P., Earley, C. J., et al. (2017). Targeting hypersensitive corticostriatal terminals in restless legs syndrome. *Annals of Neurology, 82*, 951–960.

CHAPTER TWO

D3 receptor agonist efficacy in restless legs syndrome

Francesca Casoni[a], Andrea Galbiati[a,b], Luigi Ferini-Strambi[a,b,*]

[a]Department of Clinical Neurosciences, IRCCS San Raffaele Scientific Institute, Neurology—Sleep Disorders Center, Milan, Italy

[b]Faculty of Psychology, "Vita-Salute" San Raffaele University, Milan, Italy

*Corresponding author: e-mail address: ferinistrambi.luigi@hsr.it

Contents

Abstract

Restless Legs Syndrome/Willis Ekbom Disease (RLS/WED) is a sleep related movement disorder characterized by an irresistible urge to move the limbs frequently associated with uncomfortable sensations that usually begin or worsen during inactivity and may be relieved by movement. The pathophysiology of the disorder involves several biological system; in particular, dopaminergic pathway and iron physiology have been extensively studied. Being a chronic condition, long-term treatments are required for an adequate management and strong evidence support the employment of dopamine agonists. D3 receptor agonists are of particular interest, because they act on receptors that are widely expressed in the spinal cord with an inhibitory action on sensory system. Pramipexole, rotigotine and ropinirole act on D3 receptors, even if not selectively, and are effective in reducing sensorimotor symptoms and improving sleep quality. However, despite an initial amelioration patients frequently experience augmentation, i.e., a worsening of symptoms induced by dopamine agonists. This can be explained by the activity of D1 receptor and by the non-selectiveness of D3 agonist drugs. Higher dopamine concentrations tend to activate the excitatory D1-like receptor that are associated with increased motor activity. The development of drugs that selectively target D3 receptors will be fundamental to provide alternative therapeutic strategies and to reduce the occurrence of augmentation.

Advances in Pharmacology, Volume 84
ISSN 1054-3589
https://doi.org/10.1016/bs.apha.2019.01.005

© 2019 Elsevier Inc.
All rights reserved.

Abbreviation

AC	adenylate cyclase
CNS	central nervous system
CSF	cerebrospinal fluid
D1R	dopamine D1 receptor
D2R	dopamine D2 receptor
D3KO	dopamine D3 receptor knockout mouse
D3R	dopamine D3 receptor
DA	dopamine
DAergic	dopaminergic
DDC	DOPA decarboxylase
DOPA	3,4-dihydroxyphenylalanine
DR	dopamine receptor
GPCR	G-protein-coupled receptor
IRLS	International Restless Legs Syndrome Rating Scale
Meis1KO	Meis1 knockout mouse
PD	Parkinson's disease
PET	positron emission tomography
PLMs	Periodic Limb Movement during sleep
RLS/WED	Restless Legs Syndrome/Willis Ekbom Disease
SN	*substantia nigra*
SNc	SN *pars compacta*
SNr	SN *pars reticulata*
TH	tyrosine hydroxylase
VTA	ventral tegmental area

1. Introduction

Thomas Willis, an English physician of the seventeenth century, described a pathological condition related to hyposideremia in which patients when lying at bed experienced "in the arms and legs, leapings and contractions of the tendons, and so great a restlessness and tossing of their members ensue, that the diseased are no more able to sleep than if they were in a place of the greatest torture" (Willis, 1685). After a century Theodor Wittmaack, a German neurologist, named this clinical condition *anxietas tibiarum* (Wittmaack, 1861) that is currently known with the term Restless Legs Syndrome/Willis Ekbom Disease (RLS/WED). In fact, it is only in 1945 that the Swedish neurologist Karl Axel Ekbom used the term "Restless Legs Syndrome" to describe the disorder (Ekbom, 1945).

RLS/WED is a sleep related movement disorder (American Academy of Sleep Medicine, 2014) with a prevalence in the general population that ranges from 9.4% to 15% (Ohayon, O'Hara, & Vitiello, 2012). It is characterized by an irresistible urge to move the limbs frequently associated with

Table 1 Diagnostic criteria according to the international classification of sleep disorders, third edition (American Academy of Sleep Medicine, 2014).

Diagnostic criteria **Criteria A-C must be met**
A. An urge to move the legs, usually accompanied by or thought to be caused by uncomfortable and unpleasant sensations in the legs. These symptoms must: 1. Begin or worsen during periods of rest or inactivity such as lying down or sitting; 2. Be partially or totally relieved by movement, such as walking or stretching, at least as long as the activity continues; and 3. Occur exclusively or predominantly in the evening or night rather than during the day
B. The above features are not solely accounted for as symptoms of another medical or behavioral condition
C. The symptoms of RLS/WED cause concern, distress, sleep disturbance, or impairment in mental, physical, social, occupational, educational, behavioral, or other important areas of functioning

uncomfortable sensations that usually begin or worsen during inactivity and may be relieved by movement. Even though legs are prominently affected, symptoms may also involve upper limbs (Rinaldi et al., 2016) (for diagnostic criteria according to the International Classification of Sleep Disorder see Table 1 and Allen et al., 2014 for International Restless Legs Syndrome Study Group consensus criteria). As a chronic condition, the consequences of RLS/WED extend beyond evening or night and result in sleep-onset insomnia, fatigue and decreased health related quality of life (Ohayon et al., 2012). Periodic Limb Movement during sleep (PLMs), frequently observed in RLS/WED patients, are associated with arousals from sleep that can lead to sleep disruption and to further daytime dysfunction such as daytime sleepiness and cognitive deterioration (Ferri et al., 2016; Galbiati et al., 2015).

RLS/WED may manifest in its primary form when other causes are excluded by means of instrumental examinations and is characterized by a positive familial history. On the contrary, when RLS/WED can be explained by the presence of other conditions (e.g., pregnancy, neuropathy, renal failure, ...) we can consider it as secondary (Winkelman et al., 2016).

Being a chronic condition, long-term treatments are required for an adequate management. RLS/WED has a good response to pharmacological interventions and several drugs have been studied in randomized clinical trials. Strong evidence support the employment of dopamine agonists (pramipexole, rotigotine, cabergoline, and gabapentin enacarbil) and calcium channel alpha-2-delta ligands as first line treatment. Other compounds such as opioids, benzodiazepines and iron therapy are considered treatment options (Winkelman et al., 2016).

Despite patients frequently reported an initial amelioration after pharmacologic treatment, several issues in the long-term management of RLS/WED are frequently described including loss of efficacy over time and several side effects. However, one of the main complication concerning long-term treatment with dopamine agonists is augmentation that can lead to significant problems in more than 20% of patients (Allen et al., 2011). It is defined as a worsening of symptom severity with increasing dosage of medication, with an earlier onset in the afternoon and a shorter latency at rest, a spread to other body parts, or a paradoxical response to treatment. For this reason, the therapeutic choice should be carefully tailored to the patient's risk profile and dopaminergic load must be kept as low as possible (Garcia-Borreguero et al., 2013).

It has been suggested that a breakdown of the descending A11 dopaminergic system in the hypothalamus might play a role in RLS/WED by affecting the D3 receptor system (Clemens, Rye, & Hochman, 2006). Accordingly, it has been suggested that RLS/WED might be treated with dopamine receptor agonists that target D3 receptors (Meneely et al., 2018). In the light of this evidence, in this chapter RLS/WED pathophysiology, dopaminergic receptors and the effect of D3 receptor agonist will be discussed.

2. RLS/WED pathopysiology

In the RLS/WED pathophysiology, more biological systems have been implicated: dopaminergic system, iron physiology and genetic pathways (Allen, 2015).

The dopaminergic system seems to play a central role, based on the demonstration of the efficacy of the therapy with L-Dopa and DA agonists in patients with RLS/WED (Garcia-Borreguero & Cano-Pumarega, 2017).

Anatomopathological studies (Connor et al., 2009), cerebrospinal fluid (CSF) studies (Allen, Connor, Hyland, & Earley, 2009) and brain imaging studies (Earley et al., 2011; Lin et al., 2016; Michaud, Soucy, Chabli, Lavigne, & Montplaisir, 2002; Rizzo, Li, Galantucci, Filippi, & Cho, 2017; Ruottinen et al., 2000) are consisted with overactivity of DA system in the brain.

This hyperdopaminergic state lead to a downregulation of DA receptors, but due to the circadian profile of dopamine activity, there is a relative DA deficit in the evening and during the night, that can be compensate supplying additional DA with dopaminomimetic drugs in RLS/WED patients (Khan, Ahlberg, Chow, Shah, & Koo, 2017).

It is also likely that the dopaminergic dysfunction is linked to changes in iron metabolism within the brain. Using different methods, several studies confirmed brain iron deficiency in RLS/WED patients (Allen, Barker, Wehrl, Song, & Earley, 2001; Earley, Barker, Horská, & Allen, 2006; Godau, Klose, Santo, Schweitzer, & Berg, 2008; Moon et al., 2014; Rizzo et al., 2013; Schmidauer et al., 2005) especially in the *substantia nigra*, the putamen, the caudate and also in the thalamus (Rizzo et al., 2013), and these decreases were correlated to RLS/WED symptom severity (Allen et al., 2001).

Iron deficiency may lead to an increase of tyrosine hydroxylase (TH) in the basal ganglia (Connor et al., 2009) with an increase production of extracellular DA (Beard, Chen, Connor, & Jones, 1994). Also, DA receptor density may be modified by iron deficiency, with a reduction in caudate and putamen D1 and D2 receptors (Erikson, Jones, Hess, Zhang, & Beard, 2001).

Another interesting hypothesis localized the dysfunction underlying RLS/WED pathophysiology in the spinal cord. The A11 diencephalic region is the main source of dopaminergic (DAergic) innervation for the spinal cord (Qu et al., 2006; Ondo, Zhao, & Le, 2007; Barraud et al., 2010). Clemens et al. (2006) postulated that a A11 dopamine hypofunction can lead to spinal network changes wholly consistent with RLS/WED symptoms. Based on studies on D3R knockout mouse (D3KO) and Meis1 knockout mouse (Meis1KO) it was postulated that an alteration in the D3 receptor system can produce an increased excitability of the sensory system, but the motor-associated increased activity could be due to an increased expression of the D1 receptor system in the spinal cord (Meneely et al., 2018). However, anatomopathological study failed to confirm any pathologic change in the A11 region in humans (Earley, Allen, Connor, Ferrucci, & Troncoso, 2009).

Many patients treated with DA agonist may experience *augmentation* characterized by an increase in symptom severity, an earlier onset of symptoms, a shorter latency to onset of symptoms after lying down or sitting, appearance of daytime symptoms, and spread of symptoms to other parts of the body (Allen et al., 2011). In the spinal cord low dose of DA target the D2/D3 receptor, with a inhibitory action in the dorsal spinal cord

(Keeler, Baran, Brewer, & Clemens, 2012), but high DA concentrations tend to activate the excitatory D1-like receptors (Clemens, Belin-Rauscent, Simmers, & Combes, 2012) explaining the clinical manifestation of augmentation after a long-term treatment with DA agonists (Dinkins, Lallemand, & Clemens, 2017). Moreover, it is known that with aging the expression of the D1 receptor (D1R) but not D3 receptor (D3R) is increased, supporting the role of the D1R in the emergence of RLS/WED disease and augmentation in elderly people (Samir, Yllanes, Lallemand, Brewer, & Clemens, 2017).

Furthermore, inhibitory D3R can form functional heterodimers with excitatory D1R (Guitart et al., 2014) modifying the affinity and/or intrinsic efficacy of ligands and consequently the receptor function.

Regarding genetics, several points need to be addressed. In a recent meta-analysis, new risk loci linked to RLS/WED were identified and have been found to involved in the in the development of the CNS, such as neurogenesis and neural-circuit formation, including axon guidance and synaptogenesis (Schormair et al., 2017). However, none of them contains genes directly implicated in the dopaminergic system.

3. Dopaminergic receptors

DA is the most common catecholamine in the central nervous system that can acts as a catecholamine neurotransmitter and a hormone. It is widely distributed in both the central nervous system (CNS) and peripheral nervous system, as well as in some peripheral non-neuronal areas (for example, the pituitary gland, blood vessels, human adipose tissue, and the cardiovascular and renal systems) (Rangel-Barajas, Coronel, & Florán, 2015).

DA is derived from the conversion of 2,3-dihydroxyphenylalanine (DOPA) by the enzyme DOPA decarboxylase (DDC). TH is the enzyme responsible for converting the amino acid tyrosine to DOPA, monitoring the DA amount. The synthesis of DA is localized in the DAergic neurons in the *substantia nigra pars compacta* (SNc), in the ventral tegmental area (VTA), and in the *arcuate* and periventricular nucleus of the hypothalamus.

DA can modulate different functions, like movement, cognition, reward and motivation, emotions, memory, attention and sleep regulation (Bromberg-Martin, Matsumoto, & Hikosaka, 2010; Gepshtein et al., 2014).

Three groups of dopaminergic cells give rise to three different axonal pathways with different functions: nigrostriatal, mesocorticolimbic and tuberoinfundibular system. The latter is the smallest in terms of brain DA content and controls the pituitary system, in particular, the production of prolactin. Nigrostriatal DA pathway controls voluntary movement, and dysfunction in this pathway has been implicated in movement disorder like PD. Mesocorticolimbic systems DA modulate various cognitive/emotive functions, and their degeneration may lead to some psychiatric disorder. Several studies have pointed out that mesocorticolimbic system can also modulate thalamocortical arousal state (Dauvilliers, Tafti, & Landolt, 2015; Oishi & Lazarus, 2017).

The physiological effects of DA are mediated by five G protein-coupled receptors (GPCRs) that are divided into two major subclasses: the D1-like (D1, D5) and the D2-like (D2, D3, D4) receptors (Beaulieu & Gainetdinov, 2011).

The D1-like receptors can activate the $G\alpha_{s/olf}$ family of the G proteins stimulating the production of cAMP via activation of adenylate cyclase (AC) leading to a depolarization of the neurons and are found only on the post-synaptic membrane of dopamine-receptive cells. The D2-like family can be found both postsynaptically on dopamine target cells and presynaptically on dopaminergic neurons and is coupled to $G\alpha_{i/o}$ inducing an inhibition of AC and a downregulation of the production of cAMP leading to hyperpolarization and inhibition of the neurons (Beaulieu & Gainetdinov, 2011).

These two class of receptors differ in the CNS and peripheral distribution and expression, the genetic structure, the affinity for DA, the specificity for G-protein coupling and signaling and in their regulation and desensitization (Beaulieu & Gainetdinov, 2011; Missale, Nash, Robinson, Jaber, & Caron, 1998).

D1R family are mainly implicated in the control of working memory, seeking, craving, and reward (Beninger & Gerdjikov, 2004), and D2R family are chiefly implicated in behavioral properties, such as locomotor activity, reinforcement, and reward (Sibley & Monsma, 1992).

D3R have a widespread influence on dopamine and other neurotransmitters and is an attractive target for therapeutic intervention (Gross & Drescher, 2012).

Although the D3R has a more limited pattern of distribution in the CNS, with the high density in the limbic areas (Missale et al., 1998; Sokoloff et al., 2006), comparative radioligand binding studies showed that dopamine has higher affinity for D3R than for D2R (Mach et al., 2011).

The D3R is a target of pharmacotherapeutic interest in a variety of neuropsychiatric and neurological disorders neurological and, including schizophrenia, drug addiction, Parkinson's disease (PD), depression and RLS/WED (Cortés, Moreno, Rodríguez-Ruiz, Canela, & Casadó, 2016).

4. Effects of D3 receptor agonist in RLS/WED

Dopamine agonists are recognized as first line treatment for RLS/WED as they are very effective in reducing both symptomatology and PLMs (Winkelmann et al., 2018). Dopaminergic agents for this pathology are mainly D2 and D3 receptors agonists; however, the effect on D3 seems to be more relevant in comparison to D2 in terms of treatment's efficacy, as underlined by several RLS/WED animal models (Earley, Uhl, Clemens, & Ferré, 2017; Ondo et al., 2007).

Among dopaminergic agents three of them target D3 receptor, even if not selectively: pramipexole, rotigotine and ropinirole (for a summary of efficacy and safety see Table 2).

Pramipexole is a non-ergot dopamine agonist and represents an effective treatment for RLS/WED with a level A of evidence according to the most recent guideline (Winkelmann et al., 2018). Since the first study investigating its efficacy on RLS/WED it has been reported that pramipexole is able to reduce sensorimotor discomfort and PLMs index (Montplaisir, Nicolas, Denesle, & Gomez-Mancilla, 1999). Despite it is able to successfully reduce PLMs, this amelioration is not reflected in the electroencephalographic instability (expressed by cyclic alternating pattern) and arousals that are improved by benzodiazepines (e.g., clonazepam). This would suggest the possibility of a joint treatment targeting both sensorimotor symptoms

Table 2 Efficacy, safety and side effects for D3 receptor agonists for the treatment of RLS/WED.

D3 agents	Efficacy	Safety	Side effects
Pramipexole	Efficacious at doses of 0.25, 0.50, and 0.75 mg	Acceptable risk with special monitoring for augmentation	Nausea, lightheadedness, fatigue, agumentation
Rotigotine	Efficacious at a dose of 2–3 mg	Acceptable risk with special monitoring for local site reactions and augmentation	Skin reaction, augmentation
Ropinirole	Efficacious at a dose of 0.78–4.6 mg	Acceptable risk with special monitoring for augmentation	Nausea, lightheadedness, fatigue, agumentation

Recommendations from Winkelmann, J., Allen, R. P., Högl, B., Inoue, Y., Oertel, W., Salminen, A. V., et al. (2018). Treatment of restless legs syndrome: Evidence-based review and implications for clinical practice (Revised 2017) §. *Movement Disorders, 33*(7), 1077–1091.

and sleep instability (Manconi et al., 2012). In 2006, Winkelman and collaborators assessed its effectiveness and safety in 344 patients over a period of 12 weeks in a double-blind, randomized, placebo-controlled trial with fixed doses (0.25, 0.50, and 0.75 mg/day). They demonstrated that pramipexole improved RLS/WED symptomatology with a favorable safety profile, and this ameliorement was not dose-related (Winkelman et al., 2006). In 2012, a meta-analysis of randomized controlled trials confirmed the benefit of pramipexole assessing over 1200 patients. A significant improvement was testified by an average reduction of 6.7 points at the International Restless Legs Syndrome Rating Scale (IRLS) in comparison to placebo. Furthermore, uncontrolled long-term studies lasting between 26 and 52 weeks reported a 17-point improvement in IRLS over baseline when treated with pramipexole (Aurora et al., 2012). Along with these ameliorations, it has also been reported that pramipexole has positive effects on neurocognitive functioning (Galbiati et al., 2015). Although efficacious in reducing RLS/WED symptomatology, PLMs and daytime functions, the risk of augmentation has to be taken into account. A 52-week, randomized, double-blind trial assessed the risk of augmentation in pregabalin, pramipexole and placebo. The rate of augmentation was significantly higher with pramipexole (7.7%) at a dose of 0.5 mg in comparison to pregabalin (2.1%) but not at a dose of 0.25 mg (Allen et al., 2014). Up to now it is possible to conclude that pramipexole is efficacious for the treatment of idiopathic RLS/WED at doses of 0.25, 0.50, and 0.75 mg, but given the risk of augmentation there is a need for a careful monitoring and future study should explore the possibility to reduce its occurrence (Winkelmann et al., 2018). Interestingly, it has been demonstrated that a switchover from an immediate release DA agonist to the long acting formula of pramipexole could be a therapeutic option for those patients reporting augmentation (Maestri et al., 2014).

Rotigotine is a D3 but also D1 and D2 agonist, with affinity for serotonin receptors 5-HT1A and α-adrenergic receptors (Scheller, Ullmer, Berkels, Gwarek, & Lübbert, 2009), that is available in the form of a transdermal patch (Ferini-Strambi, Marelli, & Galbiati, 2016). Rotigotine improves RLS/WED symptoms in a dose-dependent manner with a therapeutic dosage ranging from 1 to 3 mg/24 h (Hening et al., 2010; Trenkwalder et al., 2008). Rotigotine is also effective in reducing PLMs and related arousal. A significant decrease of PLMs index has been reported in RLS/WED patients treated with rotigotine in comparison to placebo. This improvement was also accompanied by a significant reduction of arousal associated with PLMs indicating a remarkable effect also in treating sleep disruption in these patients (Oertel et al., 2010). A recent study (Bauer et al., 2016) evaluated the effects of rotigotine on PLMs-associated nocturnal systolic blood pressure elevations. A significant reduction in systolic, diastolic and PLMs blood pressure elevations was found in patients treated with rotigotine indicating a possible effect in reducing cardiovascular risk. There is also evidence that the risk of augmentation is low (Oertel et al., 2011); furthermore, a recent study evaluated the effect of switching to rotigotine in augmented patients reporting an improvement of RLS/WED symptoms and augmentation over a period of 13 months (Trenkwalder et al., 2017). It is possible to conclude that rotigotine transdermal patch is an effective agents for the management of moderate and severe RLS/WED symptomatology (Winkelmann et al., 2018).

The benefit of ropinirole for the treatment of RLS/WED patients has reported by several studies (Aurora et al., 2012). In a randomized, double-blind study conducted in a population of severe RLS/WED patients (IRLS total score ≥ 24), the authors evaluated the effect of ropinirole (dosage from 0.25 to 4 mg) over 26 weeks followed by an open-label extension of 40 weeks. They found a significant effect over placebo in improving RLS/WED symptomatology, self-reported sleep and quality of life related to the disorder (Giorgi, Asgharian, & Hunter, 2013). Ropinirole is also able to reduce the presence of PLMs, arousal related to PLMs and to improve sleep by shortening sleep latency and stabilizing sleep in comparison to placebo (Allen et al., 2004). Concerning augmentation, ropinirole incidence for augmentation was found to be 4% at 26 weeks (Giorgi et al., 2013). In conclusion, it is considered efficacious for the treatment of RLS/WED at a dosage from 0.78 to 4.6 mg (Winkelmann et al., 2018).

5. Conclusion

RLS/WED is a common sensorimotor disorder with several detrimental consequences for patients' sleep and quality of life. Several biological systems are involved in the pathophysiology of this condition; in particular, dopaminergic and iron pathways have been extensively studied. Therefore, DA agonists compounds are frequently prescribed for the management of the disorder and have shown good efficacy in reducing patients' symptomatology and improving sleep and daytime functioning. DA agents, such as pramipexole, ropinirole and rotigotine, are of particular interest, because they target D3 receptors (even if not selectively) that are fundamental for the sensory symptoms as they are expressed in the spinal cord with an inhibitory action. All these compounds are efficacious in reducing sensorimotor symptoms, PLMs and improving sleep quality. However, since RLS/WED is a chronic condition, their long-term use can cause important side effects. In particular, augmentation, i.e., a severe worsening of symptoms, is frequently reported. This phenomenon can be explained by the activity of D1 receptor rather than by D3 functioning. DA acting on D3 receptors in the spinal cord has an inhibitory activity on sensorimotor symptoms; however, higher DA concentrations tend to activate the excitatory D1-like receptors, that are responsible for the increased motor activity thus explaining the clinical manifestation of augmentation after a long-term treatment with DA agonists. Moreover, D3 receptors can form functional heterodimers with excitatory D1 receptors that could again modify the effect of DA therapy. In spite of the advances on the comprehension of dopamine receptors, further work is needed for the identification of compounds with a selective action on D3 receptors. The recent findings on D3 heteromerization may provide future approaches for targeting D3 receptors by heteromer-selective drugs and identify more specific therapeutic strategies that might reduce the occurrence of augmentation.

Conflict of interest statement

The authors have no conflicts of interest to declare.

References

Allen, R. P. (2015). Restless leg syndrome/Willis-Ekbom disease pathophysiology. *Sleep Medicine Clinics*, *10*(3), 207–214.

Allen, R. P., Barker, P., Wehrl, F., Song, H., & Earley, C. (2001). MRI measurement of brain iron in patients with restless legs syndrome. *Neurology*, *56*(2), 263–265.

Allen, R. P., Becker, P. M., Bogan, R., Schmidt, M., Kushida, C. A., Fry, J. M., et al. (2004). Ropinirole decreases periodic leg movements and improves sleep parameters in patients with restless legs syndrome. *Sleep*, *27*(5), 907–914.

Allen, R. P., Chen, C., Garcia-Borreguero, D., Polo, O., DuBrava, S., Miceli, J., et al. (2014). Comparison of pregabalin with pramipexole for restless legs syndrome. *New England Journal of Medicine*, *370*(7), 621–631.

Allen, R. P., Connor, J., Hyland, K., & Earley, C. (2009). Abnormally increased CSF 3-Ortho-methyldopa (3-OMD) in untreated restless legs syndrome (RLS) patients indicates more severe disease and possibly abnormally increased dopamine synthesis. *Sleep Medicine*, *10*(1), 123–128.

Allen, R. P., Ondo, W. G., Ball, E., Calloway, M. O., Manjunath, R., Higbie, R. L., et al. (2011). Restless legs syndrome (RLS) augmentation associated with dopamine agonist and levodopa usage in a community sample. *Sleep Medicine*, *12*(5), 431–439.

Allen, R. P., Picchietti, D. L., Garcia-Borreguero, D., Ondo, W. G., Walters, A. S., Winkelman, J. W., et al. (2014). Restless legs syndrome/Willis–Ekbom disease diagnostic criteria: Updated International Restless Legs Syndrome Study Group (IRLSSG) consensus criteria–history, rationale, description, and significance. *Sleep Medicine, 15*(8), 860–873.

American Academy of Sleep Medicine. (2014). *International classification of sleep disorders* (3rd ed.). Darien, IL: American Academy of Sleep Medicine.

Aurora, R. N., Kristo, D. A., Bista, S. R., Rowley, J. A., Zak, R. S., Casey, K. R., et al. (2012). The treatment of restless legs syndrome and periodic limb movement disorder in adults—An update for 2012: Practice parameters with an evidence-based systematic review and meta-analyses: An American Academy of Sleep Medicine Clinical Practice Guideline. *Sleep, 35*(8), 1039–1062.

Barraud, Q., Obeid, I., Aubert, I., Barrière, G., Contamin, H., McGuire, S., et al. (2010). Neuroanatomical study of the A11 diencephalospinal pathway in the non-human primate. *PLoS One, 5*(10) e13306.

Bauer, A., Cassel, W., Benes, H., Kesper, K., Rye, D., Sica, D., et al. (2016). Rotigotine's effect on PLM-associated blood pressure elevations in restless legs syndrome: An RCT. *Neurology*, 10–1212.

Beard, J. L., Chen, Q., Connor, J., & Jones, B. C. (1994). Altered monamine metabolism in caudate-putamen of iron-deficient rats. *Pharmacology Biochemistry and Behavior, 48*(3), 621–624.

Beaulieu, J. M., & Gainetdinov, R. R. (2011). The physiology, signaling, and pharmacology of dopamine receptors. *Pharmacological Reviews, 63*(1), 182–217.

Beninger, R. J., & Gerdjikov, T. V. (2004). The role of signaling molecules in reward-related incentive learning. *Neurotoxicity Research, 6*(1), 91–103.

Bromberg-Martin, E. S., Matsumoto, M., & Hikosaka, O. (2010). Dopamine in motivational control: Rewarding, aversive, and alerting. *Neuron, 68*(5), 815–834. https://doi.org/10.1016/j.neuron.2010.11.022.

Clemens, S., Belin-Rauscent, A., Simmers, J., & Combes, D. (2012). Opposing modulatory effects of D1- and D2-like receptor activation on a spinal central pattern generator. *Journal of Neurophysiology, 107*(8), 2250–2259.

Clemens, S., Rye, D., & Hochman, S. (2006). Restless legs syndrome: Revisiting the dopamine hypothesis from the spinal cord perspective. *Neurology, 67*(1), 125–130.

Connor, J. R., Wang, X., Allen, R. P., Beard, J. L., Wiesinger, J. A., Felt, B. T., et al. (2009). Altered dopaminergic profile in the putamen and substantia nigra in restless leg syndrome. *Brain, 132*(9), 2403–2412.

Cortés, A., Moreno, E., Rodríguez-Ruiz, M., Canela, E. I., & Casadó, V. (2016). Targeting the dopamine D3 receptor: An overview of drug design strategies. *Expert Opinion on Drug Discovery, 11*(7), 641–664.

Dauvilliers, Y., Tafti, M., & Landolt, H. P. (2015). Catechol-O-methyltransferase, dopamine, and sleep-wake regulation. *Sleep Medicine Reviews, 22*, 47–53.

Dinkins, M., Lallemand, P., & Clemens, S. (2017). Long-term treatment with dopamine D3 receptor agonists induces a behavioral switch that can be rescued by blocking the dopamine D1 receptor. *Sleep Medicine, 40*, 47–52.

Earley, C. J., Allen, R. P., Connor, J. R., Ferrucci, L., & Troncoso, J. (2009). The dopaminergic neurons of the A11 system in RLS autopsy brains appear normal. *Sleep Medicine, 10*(10), 1155–1157.

Earley, C. J., Barker, P. B., Horská, A., & Allen, R. P. (2006). MRI-determined regional brain iron concentrations in early- and late-onset restless legs syndrome. *Sleep Medicine, 7*(5), 458–461.

Earley, C. J., Kuwabara, H., Wong, D. F., Gamaldo, C., Salas, R., Brasic, J., et al. (2011). The dopamine transporter is decreased in the striatum of subjects with restless legs syndrome. *Sleep, 34*(3), 341–347.

Earley, C. J., Uhl, G. R., Clemens, S., & Ferré, S. (2017). Connectome and molecular pharmacological differences in the dopaminergic system in restless legs syndrome (RLS): Plastic changes and neuroadaptations that may contribute to augmentation. *Sleep Medicine*, *31*, 71–77.

Ekbom, K. A. (1945). Restless Legs. *Acta Medica Scandinavica*, *158*(Suppl), 1–123.

Erikson, K. M., Jones, B. C., Hess, E. J., Zhang, Q., & Beard, J. L. (2001). Iron deficiency decreases dopamine D1 and D2 receptors in rat brain. *Pharmacology Biochemistry and Behavior*, *69*(3–4), 409–418.

Ferini-Strambi, L., Marelli, S., & Galbiati, A. (2016). Clinical pharmacology and efficacy of rotigotine (Neupro® patch) in the treatment of restless leg syndrome. *Expert Opinion on Drug Metabolism & Toxicology*, *12*(8), 967–975.

Ferri, R., Fulda, S., Allen, R. P., Zucconi, M., Bruni, O., Chokroverty, S., et al. (2016). World Association of Sleep Medicine (WASM) 2016 standards for recording and scoring leg movements in polysomnograms developed by a joint task force from the International and the European Restless Legs Syndrome Study Groups (IRLSSG and EURLSSG). *Sleep Medicine*, *26*, 86–95.

Galbiati, A., Marelli, S., Giora, E., Zucconi, M., Oldani, A., & Ferini-Strambi, L. (2015). Neurocognitive function in patients with idiopathic restless legs syndrome before and after treatment with dopamine-agonist. *International Journal of Psychophysiology*, *95*(3), 304–309.

Garcia-Borreguero, D., & Cano-Pumarega, I. (2017). New concepts in the management of restless legs syndrome. *British Medical Journal*, *356*, j104.

Garcia-Borreguero, D., Kohnen, R., Silber, M. H., Winkelman, J. W., Earley, C. J., Högl, B., et al. (2013). The long-term treatment of restless legs syndrome/Willis–Ekbom disease: Evidence-based guidelines and clinical consensus best practice guidance: A report from the International Restless Legs Syndrome Study Group. *Sleep Medicine*, *14*(7), 675–684.

Gepshtein, S., Li, X., Snider, J., Plank, M., Lee, D., & Poizner, H. (2014). Dopamine function and the efficiency of human movement. *Journal of Cognitive Neuroscience*, *26*(3), 645–657.

Giorgi, L., Asgharian, A., & Hunter, B. (2013). Ropinirole in patients with restless legs syndrome and baseline IRLS total scores $\geq$ 24: Efficacy and tolerability in a 26-week, double-blind, parallel-group, placebo-controlled study followed by a 40-week open-label extension. *Clinical Therapeutics*, *35*(9), 1321–1336.

Godau, J., Klose, U., Santo, A. D., Schweitzer, K., & Berg, D. (2008). Multiregional brain iron deficiency in restless legs syndrome. *Movement Disorders*, *23*(8), 1184–1187.

Gross, G., & Drescher, K. (2012). *The role of dopamine D3 receptors in antipsychotic activity and cognitive functions. Novel antischizophrenia treatments handbook of experimental pharmacology*. Berlin, Heidelberg: Springer, pp. 167–210.

Guitart, X., Navarro, G., Moreno, E., Yano, H., Cai, N., Sanchez-Soto, M., et al. (2014). Functional selectivity of allosteric interactions within G protein-coupled receptor oligomers: The dopamine D1-D3 receptor heterotetramer. *Molecular Pharmacology*, *86*(4), 417–429.

Hening, W. A., Allen, R. P., Ondo, W. G., Walters, A. S., Winkelman, J. W., Becker, P., et al. (2010). Rotigotine improves restless legs syndrome: A 6-month randomized, double-blind, placebo-controlled trial in the United States. *Movement Disorders*, *25*(11), 1675–1683.

Keeler, B. E., Baran, C. A., Brewer, K. L., & Clemens, S. (2012). Increased excitability of spinal pain reflexes and altered frequency-dependent modulation in the dopamine D3-receptor knockout mouse. *Experimental Neurology*, *238*(2), 273–283.

Khan, F. H., Ahlberg, C. D., Chow, C. A., Shah, D. R., & Koo, B. B. (2017). Iron, dopamine, genetics, and hormones in the pathophysiology of restless legs syndrome. *Journal of Neurology*, *264*(8), 1634–1641.

Lin, C., Fan, Y., Lin, G., Yang, F., Cheng, C., Lu, K., et al. (2016). 99mTc-TRODAT-1 SPECT as a potential neuroimaging biomarker in patients with restless legs syndrome. *Clinical Nuclear Medicine*, *41*(1), e14-7.

Mach, R. H., Tu, Z., Xu, J., Li, S., Jones, L. A., Taylor, M., et al. (2011). Endogenous dopamine (DA) competes with the binding of a radiolabeled D3 receptor partial agonist in vivo: A positron emission tomography study. *Synapse*, *65*(8), 724–732.

Maestri, M., Fulda, S., Ferini-Strambi, L., Zucconi, M., Marelli, S., Staedler, C., et al. (2014). Polysomnographic record and successful management of augmentation in restless legs syndrome/Willis–Ekbom disease. *Sleep Medicine*, *15*(5), 570–575.

Manconi, M., Ferri, R., Zucconi, M., Bassetti, C. L., Fulda, S., Aricò, D., et al. (2012). Dissociation of periodic leg movements from arousals in restless legs syndrome. *Annals of Neurology*, *71*(6), 834–844.

Meneely, S., Dinkins, M. L., Kassai, M., Lyu, S., Liu, Y., Lin, C. T., et al. (2018). Differential dopamine D1 and D3 receptor modulation and expression in the spinal cord of two mouse models of restless legs syndrome. *Frontiers in Behavioral Neuroscience*, *12*, 199.

Michaud, M., Soucy, J., Chabli, A., Lavigne, G., & Montplaisir, J. (2002). SPECT imaging of striatal pre- and postsynaptic dopaminergic status in restless legs syndrome with periodic leg movements in sleep. *Journal of Neurology*, *249*(2), 164–170.

Missale, C., Nash, S. R., Robinson, S. W., Jaber, M., & Caron, M. G. (1998). Dopamine receptors: From structure to function. *Physiological Reviews*, *78*(1), 189–225.

Montplaisir, J., Nicolas, A., Denesle, R., & Gomez-Mancilla, B. (1999). Restless legs syndrome improved by pramipexole a double-blind randomized trial. *Neurology*, *52*(5), 938–943.

Moon, H., Chang, Y., Lee, Y. S., Song, H. J., Chang, H. W., Ku, J., et al. (2014). T2 relaxometry using 3.0-tesla magnetic resonance imaging of the brain in early- and late-onset restless legs syndrome. *Journal of Clinical Neurology*, *10*(3), 197.

Oertel, W. H., Beneš, H., Garcia-Borreguero, D., Högl, B., Poewe, W., Montagna, P., et al. (2010). Rotigotine transdermal patch in moderate to severe idiopathic restless legs syndrome: A randomized, placebo-controlled polysomnographic study. *Sleep Medicine*, *11*(9), 848–856.

Oertel, W., Trenkwalder, C., Beneš, H., Ferini-Strambi, L., Högl, B., Poewe, W., et al. (2011). Long-term safety and efficacy of rotigotine transdermal patch for moderate-to-severe idiopathic restless legs syndrome: A 5-year open-label extension study. *The Lancet Neurology*, *10*(8), 710–720.

Ohayon, M. M., O'Hara, R., & Vitiello, M. V. (2012). Epidemiology of restless legs syndrome: A synthesis of the literature. *Sleep Medicine Reviews*, *16*, 283–295.

Oishi, Y., & Lazarus, M. (2017). The control of sleep and wakefulness by mesolimbic dopamine systems. *Neuroscience Research*, *118*, 66–73.

Ondo, W. G., Zhao, H. R., & Le, W. D. (2007). Animal models of restless legs syndrome. *Sleep Medicine*, *8*(4), 344–348.

Qu, S., Ondo, W. G., Zhang, X., Xie, W. J., Pan, T. H., & Le, W. D. (2006). Projections of diencephalic dopamine neurons into the spinal cord in mice. *Experimental Brain Research*, *168*(1–2), 152–156.

Rangel-Barajas, C., Coronel, I., & Florán, B. (2015). Dopamine receptors and neurodegeneration. *Aging and Disease*, *6*(5), 349.

Rinaldi, F., Galbiati, A., Marelli, S., Cusmai, M., Gasperi, A., Oldani, A., et al. (2016). Defining the phenotype of restless legs syndrome/Willis–Ekbom disease (RLS/WED): A clinical and polysomnographic study. *Journal of Neurology*, *263*(2), 396–402.

Rizzo, G., Li, X., Galantucci, S., Filippi, M., & Cho, Y. W. (2017). Brain imaging and networks in restless legs syndrome. *Sleep Medicine*, *31*, 39–48.

Rizzo, G., Manners, D., Testa, C., Tonon, C., Vetrugno, R., Marconi, S., et al. (2013). Low brain iron content in idiopathic restless legs syndrome patients detected by phase imaging. *Movement Disorders*, *28*(13), 1886–1890.

Ruottinen, H. M., Partinen, M., Hublin, C., Bergman, J., Haaparanta, M., Solin, O., et al. (2000). An FDOPA PET study in patients with periodic limb movement disorder and restless legs syndrome. *Neurology*, *54*(2), 502–504.

Samir, S., Yllanes, A. P., Lallemand, P., Brewer, K. L., & Clemens, S. (2017). Morphine responsiveness to thermal pain stimuli is aging-associated and mediated by dopamine D1 and D3 receptor interactions. *Neuroscience*, *349*, 87–97.

Scheller, D., Ullmer, C., Berkels, R., Gwarek, M., & Lübbert, H. (2009). The in vitro receptor profile of rotigotine: A new agent for the treatment of Parkinson's disease. *Naunyn-Schmiedeberg's Archives of Pharmacology*, *379*(1), 73–86.

Schmidauer, C., Sojer, M., Seppi, K., Stockner, H., Högl, B., Biedermann, B., et al. (2005). Transcranial ultrasound shows nigral hypoechogenicity in restless legs syndrome. *Annals of Neurology*, *58*(4), 630–634.

Schormair, B., Zhao, C., Bell, S., Tilch, E., Salminen, A. V., Pütz, B., et al. (2017). Identification of novel risk loci for restless legs syndrome in genome-wide association studies in individuals of European ancestry: A meta-analysis. *The Lancet Neurology*, *16*(11), 898–907.

Sibley, D. R., & Monsma, F. J. (1992). Molecular biology of dopamine receptors. *Trends in Pharmacological Sciences*, *13*, 61–69.

Sokoloff, P., Diaz, J., Le Foll, B., Guillin, O., Leriche, L., Bezard, E., et al. (2006). The dopamine D3 receptor: A therapeutic target for the treatment of neuropsychiatric disorders. *CNS & Neurological Disorders—Drug Targets*, *5*(1), 25–43.

Trenkwalder, C., Beneš, H., Poewe, W., Oertel, W. H., Garcia-Borreguero, D., de Weerd, A. W., et al. (2008). Efficacy of rotigotine for treatment of moderate-to-severe restless legs syndrome: A randomised, double-blind, placebo-controlled trial. *The Lancet Neurology*, 7(7), 595–604.

Trenkwalder, C., Canelo, M., Lang, M., Schroeder, H., Kelling, D., Berkels, R., et al. (2017). Management of augmentation of restless legs syndrome with rotigotine: A 1-year observational study. *Sleep Medicine*, *30*, 257–265.

Willis, T. (1685). *The London practice of physick*. London: Basset T. & Cooke W.

Winkelman, J. W., Armstrong, M. J., Allen, R. P., Chaudhuri, K. R., Ondo, W., Trenkwalder, C., et al. (2016). Practice guideline summary: Treatment of restless legs syndrome in adults: Report of the guideline development, dissemination, and implementation Subcommittee of the American Academy of Neurology. *Neurology*, *87*(24), 2585–2593.

Winkelman, J. W., Sethi, K. D., Kushida, C. A., Becker, P. M., Koester, J., Cappola, J. J., et al. (2006). Efficacy and safety of pramipexole in restless legs syndrome. *Neurology*, *67*(6), 1034–1039.

Winkelmann, J., Allen, R. P., Högl, B., Inoue, Y., Oertel, W., Salminen, A. V., et al. (2018). Treatment of restless legs syndrome: Evidence-based review and implications for clinical practice (revised 2017) §. *Movement Disorders*, *33*(7), 1077–1091.

Wittmaack, T. (1861). *Pathologie und Therapie der Sensibilität-Neurosen*. Lipsia: Schafer.

CHAPTER THREE

The heterotetrameric structure of the adenosine A_1-dopamine D_1 receptor complex: Pharmacological implication for restless legs syndrome

Antoni Cortés[a,b,c], Verònica Casadó-Anguera[a,b,c], Estefanía Moreno[a,b,c], Vicent Casadó[a,b,c,]*

[a]Centro de Investigación Biomédica en Red sobre Enfermedades Neurodegenerativas (CIBERNED), Madrid, Spain
[b]Institute of Biomedicine of the University of Barcelona (IBUB), Barcelona, Spain
[c]Department of Biochemistry and Molecular Biomedicine, Faculty of Biology, University of Barcelona, Barcelona, Spain
*Corresponding author: e-mail address: vcasado@ub.edu

Contents

Abstract

Dopaminergic and purinergic signaling play a pivotal role in neurological diseases associated with motor symptoms, including Parkinson's disease (PD), multiple sclerosis, amyotrophic lateral sclerosis, Huntington disease, Restless Legs Syndrome (RLS), spinal cord injury (SCI), and ataxias. Extracellular dopamine and adenosine exert their functions

Advances in Pharmacology, Volume 84
ISSN 1054-3589
https://doi.org/10.1016/bs.apha.2019.01.001
© 2019 Elsevier Inc.
All rights reserved.

interacting with specific dopamine (DR) or adenosine (AR) receptors, respectively, expressed on the surface of target cells. These receptors are members of the family A of G protein-coupled receptors (GPCRs), which is the largest protein superfamily in mammalian genomes. GPCRs are target of about 40% of all current marketed drugs, highlighting their importance in clinical medicine. The striatum receives the densest dopamine innervations and contains the highest density of dopamine receptors. The modulatory role of adenosine on dopaminergic transmission depends largely on the existence of antagonistic interactions mediated by specific subtypes of DRs and ARs, the so-called $A_{2A}R$–D_2R and A_1R–D_1R interactions. Due to the dopamine/adenosine antagonism in the CNS, it was proposed that ARs and DRs could form heteromers in the neuronal cell surface. Therefore, adenosine can affect dopaminergic signaling through receptor–receptor interactions and by modulations in their shared intracellular pathways in the striatum and spinal cord. In this work we describe the allosteric modulations between GPCR protomers, focusing in those of adenosine and dopamine within the A_1R–D_1R heteromeric complex, which is involved in RLS. We also propose that the knowledge about the intricate allosteric interactions within the A_1R–D_1R heterotetramer, may facilitate the treatment of motor alterations, not only when the dopamine pathway is hyperactivated (RLS, chorea, etc.) but also when motor function is decreased (SCI, aging, PD, etc.).

Abbreviations

A_1R adenosine A_1 receptor
$A_{2A}R$ adenosine A_{2A} receptor
BID brain iron deficiency
BiFC bimolecular fluorescence complementation
BRET bioluminescence resonance energy transfer
D_1R dopamine D_1 receptor
D_2R dopamine D_2 receptor
$D_{2S}R$ dopamine D_2 short receptor
D_3R dopamine D_3 receptor
D_4R dopamine D_4 receptor
EC extracellular
ECL extracellular loop
FRET fluorescence resonance energy transfer
GABA gamma-aminobutyric acid
GPCR G protein-coupled receptor
IC intracellular
ICL intracellular loop
L-DOPA L-3,4-dihydroxyphenylalanine
mGluR metabotropic glutamate receptor
PD Parkinson's disease
PLA proximity ligation assay
PLMS periodic leg movements during sleep
RLS Restless Legs Syndrome
SCI spinal cord injury
TM transmembrane

1. Introduction

G protein-coupled receptors (GPCRs), form the largest human membrane protein family, with 800 members overall. Many druggable targets for treatment of common diseases involve GPCRs that mediate therapeutic effects of 34% of all marketed drugs (Hauser, Attwood, Rask-Andersen, Schiöth, & Gloriam, 2017). The GPCR superfamily is classified into several classes, with rhodopsin-like class A being the largest and most studied so far. Class B includes the secretin-like and adhesion GPCRs, whereas class C contains metabotropic glutamate (mGlu), gamma-aminobutyric acid ($GABA_B$), the calcium-sensing and taste receptors. In addition, smoothened and frizzled receptors are categorized as class F (Di Pizio et al., 2016; Moller, Moreno-Delgado, Pin, & Kniazeff, 2017). GPCRs are key players in cell communication and in the transduction of sensory signals of external origin, such as light, odorants and taste molecules, and endogenous stimuli such as hormones, neurotransmitters, (neuro)peptides, chemokines, purine ligands, and calcium ions among others molecules. Recent studies shed light on the conformational changes that follow GPCR activation and the structural state of the receptor necessary for its interactions with the three classes of proteins that preferentially bind active GPCRs: G proteins, GPCR kinases and β-arrestins (Gonzalez, Cordomí, Matsoukas, Zachmann, & Pardo, 2014; Gurevich & Gurevich, 2017; Vilardaga, Agnati, Fuxe, & Ciruela, 2010; Wang, Yu, Liu, Liu, & Song, 2017).

GPCRs, also called seven-transmembrane (TM) receptors or heptahelical receptors, are cell surface proteins that share a common topology comprised by an extracellular (EC) N-terminus and seven TM α-helices connected by three intracellular (ICL) and three extracellular loops (ECL). They also have a disulphide bridge between ECL2 and TM3, and a cytoplasmic C-terminus containing an amphiphilic α-helix (H8) parallel to the cell membrane (Baltoumas, Theodoropoulou, & Hamodrakas, 2016; Gonzalez et al., 2014). The 7TM bundle can be divided into two module regions: EC and IC modules. The N-terminus ranges in length from relatively short, and often unstructured, as in many Class A members, to long and large globular domains with defined secondary structure, such as in class C GPCRs. The IC module includes the ICLs, a short helix 8 and an IC C-terminus, and is more conserved among GPCRs, compared to the EC region (Di Pizio et al., 2016; Katritch, Cherezov, & Stevens, 2012). The IC region is responsible for interaction with G proteins, β-arrestins, and other downstream effectors; in addition, it is vital for signal transduction and feedback modulation of receptor function (Moreira, 2014).

Analysis of the known crystal structures of GPCRs shows that ligand binding affinity mostly occurs in a main cavity located between the extracellular segments of TMs 3, 5, 6, and 7 or in a minor binding cavity located between the EC segments of TMs 1, 2, 3, and 7. Despite these common pockets, different ligands penetrate to different depths within the TM bundle, and this structural core binds ligands in the EC region and transduces the information to the IC module. It is the most structurally conserved component of the GPCR structure, presenting characteristic hydrophobic patterns and several functionally important signature motifs (Di Pizio et al., 2016; Katritch et al., 2012). Structural studies with class A receptors, have revealed the existence of a conformational change upon receptor activation which includes a breaking of the ionic lock formed between TM6 and the D(E)RY motif in TM3, followed by movements of the TM5 and TM6 cytoplasmic segments and the ICL3, with some minor rearrangements in the TM3 helix (Baltoumas et al., 2016).

2. GPCRs form homodimers

An emerging paradigm in GPCR research is the notion that these receptors do no act exclusively as monomers. Dimer formation has been shown to be mandatory for canonical receptor function in class C GPCRs (Kniazeff, Prézeau, Rondard, Pin, & Goudet, 2011; Moller et al., 2017). Xue et al. (2015) demonstrated that the mGluR2 dimer interface switches from TM4 to TM5 in the inactive state to TM6–TM6 interactions in the active conformation, revealing a key step in class C GPCR activation.

The quaternary structure of many of the family B members (i.e., secretin, glucagon, glucagon-like peptide and calcitonin receptors) have been actively studied and it has been demonstrated that they can form homodimers/oligomers (Gao et al., 2009; Ng & Chow, 2015; Ng, Lee, & Chow, 2013). Harikumar, Pinon, and Miller (2007) reported the existence of ligand-independent secretin receptor homodimerization; moreover, the same authors indicated that secretin and glucagon-like peptide-1 receptors form homodimeric complexes in which both protomers are associated along the lipid face of TM4 (Harikumar, Lau, Sexton, Wootten, & Miller, 2017). Very recently, Ward, Pediani, Harikumar, Miller, and Milligan (2017), using spatial intensity distribution analysis, demonstrated the existence of equilibrium between secretin receptor monomers and homodimers in CHO cells membrane, with little evidence of higher-order complexes, suggesting that there is likely a stable rate of association and dissociation of these complexes. In the same study, mutation of key residues in TM4 altered this equilibrium to greatly favor the monomeric state. Family B GPCRs also provide examples of receptors which are fully functional in their monomeric form such as the parathyroid hormone receptor and the glucagon-like peptide-1 receptors (Cai, Liu, et al., 2017; Pioszak, Harikumar, Parker, Miller, & Xu, 2010).

Concerning family A GPCRs, although it has been described that several receptors are able to operate as monomers (Arcemisbéhère et al., 2010; Bayburt et al., 2011; Chabre & le Maire, 2005; Ernst, Gramse, Kolbe, Hofmann, & Heck, 2007; Hanson et al., 2007; Kuszak et al., 2009; Whorton et al., 2007), experimental data have shown that these receptors may be expressed as a mixture of monomers and homodimers/oligomers (Nemoto, Yamanishi, Limviphuvadh, Saito, & Toh, 2016; Teichmann et al., 2014; Vischer, Castro, & Pin, 2015), and that oligomerization is required for receptor maturation, surface delivery and function (Angers et al., 2000; Angers, Salahpour, & Bouvier, 2002; Fotiadis et al., 2003; Gahbauer & Böckmann, 2016; Han, Moreira, Urizar, Weinstein, & Javitch, 2009; Herrick-Davis, Weaver, Grinde, & Mazurkiewicz, 2006; Hurevich, Talhami, Shalev, & Gilon, 2014; Jin et al., 2018; Lao et al., 2017; Liste et al., 2015; Lopez-Gimenez, Canals, Pediani, & Milligan, 2007; Ng et al., 2013; Wade et al., 2011). The existing controversy about the functionality of monomers or the dimerization requirement may come from the differences in the nature of the receptor, the experimental conditions of the assays or in the nature of the different detection technologies (Lao et al., 2017). As an example of oligomerization of class A GPCRs, using dual-color photoactivation localization microscopy with photoactivatable dyes, Jonas, Fanelli, Huhtaniemi, and Hanyaloglu (2015) reported that the luteinizing hormone receptor is organized in a mixture of monomers, dimers and higher order oligomers (<5 receptors) at the plasma membrane with distinct spatial geometries. Likewise, M1 muscarinic, dopamine D_2, β_1-adrenergic and chemokine receptors (CXCR4) can exist in a dynamic equilibrium between monomers/dimers/oligomers, that can be regulated by selective agonists, antagonists or bivalent ligands (Calebiro et al., 2013; Pediani, Ward, Godin, Marsango, & Milligan, 2016; Tabor et al., 2016). Albizu et al. (2010) demonstrated the in vivo existence of native oxytocin receptor dimers and Herrick-Davis, Grinde, Lindsley, Cowan, and Mazurkiewicz (2012);

Herrick-Davis, Grinde, Cowan, and Mazurkiewicz (2013); Herrick-Davis et al. (2015) provided strong experimental evidence that adrenergic, muscarinic, dopamine, and serotonin 5-HT_{2C} receptors form homodimers endogenously expressed in their native cellular environment. Cai, Bai, Zhang, Wang, and Chen (2017) revealed monomer-to-dimer interconversion of the apelin receptor on the cell membrane, with dimers acquiring novel functional characteristics, such as distinct G-protein binding profile and cellular responses after agonist stimulation. Very recently, Parmar, Grinde, Mazurkiewicz, and Herrick-Davis (2017), using bioluminescence resonance energy transfer (BRET), bimolecular fluorescence complementation (BiFC) and fluorescence correlation spectroscopy, indicated that β_2-adenergic receptors are predominantly homodimers. Likewise, Jastrzebska et al. (2017) demonstrated that the human red cone opsin forms stable dimers in the live cell membranes, being required for dimerization the aminoacids I230, A233 and M236. Other class A GPCRs that have been also found to form homomers, specially in the last decade, are adenosine A_1, A_{2A} and A_3, dopamine D_1 and D_3, serotonin $5HT_{1A}$, $5HT_{2A}$, and $5HT_7$, adrenergic α_{1B}, cannabinoid CB_1, angiotensin AT_1, muscarinic M_2 and M_3, δ, κ and μ opioid, melatonin MT_2, and niacin receptors (Ayoub, Levoye, Delagrange, & Jockers, 2004; Bagher, Laprairie, Toguri, Kelly, & Denovan-Wright, 2017; Bonaventura et al., 2015; Cvejic & Devi, 1997; Goin & Nathanson, 2006; Gracia et al., 2013, 2011; Guitart et al., 2014; He, Fong, von Zastrow, & Whistler, 2002; Herrick-Davis et al., 2013; Jordan & Devi, 1999; Łukasiewicz et al., 2007; Mandrika, Petrovska, & Klovins, 2010; May, Bridge, Stoddart, Briddon, & Hill, 2011; Pou, Mannoury la Cour, Stoddart, Millan, & Milligan, 2012; Szalai et al., 2012; Teitler, Toohey, Knight, Klein, & Smith, 2010).

In general, the ongoing development and improvement of membrane protein crystallography allowed resolving several crystal structures of GPCRs (Ghosh, Kumari, Jaiman, & Shukla, 2015). Several dimer interfaces have been found for class A receptors. One of the most frequent dimer interfaces involves symmetrical regions of TM1 and TM2 and H8 (rhodopsin, opsin, μ and k opioid and β_1-adrenergic receptors). Other dimeric interfaces found are TM1–TM1, TM1–H8 (β_1- and β_2-adrenergic and dopamine D_2 receptors) and TM4–TM5 or TM5–TM6 (rhodopsin, opsin, adenosine A_{2A}, CXCR4, β_1 and β_2 receptors) (Baltoumas et al., 2016; Gonzalez et al., 2014). These GPCR dimer interfaces are similar to those predicted by mutagenesis, cross-linking and computational modeling (Provasi, Boz, Johnston, & Filizola, 2015), suggesting that they may have physiological relevance. Moreover, Baltoumas et al. (2016), using molecular dynamics and interface analysis, suggested the presence of conserved structural features in TM1–TM2–TM8, TM4–TM5 and TM5–TM6 of different GPCR dimers, despite the low sequence similarity usually found between the receptors. By using BiFC, proximity ligation assay (PLA) and radioligand binding techniques in the absence or presence of TM peptides that mimic specific TM domains of the receptors, disturbing the dimer interface, it has been reported the involvement of TM6–TM6 in D_2R homodimers (Navarro et al., 2018; Pulido et al., 2018), TM6–TM6 in $A_{2A}R$ homodimers if D_2Rs are present in the complex (Navarro et al., 2018) or TM4–TM5 in $A_{2A}R$ homodimers in the presence of A_1Rs (Navarro et al., 2016).

3. GPCRs form heteromers

GPCRs are not only present as monomers and homomers but also form heteromers with other GPCRs (Ferré et al., 2014; Smith & Milligan, 2010). GPCR heteromers are macromolecular complexes, composed of at least two receptor units (protomers), with biochemical properties that are demonstrably different from those of their individual components (Ferré et al., 2009, 2014; Gomes, Ayoub, et al., 2016). Three consensus criteria were published by the International Union of Basic and Clinical Pharmacology to facilitate the classification of true GPCR heteromers (Kenakin et al., 2010). The first of these criteria indicates that heteromer components not only must co-localize in the same subcellular compartment but also physically interact in native tissues (Albizu et al., 2010; Gomes, Ayoub, et al., 2016; Hounsou et al., 2015). The second consensus criteria requires that the heteromers must exhibit specific properties, which have to differ from those associated with the individual protomers, such as trafficking, ligand binding and signaling (biochemical fingerprint) (Bellot et al., 2015; Gomes, Ayoub, et al., 2016; Gomes, Ijzerman, Ye, Maillet, & Devi, 2011; González et al., 2012; Hillion et al., 2002; Jonas et al., 2018; Jordan & Devi, 1999; Kern, Albarran-Zeckler, Walsh, & Smith, 2012; Sohy, Parmentier, & Springael, 2007; Terrillon, Barberis, & Bouvier, 2004). Finally, criterion 3 postulates that heteromer disruption must lead to a loss of interaction and, consequently, a loss of its unique biochemical fingerprint (Baba et al., 2013; Fujita, Gomes, & Devi, 2015; Gomes, Ayoub, et al., 2016).

Although many GPCR heteromers have been identified using heterologous cell lines, only very few fit all three criteria. This is mainly due to the difficulties to study these structures in native tissues because of the lack of sensitive and selective tools, not only capable of detecting in vivo evidence of these endogenous heteromers, but also of demonstrating that they are close enough to interact (Gomes, Sierra, & Devi, 2016). Therefore, it was agreed that the fulfillment of two out of three of the criteria is sufficient for the acceptance of a GPCR heteromer (Jonas & Hanyaloglu, 2017). The most widely used methods to detect heteromers are resonance energy transfer based techniques, which involve either fluorescence or bioluminescence resonance energy transfer (FRET or BRET) between a donor and an acceptor molecule fused to two proteins within the heteromer complex, such as BRET saturation assays (Mercier, Salahpour, Angers, Breit, & Bouvier, 2002) or the GPCR heteromer identification technology (Mustafa & Pfleger, 2011). Another extensively used technique is the proximity ligation assay, which is an immunochemical based technique that allows the detection of molecular interactions between two endogenous or transfected proteins. If these proteins are separated <17 nm, heteromers will be observed as red dots in a confocal microscope (Gomes, Sierra, et al., 2016; Söderberg et al., 2008; Taura, Fernández-Dueñas, & Ciruela, 2015). Alternative strategies to target GPCR heteromers are the generation of selective compounds (bivalent, multifunctional or small molecule ligands), which exhibit higher efficacy in cells expressing both receptors and in tissues from wild type animals, as compared with cell expressing individual receptors or tissues from animals lacking the individual receptors (Akgün et al., 2013; Gomes, Gupta, & Devi, 2013; Molero et al., 2015; Nimczick & Decker, 2015; Peterson et al., 2017; Qian, Vasudevan, et al., 2018; Qian, Wouters, et al., 2018).

Likewise, the use of membrane-permeable peptides that target the dimerization interface or heteromer-selective antibodies that can recognize an epitope in the heteromer but not in the individual protomers, have been emerged as useful tools to detect the presence of GPCR heteromers in vivo (Gupta et al., 2010; He et al., 2011; Jacobs et al., 2018; Moreno et al., 2017; Navarro et al., 2015; Rivera-Oliver et al., 2018; Viñals et al., 2015). Finally, it is important to note the existence of single-molecule techniques, which are ideally designed to understand the dynamic signaling and conformational complexity of GPCRs (Tian, Fürstenberg, & Huber, 2017). Their application can provide tools to directly visualize individual receptors forming homomers and heteromers and how GPCRs can move and interact in living cells; in addition, they are useful to study the effects in their mobility and interactions caused by different ligands that can alter this dynamics, stabilizing preexisting dimers prolonging their lifetime (Calebiro & Sungkaworn, 2018; Jonas, Huhtaniemi, & Hanyaloglu, 2016; Scarselli et al., 2016; Tabor et al., 2016).

The class C $GABA_B$ receptor is the first known GPCR that was demonstrated to require heterodimerization for functioning. In fact, it is called an obligatory heterodimer (or heteromeric receptor; Ferré et al., 2009) composed by two subunits, GBR_1 and GBR_2, that have complementary functions in signal transmission (Kniazeff et al., 2011; Moller et al., 2017). While the extracellular domain of GBR_1 is responsible for ligand recognition, the transmembrane domain of GBR_2 is required for G-protein activation. In addition, GBR_2 facilitates the cell surface expression of GBR_1 through coiled-coil interactions in the cytoplasmic region. This heteromer has been crystallized bound to different agonists and antagonists (Geng, Bush, Mosyak, Wang, & Fan, 2013). On the other hand, mGluRs, another members of family C GPCRs, can form non-obligatory heterodimers (or receptor heteromers; Ferré et al., 2009), being the mGlu2-4 the most studied pair due to its physiological interest; concretely, they are involved in control synaptic activity at the level of the cortico-striatal terminals in the striatum (Yin et al., 2014) and at the level of lateral performant path terminals in the dendate gyrus (Moreno-Delgado et al., 2017). Recently, Liu et al. (2017) reported an oriented asymmetry in the activation of this heterodimer that can be controlled with allosteric modulators.

The first ones class A receptors found as heterodimers were reported by Gomes et al. (2000), who identified a heteromer constituted by two subtypes of opioid receptors (μ and δ) in heterologous cells. The same year, Ginés et al. (2000) showed the first heteromer composed of two different receptors, the adenosine A_1 and dopamine D_1 receptors, in cotransfected fibroblast cells. It is important to mention that many of the heterooligomeric assemblies that have been detected in vivo so far, demonstrate the preponderance of dopamine- and adenosine-containing receptors, indicating their major contribution to various neurological conditions and the full breadth of their therapeutic potential (Farran, 2017).

4. Dopamine and adenosine in CNS

Dopaminergic and purinergic signaling play a pivotal role in neurological diseases with motor symptoms, including Parkinson's disease (PD), motor neuron diseases, multiple sclerosis, amyotrophic lateral sclerosis, Huntington disease, Restless Legs Syndrome (RLS) and ataxias (Oliveira-Giacomelli et al., 2018).

Dopamine is a pleiotropic compound that acts as a neurotransmitter and a hormone (Borcherding et al., 2011), and plays a key role in numerous CNS processes including attention, behavior and cognition, motor control, motivation and reward, mood, sleep, learning and memory (Puig, Rose, Schmidt, & Freund, 2014; Rubí & Maechler, 2010). Dopamine acts on specific receptors (DRs) belonging to the GPCR family A, which are categorized in two main groups: D1-like (D_1R and D_5R) and D2-like (D_2R, D_3R and D_4R), that are linked to stimulation (D_1R-like) or inhibition (D_2R-like) of adenylate cyclase (Cortés, Moreno, Rodríguez-Ruiz, Canela, & Casadó, 2016). DRs directly regulate neurotransmission of other neurotransmitters, release of cAMP, and also cell proliferation and differentiation (Mishra, Singh, & Shukla, 2018). The striatum receives the densest dopamine innervation and contains the highest density of DRs in the brain. D_1Rs are expressed selectively by the direct pathway GABAergic spiny projection neurons, whereas D_2Rs are expressed by the indirect pathway. Striatal direct and indirect pathways form the functional backbone of the basal ganglia circuit. Both D_1R and D_2R have distinctive linkages to intracellular signaling cascades and targets, leading to fundamentally different cellular responses to extracellular dopamine (Gerfen & Surmeier, 2011).

Adenosine is a naturally occurring purine nucleoside that is distributed ubiquitously throughout the body as a metabolic intermediary. In the brain, adenosine functions as an important upstream neuromodulator of a broad spectrum of neurotransmitters, receptors and signaling pathways. By acting through four family A GPCRs (A_1R, $A_{2A}R$, $A_{2B}R$ and A_3R), adenosine contributes critically to homeostasis and neuromodulatory control of a variety of normal and abnormal brain functions, ranging from synaptic plasticity to cognition, motor activity, neuroinflammation and cell death (Chen, Lee, & Chern, 2014). In addition, adenosine is a main endogenous homeostatic sleep-promoting substance and plays a very significant role in the modulation of dopaminergic transmission, with implications for psychomotor activity and reinforcement (Ferré, 2016; Nunes, Randall, Podurgiel, Correa, & Salamone, 2013). The two main ARs in the CNS are A_1R and $A_{2A}R$. A_1R is predominantly present in cortex, hippocampus, cerebellum, nerve terminals, spinal cord and glia (Ballesteros-Yáñez, Castillo, Merighi, & Gessi, 2018; Chen et al., 2014; Fuxe et al., 2010). $A_{2A}R$ is mainly expressed in the striatum, but it is also detectable in the olfactory tubercle, hippocampus, glial cells and cerebral cortex (Ballesteros-Yáñez et al., 2018; de Lera Ruiz, Lim, & Zheng, 2014).

5. Restless legs syndrome

RLS, also known as Willis-Ekbom disease, is a very prevalent neurologic disorder with unique clinical features, characterized by a periodic, rest-induced, mostly nocturnal, movement-responsive urge to move the legs or periodic leg movements during sleep (PLMS) and hyperarousal (Allen, Stillman, & Myers, 2010; Ferré, Quiroz, et al., 2018; Ferri et al., 2015). Several neuropsychological studies have shown that RLS is associated with deficits in cognitive functions, such as attention, working memory and frontal executive functions (Cha, Choi, Jung, & Kim, 2017). Moreover, it has been indicated that RLS is a multifactorial network disorder involving many regions of the nervous system, from the spinal cord and peripheral nerves to the dopaminergic and glutamatergic nuclei of the CNS (Earley et al., 2014; Hartmann, Pfister, & Pfadenhauer, 1999; Paulus & Schomburg, 2006; Pitarokoili et al., 2018). RLS symptoms follow a circadian pattern becoming worse in the evening. This disease affects 5–10% of European and North American with 2–3% experiencing moderate to severe symptoms, it occurs twice as often in women as in men, and has a mean onset age between 30 and 40 years (Allen et al., 2014; Garcia-Borreguero & Cano-Pumarega, 2017; Hening et al., 1999; Kim & Deeks, 2016). Modifiable lifestyle factors can influence the risk of RLS; as an example, patients who are physically active, nonsmokers, with healthy weight and moderate alcohol consumption, are less likely to develop RLS (Batool-Anwar et al., 2016).

RLS is a genetically complex disorder in which genetic and environmental factors contribute to the phenotype (Trenkwalder, Allen, Högl, Paulus, & Winkelmann, 2016). This disease is highly familial and six genetic variants with single nucleotide polymorphisms have been identified by genome-wide association studies (Scholz, 2017; Winkelman et al., 2011, 2007). It is interesting to notice that the products of three of these genes (BTBD9, MAP2K5 and MEIS1) are highly expressed in the basal ganglia, red nucleus, cerebral cortex and spinal cord (Guo et al., 2017; Winkelman, 2008). Recently, Schormair et al. (2017) described a meta-analysis of genome-wide association studies of RLS in which they demonstrated strong and reproducible evidence for 13 new genetic loci that contribute to risk of RLS and have provided further insights into the molecular mechanisms underlying the disorder, evidencing possible novel therapeutic targets or avenues for the repurposing of existing drugs.

Although the pathophysiology of RLS is not fully understood, evidence indicates that both iron deficiency and dopaminergic abnormalities are involved in its etiology. As iron is a major cofactor in dopaminergic neurotransmission, iron deficits may produce dopaminergic changes that exacerbate RLS symptoms (Allen & Earley, 2007; Becker & Novak, 2014). However, the fact that there is an overall increase in severity of symptoms after long-term dopaminergic therapy is leading to a shift towards non-dopaminergic alternatives such as calcium channel $\alpha 2\delta$ ligands (i.e., gabapentin, gabapentin enacarbil and pregabalin), opioids (i.e., oxycodone and methadone), and substances that act on glutamate and adenosine systems (Anguelova, Vlak, Kurvers, & Rijsman, 2018; Faulkner, 2018; Garcia-Borreguero & Cano-Pumarega, 2017; Garcia-Borreguero et al., 2018; Quiroz et al., 2016; Silber et al., 2018; Trenkwalder, Zieglgänsberger, Ahmedzai, & Högl, 2017) (see Table 1).

6. Dopaminergic abnormalities in RLS and treatments

Tyrosine hydroxylase is the rate-limiting enzyme in the biosynthesis of dopamine, which catalyzes the non-heme ferrous-mediate incorporation of one atom of molecular oxygen into both the amino acid substrate and the reducing cofactor 6R-tetrahydrobiopterin. The reaction produces the catechol amino acid L-3,4-dihydroxyphenylalanine (L-DOPA) and the pterin product via an electrophilic aromatic substitution (Roberts & Fitzpatrick, 2013). As iron is a cofactor of this enzyme, iron deficiency may affect dopamine production indirectly and can alter the dopaminergic system in the brain (Dauvilliers & Winkelmann, 2013). Moreover, iron deficiency has been shown to alter the expression of dopamine-related genes, including a ferritin regulatory gene SDF-1 (Hare, Ayton, Bush, & Lei, 2013; Jellen et al., 2013). In addition, a preclinical study found that loss of the transferrin receptor causes neuronal iron deficiency and dopaminergic neurodegeneration (Matak et al., 2016). Altered dopamine function plays an important role in PLMS symptomatology of RLS. The most compelling argument that supports this idea is that RLS symptoms are strikingly improved after the treatment with dopaminergic drugs that target D_2R/D_3R, and it is also in agree with the repeated demonstration of biochemical changes related to the dopaminergic system (Earley et al., 2014; Garcia-Borreguero et al., 2013; Yepes et al., 2017). The dopaminergic profile in RLS includes abnormally high levels of the dopamine metabolites 3-ortho-methyldopa and homovanillic acid in the

Table 1 Summary of pharmacological therapies for RLS in humans.

Target protein	Ligand type	Compound	Brand name	Company	Usual dose range (mg/day)	Clinical status
D_1R-like D_2R-like	Precursor of endogenous agonist	Levodopa/Carbidopa	Sinemet Bidopal Carbidopa/levodopa	Merck GlaxoSmithKline Mylan, Actavis	100–300/ 25–100	Not approved
		Levodopa/Benserazide	Madopar, Prolopa Numient	Roche Amneal	100–300/ 25–75	
D_2R-like	Non-ergot full agonists	Pramipexole	Mirapex	Boehringer, Ingelheim	0.25–0.5	FDA 1997 approval
			Pramipexole	Barr, Apotex, Mylan, Sandoz, etc.		FDA 2008 approval
		Ropinirole	Requip	GlaxoSmithKline	0.25–4	FDA 1997 approval
			Ropinirole	G and W, Apotex, Mylan, Sandoz, Watson, etc.		FDA 2008 approval
		Rotigotine	Neupro, Leganto	UCB	1–3	FDA 2007 approval
	Ergot agonists	Cabergoline	Dostinex, Cabaser	Pfizer	0.3	Not approved
		Pergolide	Permax	Valeant, Eli Lilly	3	Not approved
		Lisuride	Dopergin; Dipergon	Bayer	0.3–4	Not approved

Continued

Table 1 Summary of pharmacological therapies for RLS in humans.—cont'd

Target protein	Ligand type	Compound	Brand name	Company	Usual dose range (mg/day)	Clinical status
DR indirectly	DAT Na^+ depend. inhibitor	Bupropion	Aplenzin	Sanofi, Valeant	150–300	Not approved
ADR α_2	Partial agonist	Clonidine	Catapres	Boehringer	0.2–0.6	Not approved
Opioid receptors	μ-δ-κ-agonist/ μ-δ-κ-antagonist	Oxycodone/naloxone	Targin	Purdue, Mundipharma	10–40/ 5–20	EMA 2014 approval
	μ-δ-agonist NMDA antagonist nAchR antagonist	Methadone	Metadol Methadone	Paladin	10–40	Not approved
		Morphine	–	–	15–45	Not approved
	μ-agonist	Tramadol	ConZip Tramal	Vertical Grünenthal	100–200	Not approved
	μ-δ-κ-agonist	Codeine	Codeine	Riva, Purdue, Hospira, Roxane	15–120	Not approved
	μ-δ-agonist	Hydrocodone	Hycodan	Bristol Myers S.	20–30	Not approved
		Dextropropoxyphene	Darvon Depronal	Eli Lilly Pfizer	65–400	Not approved
AR indirectly	ENT1/2 inhibitor ADA inhibitor	Dipyridamole	Dipyridamole	Hospira, Pro Doc	280	Not approved
Nicotinic AchR	Inhibitor	Carbamazepine	Apo-carbamazepine Carbamazepine	Apotex Caraco	400–1200	Not approved

GABAR	Positive allosteric modulator	Clonazepam	Clonazepam Klonopin	Valeant Roche	0.25–2	Not approved
		Eszopiclone	Lunesta	Physicians Total Care	1–3	Not approved
		Temazepam	Restoril	Physicians Total Care	15–30	Not approved
		Zolpidem	Ambien	Physicians Total Care, Sanofi	5–10	Not approved
		Zaleplon	Sonata	Pfizer	5–10	Not approved
AMPAR	Noncompetitive antagonists	Perampanel	Fycompa	Eisai	2–4	Not approved
VSCC	α_{1B} inhibitor	Levetiracetam	Keppra	Ucb	1000	Not approved
	$\alpha 2\delta$ inhibitor	Gabapentin	Neurotin	Pfizer	300–2400	Not approved
		Gabapentin enacarbil	Horizant	Arbor	800–1200	FDA 2011 approval
		Pregabalin	Lyrica	Pfizer	75–450	Not approved
–	Iron	$FeSO_4$	–	–	650–975	Not approved
		IV ferric carboxymaltose	Injectafer	Daiichi Sankyo	1000	Not approved
		Iron sucrose	Venofer	American Reagent Fresenius Med.	400–1000	Not approved

ADA, adenosine deaminase; ADR, adrenoceptor; AMPAR, AMPA receptor; AR, adenosine receptor; DAT, dopamine transporter; DR, dopamine receptor; ENT, equilibrative nucleoside transporter; GABAR, GABA receptor; nAchR, nicotinic acetylcholine receptor; VSCC, voltage-sensitive calcium channel. Based on the following references: Anguelova et al. (2018); Becker and Novak (2014); García-Borreguero et al. (2018); Sales, Sanghera, Klocko, & Stewart (2016); Silber et al. (2018); Trenkwalder, Winkelmann, Inoue, & Paulus (2015); Wijemanne and Ondo (2017); Winkelman et al. (2016); https://www.accessdata.fda.gov; https://clinicaltrials.gov; https://www.drugbank.ca; https://www.drugs.com/dosage; https://www.ema.europa.eu.

cerebrospinal fluid, a decrease in the density of striatal D_2R and in the mesolimbic D_2R/D_3R and dopamine transporters (mostly membrane-bound transporters) and a pronounced increase in tyrosine hydroxylase activity in the striatum and substantia nigra (Earley et al., 2011; Ferré, Quiroz, et al., 2018; Garcia-Borreguero & Cano-Pumarega, 2017; Oboshi et al., 2012; Wijemanne & Ondo, 2017). These data, when taken together, would be mostly compatible with a hyperdopaminergic-presynaptic state: increased synthesis and release and a decreased uptake of dopamine, leading to an increase in synaptic dopamine (Earley et al., 2014). In addition, the findings also predict the existence of a hypodopaminergic-postsynaptic state with decreased D_2R/D_3R. Overall, these data suggest that a hyperdopaminergic-presynaptic state in RLS is in balance or in opposition to a hypodopaminergic-postsynaptic state (Earley et al., 2014; Earley, Uhl, Clemens, & Ferré, 2017). Recently, Rizzo, Li, Galantucci, Filippi, and Cho (2017) indicated the existence of an even more complex dopaminergic change in RLS, with different dopamine levels depending on the disease duration and clinical severity, and with some brain regions presenting hyperdopaminergic and other hypodopaminergic activity.

Until recently, the first line treatment of RLS was the administration of low dose of three dopaminergic drugs, which has been approved by the US Food and Drug Administration and the European Medicines Agency for the treatment of moderate to severe RLS. These compounds are pramipexole (Mirapex), ropinirole (Requip) and rotigotine transdermal patch (Neupro), which act as agonists that mainly target the D_3R (Cortés, Moreno, et al., 2016; Dinkins, Lallemand, & Clemens, 2017). While initially highly effective, these compounds lose their efficacy over time, and long-term therapy regularly leads to a worsening of the RLS symptoms. In fact, augmentation is the main complication of long-term dopaminergic therapy and was first reported with the dopamine precursor L-DOPA (Becker & Novak, 2014). Characteristic features of augmentation include an increase in RLS symptom intensity, the onset of symptoms earlier in the day, a shorter time to symptom onset during periods of rest, spread of symptoms to previously unaffected body parts and a shorter period of relief following the administration of medication (Anguelova et al., 2018; Becker & Novak, 2014; García-Borreguero et al., 2007). Recent experimental data indicate that the mechanisms leading to augmentation in RLS patients after long-term use of D_3R drugs may be related to a parallel D_3R-induced upregulation of the D_1R system, suggesting that this receptor might serve as a target for the treatment of augmentation. Therefore, a combination therapy of activating the D_3R system and adjuvant blocking of the D_1R system may provide the initial relief sought by patients and also may maintain the efficacy of the treatment over time (Dinkins et al., 2017).

Yepes et al. (2017) showed the existence of hypersensitivity of corticostriatal glutamatergic terminals in rodents with brain iron deficiency, which were targeted for locally perfused pramipexole, ropinirole and gabapentin. Furthermore, using selective antagonists they demonstrated that there was an involvement of D_2R and D_4R subtypes in the effects of pramipexole. The dopamine D_2 short receptor ($D_{2S}R$) and the D_4R are preferentially localized in corticostriatal glutamatergic terminals and are involved in the direct modulation of striatal glutamate release (Bonaventura et al., 2017; Centonze et al., 2004; González et al., 2012). Therefore, more selective $D_{2S}R$ and D_4R agonists could be potential medications for RLS. D_4R can be particularly seen as the main therapeutic target, because it is more selectively expressed by corticostriatal neurons than $D_{2S}R$ and it has been recently shown to play a main role as a mediator of dopamine modulation of corticostriatal neurotransmission (Bonaventura et al., 2017). These data support a switch in the dopamine receptor subtype as a therapeutic target for RLS from the D_3R to the D_4R, with fewer secondary effects (Yepes et al., 2017).

7. Adenosinergic neuromodulation and RLS

In three separate studies Ferré's group pointed at a relation between adenosine and its two main receptor subtypes in the brain (A_1R and $A_{2A}R$) and brain iron deficiency (BID) in RLS. These authors found a consistent upregulation of striatal $A_{2A}R$ in rats and rodents with severe BID (Gulyani et al., 2009; Quiroz et al., 2016, 2010). In the same animal model, A_1R density was found decreased in animals with mild, moderate and severe deficiency accompanied by dopaminergic D_2R downregulation and an increased presynaptic $A_{2A}R$ density in animals submitted to a more iron deficient diet (Quiroz et al., 2016). These results indicate that downregulation of A_1R might constitute a more significant correlate of BID in RLS, while changes on $A_{2A}R$ density would be only observed with severe BID (Ferré, Earley, Gulyani, & Garcia-Borreguero, 2017).

There is increasing evidence from preclinical and clinical studies that links BID and impairments in glutamatergic and adenosinergic neurotransmission as pathogenetic mechanisms involved in RLS (Ferré et al., 2017; Garcia-Borreguero & Cano-Pumarega, 2017). A single alteration in the adenosinergic system, such as an A_1R downregulation-mediated increased sensitivity of corticostriatal terminals, could produce presynaptic striatal hyperglutamatergic and hyperdopaminergic states, which could be a sufficient pathophysiological mechanism to explain PLMS in RLS. Downregulation of presynaptic D_2R localized in glutamatergic and dopaminergic terminals could also be a significant contributing factor. Therefore, adenosine neurotransmission can provide the link between dopamine and glutamate mechanisms in RLS and a hypoadenosinergic state can explain the hyperdopaminergic and hyperglutamatergic state of RLS (Ferré, Quiroz, et al., 2018).

8. Dopamine D_1 and adenosine A_1 receptor heteromers

8.1 A_1R–D_1R heteromers in brain striatum

The modulatory role of adenosine on dopaminergic transmission depends largely on the existence of antagonistic interactions mediated by specific subtypes of adenosine and dopamine receptors, the so-called $A_{2A}R$–D_2R interactions and the A_1R–D_1R interactions (Ferré, Fredholm, Morelli, Popoli, & Fuxe, 1997). Apart from the endogenous neurotransmitters, these specific ARs-DRs interactions are involved in the central effects of caffeine, the most consumed psychoactive drug in the world, which acts as a nonselective A_1R and $A_{2A}R$ competitive antagonist (Acevedo et al., 2016; Cortés, Casadó-Anguera, Moreno, & Casadó, 2016; Ferré, 2016; Ferré et al., 2008). A large amount of data indicates that adenosine antagonizes D_1R-mediated transmission via stimulation of A_1Rs (Ferré et al., 1997, 2001). Moreover, it has been shown that A_1Rs and D_1Rs are colocalized in the striatum and A_1Rs antagonistically modulate D_1Rs at the level of receptor binding and second messengers (Ferré et al., 1997). Due to the dopamine/adenosine antagonism in the CNS, it was suspected that ARs and DRs could form heteromers in the cell surface of the neuron. Therefore, adenosine can affect dopaminergic signaling through receptor heteromer formations and shared intracellular pathways (Nazario, da Silva, & Bonan, 2017).

The first evidence of the existence of a receptor-receptor interaction between A_1R and D_1R was provided by means of co-immunoprecipitation experiments and confocal microscopy analysis in co-transfected mouse fibroblasts Lkt^- cells with human A_1R and D_1R cDNAs and in cortical neurons in culture (Ginés et al., 2000). Similarly, by means of double immunofluorescence experiments with confocal microscopy, Toda, Alguacil, and Kalivas (2003) found a high degree of A_1R and D_1R co-localization in both cotransfected fibroblast cells and in rat nucleus accumbens.

This co-localization disappeared after pretreatment with a selective D_1R agonist, but not after combined pretreatment with D_1R and A_1R agonists. Functional experiments on the D_1R agonist-induced cAMP production suggested that coactivation of A_1R and D_1R in the heteromeric complex leads to an uncoupling of D_1R from Gi (Ginés et al., 2000). In addition, Le Crom, Prou, and Vernier (2002) reported that the A_1R selective antagonist DPCPX had an effect on the affinity value of the D_1R selective agonist SKF 38393 in cells transfected with A_1R and D_1R; thus adenosine would exert a tonic inhibition of dopamine in the D_1R mediated function through the A_1R–D_1R complex. The presence of adenosine deaminase is important in the A_1R–D_1R interaction, probably by providing the high affinity binding state of the A_1R (Torvinen et al., 2002). It is now well accepted that the simultaneous activation of both receptors may allow the antagonistic intramembrane receptor-receptor interaction to take place, and it has been suggested that one functional meaning of this interaction is the uncoupling of the D_1R from the Gs protein with the consequent disappearance of the D_1R high affinity state (Ciruela et al., 2011; Franco et al., 2007).

It has been demonstrated that the pretreatment with an A_1R agonist caused co-clustering (coaggregation) of A_1Rs and D_1Rs, which was blocked by combined pretreatment with A_1Rs and D_1Rs agonists (Ciruela et al., 2011; Ginés et al., 2000). These results indicated that the movement of the heteromer and/or clusters of heteromers in the plasma membrane could be agonist-dependent, and that receptor trafficking may depend on the activity of the two receptors of the heteromer. Moreover, radioligand binding experiments performed in cotransfected A_1R/D_1R cells showed that the A_1R activation induced a concentration-dependent decrease in the affinity for the D_1R agonist SKF38393 and inhibit the effect induced by D_1R activation at the second messenger level generation (Cao, Sun, Jin, Xie, & Zhu, 2006). The same authors showed that long term exposure of HEK 293 cells to the D_1R agonist SKF38393 caused a rapid desensitization of D_1R, and that this effect is potentiated by coadministration of the A_1R agonist CPA (Cao, Xie, & Zhu, 2007). This enhancement effect of CPA was mediated by the A_1R and was Gi protein independent, demonstrating that A_1R plays an important role in the regulation of D_1R by potentiating ligand-induced desensitization. Therefore, the neurochemical and behavioral findings showing different interactions between A_1R and D_1R, can be explained by the existence of A_1R–D_1R heteromers in striatal and prefrontal cortex (Fuxe, Ferré, Genedani, Franco, & Agnati, 2007; Fuxe et al., 2010).

Shen et al. (2013) evidenced for the existence of striatal $A_1R–D_1R$ dimerization ex vivo. These authors designed and synthesized a group of bivalent ligands containing a D_1R agonist (SKF38393) and an A_1R antagonist (a naphthylxantine derivative), linked by different lengths of polyethylene glycol linkers. The binding affinities of these compounds were determined by radioligand binding studies in membrane preparations from brain striatum, and fluorescence resonance energy transfer (FRET) experiments were performed to test if these bivalent ligands were able to promote the formation of $A_1R–D_1R$ heterodimers. Two of these compounds were able to induce the formation of $A_1R–D_1R$ heteromers, detected by FRET techniques, showing affinities for the A_1R 10–100 times higher than those of the corresponding monovalent ligands. Moreover, these authors proposed a heterodimer model with the interface of helixes 3, 4 and 5 of the A_1R and helixes 1, 6 and 7 from the D_1R was established with molecular modeling. With this model they confirmed that the distance between the two ligand binding sites in the heterodimer model was shorter than the length of the bivalent ligands. In addition, the ligand docking studies confirmed that the bivalent ligand was able bind to both binding sites in the heterodimer (Shen et al., 2013).

Using cell patch-clamp recordings, Mango et al. (2014) demonstrated that the A_1R stimulation by the selective agonist 5′Cl5′d-ENBA reduces D_1R-mediated GABAergic transmission from striato-nigral terminals and attenuates L-DOPA-induced dyskinesia in dopamine-denervate mice. These results can only be explained by the existence of $A_1R–D_1R$ heteromers, and suggest the potential benefit of A_1R agonists like 5′Cl5′d-ENBA, that have reduced cardiovascular effects and may ameliorate dyskinetic and hyperkinetic movements associated with L-DOPA treatment of PD patients, providing a mechanistic framework for the study of the interaction between dopamine and adenosine in the striatonigral system (Mango et al., 2014).

In summary, the $A_1R–D_1R$ heteromeric complex may give the molecular basis for the well documented antagonistic $A_1R–D_1R$ interactions found in the neuronal networks of the brain (see above). Therefore, the understanding of the $A_1R–D_1R$ interactions within this heteromer is of significant functional and pharmacologic importance and has been useful for the development of novel treatments for some neuropathologies that include attention deficit hyperactivity disorder, PD, dyskinesias, schizophrenia and drug addiction (Ciruela et al., 2011; Fuxe et al., 2007; Hobson et al., 2013; Mango et al., 2014; Mioranzza et al., 2011).

8.2 $A_1R–D_1R$ heteromers in spinal cord

The spinal cord, which extends from the base of the brain to the upper lumbar region, is the main information pathway connecting the brain and the peripheral nervous system. Together with brain, it forms the CNS and functions primarily in the modulation and transmission of neural signals traveling between the body and the brain (Weber et al., 2018). Adenosinergic modulation has been detected in motor networks of the spinal cord and brainstem. By acting on A_1R, adenosine reduce the frequency of locomotor-related bursting in the spinal locomotor central pattern generators of postnatal mice (Witts, Nascimento, & Miles, 2015) and it has been suggested that adenosine is the primary glial cell-derived modulator of spinal motor networks and of locomotor behavior (Acton & Miles, 2015). Likewise, it has been reported that A_1R may be one of the most promising targets for the development of new anxiolytic drugs and that their activation may reduce pain signaling in the spinal cord (Varani, Vincenzi, Merighi, Gessi, & Borea, 2017). On the other hand, spinal dopaminergic neurotransmission, and more specifically D_1R, is also being considered as a potential new target to promote recovery of locomotor function after spinal cord injury (SCI) (Sharples, Koblinger, Humphreys, & Whelan, 2014), the main cause of disability worldwide produced mainly by mechanical and physical damage (Palacios et al., 2012). Moreover, D1-like receptors are highly expressed in the ventral horn, in lamina IX, including the motoneurons, where they mediate motor excitatory effects (Clemens, Belin-Rauscent, Simmers, & Combes, 2012; Sharples et al., 2014).

Interestingly, the blockade of A_1R by caffeine has been involved in mediating neuroprotective effects against SCI, including reduction of hyperalgesia, which involves an attenuation of hypersensitivity to pain, usually caused by damage to nociceptors (pain receptors) and/or peripheral nerves after injury (Palacios et al., 2012; Stone, Ceruti, & Abbracchio, 2009). Furthermore, daily caffeine intake in mice has been shown to inhibit the process of antinociception (increased tolerance to pain) by modulation of A_1Rs, as demonstrated using the specific A_1R antagonist DPCPX, which mimicked the effects of caffeine (Salvemini, Kim, & Mollace, 2013). In addition, caffeine application to the spinal cord of guinea pigs after SCI induced an up-regulation of the A_1R and of tissue growth factor-beta mRNAs, which has been shown to provide immune regulation of inflammation further supporting a neuroprotective role of caffeine (Chen et al., 2010; Rivera-Oliver & Díaz-Ríos, 2014; Salvemini et al., 2013).

Recently, the effects of caffeine on the locomotor function of the spinal central pattern generators network via extracellular ventral root recording has been assessed by Acevedo et al. (2016), using isolated neonatal mouse spinal cord preparations. The addition of 50 μM caffeine or of a selective A_1R antagonist (DPCPX) significantly decreased the cycle period accelerating the ongoing locomotor rhythm while decreasing burst duration reversibly in most preparations, suggesting the role of A_1R as the primary target of caffeine. Additionally, the use of caffeine or an A_1R antagonist failed to stimulate ongoing locomotor activity in the absence of dopamine or in the presence of a D_1R but not a D_2R antagonist, supporting the A_1R–D_1R dependent mechanism of action (Acevedo et al., 2016). These results support a stimulant effect of caffeine on the lumbar spinal network controlling hindlimb locomotion through the inhibition of A_1Rs and subsequent activation of D_1Rs via a PKA-dependent mechanism (Acevedo et al., 2016). The cessation of locomotor activity at higher concentrations of caffeine raises the possibility that caffeine can have an "inverted U shape" dose-dependent-effect in the spinal locomotor function, similar to reported effects of systemic application of this drug in freely behaving animals (Soares et al., 2009). These studies suggested that caffeine exerts a stimulating effect on locomotor activity at low moderate doses, but less stimulating and even depressive effects at higher doses (Gracia et al., 2013; Zhang et al., 2011).

The same authors (Rivera-Oliver et al., 2018), combining a selective destabilizing peptide strategy with BRET, BiFC, PLA (Fig. 1) and patch-clamp electrophysiology in slices from male mouse lumbar spinal cord, identified A_1R–D_1R heteromers in the spinal motoneuron (with TM5 of D_1R forming part of the heteromeric interface). These studies have demonstrated that A_1R–D_1R heteromers mediate the ability of adenosine to exert a tonic inhibitory modulation of dopamine-mediated increase in neuronal excitability. Likewise, the psychostimulant effects of caffeine in spinal motoneurons depends on its ability to counteract the tonic inhibitory effect of endogenous adenosine via A_1R–D_1R heteromers, which extends to the spinal cord the previously established supraspinal mechanism of these psychostimulant effects (Acevedo et al., 2016). Acton, Broadhead, and Miles (2018) provided evidence that adenosine produced upon stimulation of astrocytes within the spinal cord, acts via A_1Rs to inhibit signaling through D_1Rs and does not act by previously described dopamine-independent pathways (Carlsen & Perrier, 2014). These data support a novel form of

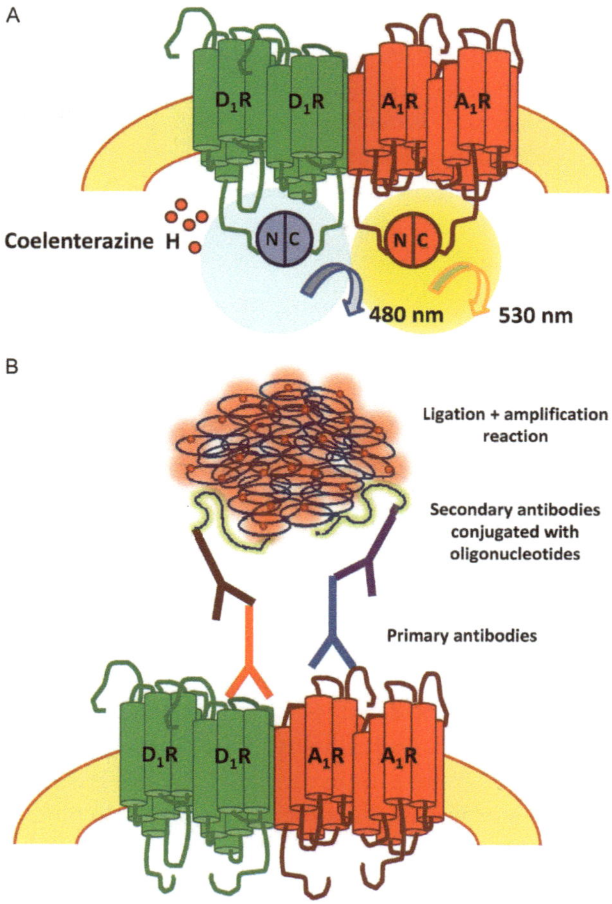

Fig. 1 Methods for detecting $A_1R–D_1R$ heteromers. (A) Recognition in vitro using biophysical methods as BRET after luminescence and fluorescence complementation of the different protomers within the heterotetramer. (B) In situ detection of heteromers by PLA.

metamodulation within the mammalian spinal cord, enhancing the understanding of neuron-astrocyte interactions and their importance in shaping network activity.

It has been recently suggested that normal aging is associated with a D_1R upregulation in the spinal cord with a lack of concomitant increased expression of inhibitory receptors (Keeler, Lallemand, Patel, de Castro Brás, & Clemens, 2016). Moreover, recent preclinical evidence indicates that alterations in the adenosinergic system, and particularly downregulation of A_1R, play a key pathogenetic role in RLS (Ferré, Quiroz, et al., 2018; Quiroz et al., 2016). Therefore, the spinal $A_1R–D_1R$ heteromer can explain the recently demonstrated spinally-generated caffeine-induced locomotor activation in rats (Acevedo et al., 2016) and can constitute a new target for the pharmacological therapy after SCI, motor aging-associated disorders and the spinal component of RLS (Rivera-Oliver et al., 2018; Trenkwalder & Paulus, 2010), also associated to SCI (Hartmann et al., 1999).

9. GPCRs form heterotetramers

In addition to homodimers and heterodimers, for several family A receptor heteromers, experimental evidence supports the presence of higher order rearrangements as tetrameric structures, comprised of two different homodimers, each able to signal with its preferred G protein, that can act as the conduit of allosteric interactions between orthosteric ligands (Ferré, 2015; Ferré et al., 2016). As an example, Guitart et al. (2014), by combining BiFC and luminescence complementation with BRET and complemented donor-acceptor resonance energy transfer (CODA-RET) assays, demonstrated the existence of a tetrameric D_1R-D_3R heteromer, comprised of D_1R and D_3R homodimers able to couple to G_s and G_i proteins, respectively. Moreover, these authors identified that the TM5–TM6 interface is essential for the stability of this structure and also demonstrated ligand-induced allosteric interactions, such as positive cross-talk and cross-antagonism, which constitute specific biochemical characteristics of the D_1R-D_3R heteromer. These allosteric modulations may have implications for the treatment of several neuropsychiatric disorders, because this heteromer is being considered as a target for drug development in L-DOPA-induced dyskinesia and drug addiction (Cortés, Moreno, et al., 2016; Ferré, Lluis, Lanciego, & Franco, 2010; Fiorentini, Busi, Spano, & Missale, 2010).

Another example of tetrameric structures emerged from a study on $A_1R–A_{2A}R$ heteromers in primary cultures of rat astrocytes. This complex was found to couple to both $G_{i/o}$ and G_s proteins, resulting in cross-antagonism. The A_1R agonist increased $G_{i/o}$ activity, which was suppressed by an $A_{2A}R$ agonist. Reciprocally, G_s activation was restricted to $A_{2A}R$ and was abolished by the binding of an A_1R antagonist, consisting with the existence of $A_1R–A_{2A}R$ heteromers of two homodimers, thus enabling the binding of two distinct G proteins (Cristóvão-Ferreira et al., 2013). BRET assays and computer modeling to monitor receptor oligomerization revealed 2:2 receptor heteromers, suggesting a rhombus-shaped tetramer arrangement connected by a TM4–TM5 interface for homodimerization and a TM5–TM6 for heterodimerization (Navarro et al., 2016). In this heterotetramer are bound two different interacting G proteins, G_i and G_s, highlighting the function of the tetramer as a possible G_s/G_i mediated switching mechanism by which low and high concentrations of adenosine fine-tune glutamate release (Farran, 2017).

In the case of the $A_{2A}R$–D_2R tetrameric complex, $A_{2A}R$ and D_2R preferentially couple to G_s and G_i proteins, respectively. This heterotetramer has been detected in transfected cells and mammalian striatum, and has been found to be implicated in PD, schizophrenia and drug abuse (Ferré, 2015; Trifilieff et al., 2011). In this heteromeric complex, D_2R agonists exert a negative allosteric modulation, decreasing the affinity and intrinsic efficacy of $A_{2A}R$ ligands (Trincavelli et al., 2012). Reciprocally, any orthosteric $A_{2A}R$ ligand, agonist or antagonist, including the well-known caffeine, exerts a negative allosteric modulation, decreasing the affinity and intrinsic efficacy of any orthosteric D_2R ligand, agonist or antagonist (Azdad et al., 2009; Bonaventura et al., 2015). This could explain the behavioral depressant effects of adenosine analogues and the psychostimulant effects of caffeine on $[^{11}C]$ raclopride binding in human striatum (Casadó-Anguera et al., 2016; Ferré, 2016; Gaitonde & González-Maeso, 2017; Volkow et al., 2015). Altogether, different experimental results on $A_{2A}R$–D_2R heteromer can be better explained by the heterotetrameric model, a necessary frame for the canonical antagonistic G_s-G_i interaction (Ferré, 2015; Ferré et al., 2016). Very recently, in mammalian transfected cells, using synthetic peptides with amino acid sequences of all TM domains of $A_{2A}R$ and D_2R and the putative TMs of AC5, we have provided clear evidence for the existence of functional pre-coupled complexes of $A_{2A}R$ and D_2R homodimers, their cognate G_{olf} and G_i proteins and AC5 (Navarro et al., 2018). We first identified a symmetrical TM6 interface for the $A_{2A}R$ and D_2R homodimers and a symmetrical TM4–TM5 $A_{2A}R$–D_2R heteromeric interface. Likewise, we also found asymmetrical interfaces formed by TMs of the receptors and putative TMs of AC5 which rearrange upon agonist exposure. Computational analysis indicated the existence of a minimal functional complex formed by two $A_{2A}R$–D_2R heterotetramers and two AC5 molecules (Ferré, Bonaventura, et al., 2018). In fact, this quaternary structure suggests the possible formation of zig-zagged arranged higher-order oligomeric structures, a higher-order linear arrangement of GPCR heteromers and effectors (Navarro et al., 2018). Finally, we could demonstrate that this macromolecular complex allows the canonical G_s-G_i antagonistic interaction at the level of AC5, and acts as an integrative device of adenosine and dopamine neurotransmission (Ferré, Bonaventura, et al., 2018).

Lately, using receptor TM peptides, BiFC and PLA experiments, we have also obtained experimental evidence for the tetrameric structure of A_1R–D_1R, which explains the canonical interaction on G_i and G_s, respectively (Fig. 2). We have demonstrated for the first time the presence of this heterotetramer in striatal tissue (manuscript in preparation), in addition to in spinal motoneurons (Ferré, Quiroz, et al., 2018; Rivera-Oliver et al., 2018). The spinal A_1R–D_1R heterotetramer could explain the recently demonstrated spinally-generated caffeine-induced locomotor activation in rats (Acevedo et al., 2016), and highlights the mechanism involved in the spinal component of RLS (Trenkwalder & Paulus, 2010).

Interestingly, Cordomí, Navarro, Aymerich, and Franco (2015) previously proposed for several tetrameric GPCRs heteromers coupled to two G proteins, the existence of "linear" and "zig-zagged" tetramers. In these structures the two G proteins may potentially bind either to the inner or outer protomers, giving rise to "in–in," "in–out," or "out–out" possibilities. These arrangements are compatible with available structural data and current knowledge of signal transduction, and are more permissive than the formation of "compact" tetramers that obstruct G protein binding due to excessive crowding at the cytoplasmic region. Moreover, these structures may be useful to reveal how one receptor may allosterically modulate another receptor,

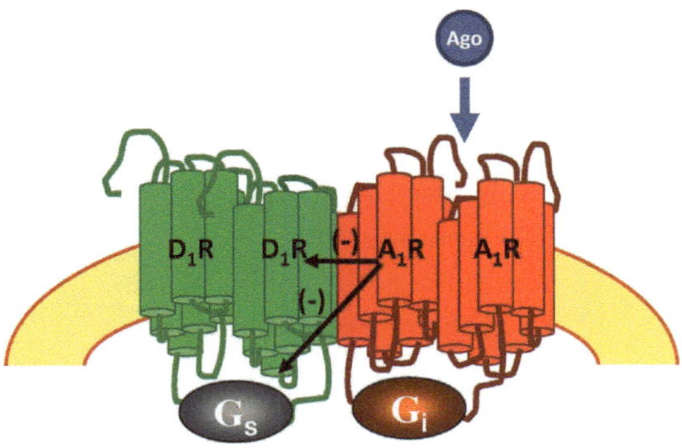

Fig. 2 A_1R–D_1R heterotetramer coupled to the respective G proteins showing the antagonistic allosteric interactions of A_1R agonist on drug binding to D_1R and on its signaling.

and can explain how two G proteins can communicate with each other and affect heteromer-mediated signaling (Cordomí et al., 2015).

The current accumulated knowledge of the biochemical properties of the recently detected $A_{2A}R$–D_2R heterotetramer-AC5 complex offers new therapeutic possibilities for PD, schizophrenia, substance use disorder and other neuropsychiatric disorders with dysfunction of dorsal or ventral striatopallidal neurons (Ferré, Bonaventura, et al., 2018). Moreover, given their involvement in the modulation of crucial physiological processes, GPCR heteromers could constitute important therapeutic targets for a wide range of diseases including obesity, pre-eclampsia, pain, alterations of endocrine regulation, liver fibrosis, acromegaly, pancreatic cancer, and several CNS disorders with abnormal movements such as RLS and SCI.

10. Conclusion

There are accumulating evidences indicating the involvement of dopaminergic and adenosinergic abnormalities in the pathophysiology of RLS, some of them clearly related with iron deficiency. Thereby, several effects suggesting a hyperdopaminergic-presynaptic state responsible of the PLMS symptomatology have been described. Furthermore, it has been correlated BID present in RLS with alterations in adenosinergic system. In addition, a hypoadenosinergic state has been proposed to explain the hyperdopaminergic and hyperglutamatergic states of RLS.

Two decades ago, it was described the antagonistic modulatory role of adenosine on dopaminergic transmission, which was largely dependent on the allosteric interactions between specific subtypes of adenosine and dopamine GPCRs. Nowadays, the modulations between $A_{2A}R$ and D_2R and between A_1R and D_1R are well established in the brain striatum, where these receptors have been detected in situ forming heteromeric complexes. These GPCR heteromers are between the very few that fit to all three criteria to be considered true heteromers. All of these facts suggest that AR-DR heteromers are potential therapeutic targets for the treatment of motor dysfunctions in aging, PD, SCI or PLMS in RLS.

We have focused this essay on the A_1R–D_1R heteromer as a potential target for RLS treatment not only because it has been reported an A_1R downregulation in animals with BID but also since there is an up-regulation of the D_1R system after long-term use of D_3R drugs that leads to augmentation in RLS patients and, in addition, due to the fact that this heteromer is also expressed in spinal cord motoneurons. The A_1R–D_1R heteromer, as reported for other receptors, has a basic heterotetrameric structure formed by a homodimer of A_1R coupled to G_i and a homodimer of D_1R coupled to G_s. A good knowledge about the allosteric interactions within this complex would allow the pharmacological control of the dopamine-adenosine modulations found altered in several motor pathologies as PLMS in RLS. Thus, depending on the striatal or spinal cord pathology, different drugs acting on the A_1R–D_1R heterotetramer could modulate D_1R-mediated excitability of the direct-pathway in striatal spiny neurons or of the spinal motoneurons. In this context, A_1R agonists may counteract D_1R activation and this could be useful for the treatment of RLS and other hyperactivity-like diseases (Fig. 2). In contrast, A_1R antagonists may promote a better D_1R activation and could be useful for the treatment of PD, SCI and aging motor deficits.

In summary, we hypothesize that targeting the A_1R–D_1R heterotetramer with heteromer-selective drugs might improve safety and efficacy of the pharmacological therapy for RLS and other motor diseases, resulting in fewer side effects than classical drugs developed for targeting monomeric A_1R or D_1R.

Acknowledgments

This work was supported by "Ministerio de Economía y Competitividad" and European Regional Development Funds of the European Union (Grant SAF2017-87629-R), the "Fundació La Marató de TV3" (Grant 20140610), "Generalitat de Catalunya" (Grant 2017-SGR-1497).

Conflict of interest

The authors have no conflict of interest to declare.

References

Acevedo, J., Santana-Almansa, A., Matos-Vergara, N., Marrero-Cordero, L. R., Cabezas-Bou, E., & Díaz-Ríos, M. (2016). Caffeine stimulates locomotor activity in the mammalian spinal cord via adenosine A_1 receptor-dopamine D_1 receptor interaction and PKA-dependent mechanisms. *Neuropharmacology*, *101*, 490–505.

Acton, D., Broadhead, M. J., & Miles, G. B. (2018). Modulation of spinal motor networks by astrocyte-derived adenosine is dependent on D_1-like dopamine receptor signaling. *Journal of Neurophysiology*, *120*(3), 998–1009.

Acton, D., & Miles, G. B. (2015). Stimulation of glia reveals modulation of mammalian spinal motor networks by adenosine. *PLoS One*, *10*(8), e0134488.

Akgün, E., Javed, M. I., Lunzer, M. M., Smeester, B. A., Beitz, A. J., & Portoghese, P. S. (2013). Ligands that interact with putative MOR-mGluR5 heteromer in mice with inflammatory pain produce potent antinociception. *Proceedings of the National Academy of Sciences of the United States of America*, *110*(28), 11595–11599.

Albizu, L., Cottet, M., Kralikova, M., Stoev, S., Seyer, R., Brabet, I., et al. (2010). Time-resolved FRET between GPCR ligands reveals oligomers in native tissues. *Nature Chemical Biology*, *6*(8), 587–594.

Allen, R. P., & Earley, C. J. (2007). The role of iron in restless legs syndrome. *Movement Disorders*, *22*(Suppl. 18), S440–S448.

Allen, R. P., Picchietti, D. L., Garcia-Borreguero, D., Ondo, W. G., Walters, A. S., Winkelman, J. W., et al. (2014). Restless legs syndrome/Willis-Ekbom disease diagnostic criteria: Updated international restless legs syndrome study group (IRLSSG) consensus criteria—History, rationale, description, and significance. *Sleep Medicine*, *15*(8), 860–873.

Allen, R. P., Stillman, P., & Myers, A. J. (2010). Physician-diagnosed restless legs syndrome in a large sample of primary medical care patients in western Europe: Prevalence and characteristics. *Sleep Medicine*, *11*(1), 31–37.

Angers, S., Salahpour, A., & Bouvier, M. (2002). Dimerization: An emerging concept for G protein-coupled receptor ontogeny and function. *Annual Review of Pharmacology and Toxicology*, *42*, 409–435.

Angers, S., Salahpour, A., Joly, E., Hilairet, S., Chelsky, D., Dennis, M., et al. (2000). Detection of beta 2-adrenergic receptor dimerization in living cells using bioluminescence resonance energy transfer (BRET). *Proceedings of the National Academy of Sciences of the United States of America*, *97*(7), 3684–3689.

Anguelova, G. V., Vlak, M. H. M., Kurvers, A. G. Y., & Rijsman, R. M. (2018). Pharmacologic and nonpharmacologic treatment of restless legs syndrome. *Sleep Medicine Clinics*, *13*(2), 219–230.

Arcemisbéhère, L., Sen, T., Boudier, L., Balestre, M. N., Gaibelet, G., Detouillon, E., et al. (2010). Leukotriene BLT2 receptor monomers activate the G(i2) GTP-binding protein more efficiently than dimers. *Journal of Biological Chemistry*, *285*(9), 6337–6347.

Ayoub, M. A., Levoye, A., Delagrange, P., & Jockers, R. (2004). Preferential formation of MT1/MT2 melatonin receptor heterodimers with distinct ligand interaction properties compared with MT2 homodimers. *Molecular Pharmacology*, *66*(2), 312–321.

Azdad, K., Gall, D., Woods, A. S., Ledent, C., Ferré, S., & Schiffmann, S. N. (2009). Dopamine D_2 and adenosine A_{2A} receptors regulate NMDA-mediated excitation in accumbens neurons through A_{2A}-D_2 receptor heteromerization. *Neuropsychopharmacology*, *34*(4), 972–986.

Baba, K., Benleulmi-Chaachoua, A., Journé, A. S., Kamal, M., Guillaume, J. L., Dussaud, S., et al. (2013). Heteromeric MT1/MT2 melatonin receptors modulate photoreceptor function. *Science Signaling*, *6*(296), ra89.

Bagher, A. M., Laprairie, R. B., Toguri, J. T., Kelly, M. E. M., & Denovan-Wright, E. M. (2017). Bidirectional allosteric interactions between cannabinoid receptor 1 (CB1) and dopamine receptor 2 long (D2L) heterotetramers. *European Journal of Pharmacology*, *813*, 66–83.

Ballesteros-Yáñez, I., Castillo, C. A., Merighi, S., & Gessi, S. (2018). The role of adenosine receptors in psychostimulant addiction. *Frontiers in Pharmacology*, *8*, 985.

Baltoumas, F. A., Theodoropoulou, M. C., & Hamodrakas, S. J. (2016). Molecular dynamics simulations and structure-based network analysis reveal structural and functional aspects of G-protein coupled receptor dimer interactions. *Journal of Computer-Aided Molecular Design*, *30*(6), 489–512.

Batool-Anwar, S., Li, Y., De Vito, K., Malhotra, A., Winkelman, J., & Gao, X. (2016). Lifestyle factors and risk of restless legs syndrome: Prospective cohort study. *Journal of Clinical Sleep Medicine*, *12*(2), 187–194.

Bayburt, T. H., Vishnivetskiy, S. A., McLean, M. A., Morizumi, T., Huang, C. C., Tesmer, J. J., et al. (2011). Monomeric rhodopsin is sufficient for normal rhodopsin kinase (GRK1) phosphorylation and arrestin-1 binding. *Journal of Biological Chemistry*, *286*(2), 1420–1428.

Becker, P. M., & Novak, M. (2014). Diagnosis, comorbidities, and management of restless legs syndrome. *Current Medical Research and Opinion*, *30*(8), 1441–1460.
Bellot, M., Galandrin, S., Boularan, C., Matthies, H. J., Despas, F., Denis, C., et al. (2015). Dual agonist occupancy of AT1-R-α2C-AR heterodimers results in atypical Gs-PKA signaling. *Nature Chemical Biology*, *11*(4), 271–279.
Bonaventura, J., Navarro, G., Casadó-Anguera, V., Azdad, K., Rea, W., Moreno, E., et al. (2015). Allosteric interactions between agonists and antagonists within the adenosine A_{2A} receptor-dopamine D_2 receptor heterotetramer. *Proceedings of the National Academy of Sciences of the United States of America*, *112*(27), E3609–E3618.
Bonaventura, J., Quiroz, C., Cai, N. S., Rubinstein, M., Tanda, G., & Ferré, S. (2017). Key role of the dopamine D_4 receptor in the modulation of corticostriatal glutamatergic neurotransmission. *Science Advances*, *3*(1), e1601631.
Borcherding, D. C., Hugo, E. R., Idelman, G., De Silva, A., Richtand, N. W., Loftus, J., et al. (2011). Dopamine receptors in human adipocytes: Expression and functions. *PLoS One*, *6*, e25537.
Cai, X., Bai, B., Zhang, R., Wang, C., & Chen, J. (2017). Apelin receptor homodimer-oligomers revealed by single-molecule imaging and novel G protein-dependent signaling. *Scientific Reports*, *7*, 40335.
Cai, Y., Liu, Y., Culhane, K., DeVree, B. T., Yang, Y., Sunahara, R. K., et al. (2017). Purification of family B G protein-coupled receptors using nanodiscs: Application to human glucagon-like peptide-1 receptor. *PLoS One*, *12*(6), e0179568.
Calebiro, D., Rieken, F., Wagner, J., Sungkaworn, T., Zabel, U., Borzi, A., et al. (2013). Single-molecule analysis of fluorescently labeled G-protein-coupled receptors reveals complexes with distinct dynamics and organization. *Proceedings of the National Academy of Sciences of the United States of America*, *110*(2), 743–748.
Calebiro, D., & Sungkaworn, T. (2018). Single-molecule imaging of GPCR interactions. *Trends in Pharmacological Sciences*, *39*(2), 109–122.
Cao, Y., Sun, W. C., Jin, L., Xie, K. Q., & Zhu, X. Z. (2006). Activation of adenosine A_1 receptor modulates dopamine D_1 receptor activity in stably cotransfected human embryonic kidney 293 cells. *European Journal of Pharmacology*, *548*(1–3), 29–35.
Cao, Y., Xie, K. Q., & Zhu, X. Z. (2007). The enhancement of dopamine D_1 receptor desensitization by adenosine A1 receptor activation. *European Journal of Pharmacology*, *562*(1–2), 34–38.
Carlsen, E. M., & Perrier, J. F. (2014). Purines released from astrocytes inhibit excitatory synaptic transmission in the ventral horn of the spinal cord. *Frontiers in Neural Circuits*, *8*, 60.
Casadó-Anguera, V., Bonaventura, J., Moreno, E., Navarro, G., Cortés, A., Ferré, S., et al. (2016). Evidence for the heterotetrameric structure of the adenosine A_{2A}-dopamine D_2 receptor complex. *Biochemical Society Transactions*, *44*(2), 595–600.
Centonze, D., Gubellini, P., Usiello, A., Rossi, S., Tscherter, A., Bracci, E., et al. (2004). Differential contribution of dopamine D2S and D2L receptors in the modulation of glutamate and GABA transmission in the striatum. *Neuroscience*, *129*(1), 157–166.
Cha, K. S., Choi, J. W., Jung, K. Y., & Kim, K. H. (2017). Frontal dysfunction in patients with restless legs syndrome performing a visual oddball task: An event-related potential source imaging study. *Sleep Medicine*, *36*, 48–54.
Chabre, M., & le Maire, M. (2005). Monomeric G-protein-coupled receptor as a functional unit. *Biochemistry*, *44*(27), 9395–9403.
Chen, G. Q., Chen, Y. Y., Wang, X. S., Wu, S. Z., Yang, H. M., Xu, H. Q., et al. (2010). Chronic caffeine treatment attenuates experimental autoimmune encephalomyelitis induced by guinea pig spinal cord homogenates in Wistar rats. *Brain Research*, *1309*, 116–125.

Chen, J. F., Lee, C. F., & Chern, Y. (2014). Adenosine receptor neurobiology: Overview. *International Review of Neurobiology*, *119*, 1–49.
Ciruela, F., Gomez-Soler, M., Guidolin, D., Borroto-Escuela, D. O., Agnati, L. F., Fuxe, K., et al. (2011). Adenosine receptor containing oligomers: Their role in the control of dopamine and glutamate neurotransmission in the brain. *Biochimica et Biophysica Acta*, *1808*, 1245–1255.
Clemens, S., Belin-Rauscent, A., Simmers, J., & Combes, D. (2012). Opposing modulatory effects of D_1- and D_2-like receptor activation on a spinal central pattern generator. *Journal of Neurophysiology*, *107*(8), 2250–2259.
Cordomí, A., Navarro, G., Aymerich, M. S., & Franco, R. (2015). Structures for G-protein-coupled receptor tetramers in complex with G proteins. *Trends in Biochemical Sciences*, *40*(10), 548–551.
Cortés, A., Casadó-Anguera, V., Moreno, E., & Casadó, V. (2016). Caffeine, adenosine A_1 receptors, and the brain cortex. Molecular aspects. Chapter 74. In V. R. Preedy (Ed.), *Vol. 3. Neuropathology of drug addictions and substance misuse* (pp. 741–752).
Cortés, A., Moreno, E., Rodríguez-Ruiz, M., Canela, E. I., & Casadó, V. (2016). Targeting the dopamine D_3 receptor: An overview of drug design strategies. *Expert Opinion on Drug Discovery*, *11*(7), 641–664.
Cristóvão-Ferreira, S., Navarro, G., Brugarolas, M., Pérez-Capote, K., Vaz, S. H., Fattorini, G., et al. (2013). A_1R-$A_{2A}R$ heteromers coupled to Gs and G i/0 proteins modulate GABA transport into astrocytes. *Purinergic Signalling*, *9*(3), 433–449.
Cvejic, S., & Devi, L. A. (1997). Dimerization of the delta opioid receptor: Implication for a role in receptor internalization. *Journal of Biological Chemistry*, *272*, 26959–26964.
Dauvilliers, Y., & Winkelmann, J. (2013). Restless legs syndrome: Update on pathogenesis. *Current Opinion in Pulmonary Medicine*, *19*(6), 594–600.
de Lera Ruiz, M., Lim, Y. H., & Zheng, J. (2014). Adenosine A2A receptor as a drug discovery target. *Journal of Medicinal Chemistry*, *57*(9), 3623–3625.
Di Pizio, A., Levit, A., Slutzki, M., Behrens, M., Karaman, R., & Niv, M. Y. (2016). Comparing class a GPCRs to bitter taste receptors: Structural motifs, ligand interactions and agonist-to-antagonist ratios. *Methods in Cell Biology*, *132*, 401–427.
Dinkins, M. L., Lallemand, P., & Clemens, S. (2017). Long-term treatment with dopamine D_3 receptor agonists induces a behavioral switch that can be rescued by blocking the dopamine D1 receptor. *Sleep Medicine*, *40*, 47–52.
Earley, C. J., Connor, J., Garcia-Borreguero, D., Jenner, P., Winkelman, J., Zee, P. C., et al. (2014). Altered brain iron homeostasis and dopaminergic function in restless legs syndrome (Willis-Ekbom disease). *Sleep Medicine*, *15*(11), 1288–1301.
Earley, C. J., Kuwabara, H., Wong, D. F., Gamaldo, C., Salas, R., Brasic, J., et al. (2011). The dopamine transporter is decreased in the striatum of subjects with restless legs syndrome. *Sleep*, *34*(3), 341–347.
Earley, C. J., Uhl, G. R., Clemens, S., & Ferré, S. (2017). Connectome and molecular pharmacological differences in the dopaminergic system in restless legs syndrome (RLS): Plastic changes and neuroadaptations that may contribute to augmentation. *Sleep Medicine*, *31*, 71–77.
Ernst, O. P., Gramse, V., Kolbe, M., Hofmann, K. P., & Heck, M. (2007). Monomeric G protein-coupled receptor rhodopsin in solution activates its G protein transducin at the diffusion limit. *Proceedings of the National Academy of Sciences of the United States of America*, *104*(26), 10859–10864.
Farran, B. (2017). An update on the physiological and therapeutic relevance of GPCR oligomers. *Pharmacological Research*, *117*, 303–327.
Faulkner, M. A. (2018). Use of $\alpha 2\delta$ ligands for restless legs syndrome/Willis Ekbom disease. *CNS Drugs*, *32*(2), 149–159.

Ferré, S. (2015). The GPCR heterotetramer: Challenging classical pharmacology. *Trends in Pharmacological Sciences*, *36*(3), 145–152.
Ferré, S. (2016). Mechanisms of the psychostimulant effects of caffeine: Implications for substance use disorders. *Psychopharmacology (Berlin)*, *233*(10), 1963–1979.
Ferré, S., Baler, R., Bouvier, M., Caron, M. G., Devi, L. A., Durroux, T., et al. (2009). Building a new conceptual framework for receptor heteromers. *Nature Chemical Biology*, *5*(3), 131–134.
Ferré, S., Bonaventura, J., Tomasi, D., Navarro, G., Moreno, E., Cortés, A., et al. (2016). Allosteric mechanisms within the adenosine A_{2A}-dopamine D_2 receptor heterotetramer. *Neuropharmacology*, *104*, 154–160.
Ferré, S., Bonaventura, J., Zhu, W., Hatcher-Solis, C., Taura, J., Quiroz, C., et al. (2018). Essential control of the function of the striatopallidal neuron by pre-coupled complexes of adenosine A_{2A}-dopamine D_2 receptor heterotetramers and adenylyl cyclase. *Frontiers in Pharmacology*, *9*, 243.
Ferré, S., Casadó, V., Devi, L. A., Filizola, M., Jockers, R., Lohse, M. J., et al. (2014). G protein-coupled receptor oligomerization revisited: Functional and pharmacological perspectives. *Pharmacological Reviews*, *66*(2), 413–434.
Ferré, S., Ciruela, F., Borycz, J., Solinas, M., Quarta, D., Antoniou, K., et al. (2008). Adenosine A_1-A_{2A} receptor heteromers: New targets for caffeine in the brain. *Frontiers in Bioscience*, *13*, 2391–2399.
Ferré, S., Earley, C., Gulyani, S., & Garcia-Borreguero, D. (2017). In search of alternatives to dopaminergic ligands for the treatment of restless legs syndrome: Iron, glutamate, and adenosine. *Sleep Medicine*, *31*, 86–92.
Ferré, S., Fredholm, B. B., Morelli, M., Popoli, P., & Fuxe, K. (1997). Adenosine-dopamine receptor-receptor interactions as an integrative mechanism in the basal ganglia. *Trends in Neurosciences*, *20*, 482–487.
Ferré, S., Lluis, C., Lanciego, J. L., & Franco, R. (2010). Prime time for G-protein-coupled receptor heteromers as therapeutic targets for CNS disorders: The dopamine D_1-D_3 receptor heteromer. *CNS & Neurological Disorders Drug Targets*, *9*(5), 596–600.
Ferré, S., Popoli, P., Giménez-Llort, L., Rimondini, R., Müller, C. E., Strömberg, I., et al. (2001). Adenosine/dopamine interaction: Implications for the treatment of Parkinson's disease. *Parkinsonism & Related Disorders*, 7(3), 235–241.
Ferré, S., Quiroz, C., Guitart, X., Rea, W., Seyedian, A., Moreno, E., et al. (2018). Pivotal role of adenosine neurotransmission in restless legs syndrome. *Frontiers in Neuroscience*, *11*, 722.
Ferri, R., Rundo, F., Zucconi, M., Manconi, M., Bruni, O., Ferini-Strambi, L., et al. (2015). An evidence-based analysis of the association between periodic leg movements during sleep and arousals in restless legs syndrome. *Sleep*, *38*(6), 919–924.
Fiorentini, C., Busi, C., Spano, P., & Missale, C. (2010). Dimerization of dopamine D_1 and D_3 receptors in the regulation of striatal function. *Current Opinion in Pharmacology*, *10*(1), 87–92.
Fotiadis, D., Liang, Y., Filipek, S., Saperstein, D. A., Engel, A., & Palczewski, K. (2003). Atomic-force microscopy: Rhodopsin dimers in native disc membranes. *Nature*, *421*(6919), 127–128.
Franco, R., Lluis, C., Canela, E. I., Mallol, J., Agnati, L., Casadó, V., et al. (2007). Receptor-receptor interactions involving adenosine A_1 or dopamine D_1 receptors and accessory proteins. *Journal of Neural Transmission (Vienna)*, *114*(1), 93–104.
Fujita, W., Gomes, I., & Devi, L. A. (2015). Heteromers of μ-δ opioid receptors: New pharmacology and novel therapeutic possibilities. *British Journal of Pharmacology*, *172*(2), 375–387.
Fuxe, K., Ferré, S., Genedani, S., Franco, R., & Agnati, L. F. (2007). Adenosine receptor-dopamine receptor interactions in the basal ganglia and their relevance for brain function. *Physiology and Behavior*, *92*, 210–217.

Fuxe, K., Marcellino, D., Borroto-Escuela, D. O., Guescini, M., Fernández-Dueñas, V., Tanganelli, S., et al. (2010). Adenosine-dopamine interactions in the pathophysiology and treatment of CNS disorders. *CNS Neuroscience & Therapeutics*, *16*(3), e18–e42.

Gahbauer, S., & Böckmann, R. A. (2016). Membrane-mediated oligomerization of G protein coupled receptors and its implications for GPCR function. *Frontiers in Physiology*, *7*, 494.

Gaitonde, S. A., & González-Maeso, J. (2017). Contribution of heteromerization to G protein-coupled receptor function. *Current Opinion in Pharmacology*, *32*, 23–31.

Gao, F., Harikumar, K. G., Dong, M., Lam, P. C., Sexton, P. M., Christopoulos, A., et al. (2009). Functional importance of a structurally distinct homodimeric complex of the family B G protein-coupled secretin receptor. *Molecular Pharmacology*, *76*(2), 264–274.

García-Borreguero, D., Allen, R. P., Kohnen, R., Högl, B., Trenkwalder, C., Oertel, W., et al. (2007). Diagnostic standards for dopaminergic augmentation of restless legs syndrome: Report from a world Association of Sleep Medicine-International Restless Legs Syndrome Study Group consensus conference at the Max Planck institute. *Sleep Medicine*, *8*(5), 520–530.

Garcia-Borreguero, D., & Cano-Pumarega, I. (2017). New concepts in the management of restless legs syndrome. *BMJ*, *356*. j104.

Garcia-Borreguero, D., Guitart, X., Garcia Malo, C., Cano-Pumarega, I., Granizo, J. J., & Ferré, S. (2018). Treatment of restless legs syndrome/Willis-Ekbom disease with the non-selective ENT1/ENT2 inhibitor dipyridamole: Testing the adenosine hypothesis. *Sleep Medicine*, *45*, 94–97.

Garcia-Borreguero, D., Kohnen, R., Silber, M. H., Winkelman, J. W., Earley, C. J., Högl, B., et al. (2013). The long-term treatment of restless legs syndrome/Willis-Ekbom disease: Evidence-based guidelines and clinical consensus best practice guidance: A report from the international restless legs syndrome study group. *Sleep Medicine*, *14*(7), 675–684.

Geng, Y., Bush, M., Mosyak, L., Wang, F., & Fan, Q. R. (2013). Structural mechanism of ligand activation in human GABA(B) receptor. *Nature*, *504*(7479), 254–259.

Gerfen, C. R., & Surmeier, D. J. (2011). Modulation of striatal projection systems by dopamine. *Annual Review of Neuroscience*, *34*, 441–466.

Ghosh, E., Kumari, P., Jaiman, D., & Shukla, A. K. (2015). Methodological advances: The unsung heroes of the GPCR structural revolution. *National Reviews Molecular Cell Biology*, *16*(2), 69–81.

Ginés, S., Hillion, J., Torvinen, M., Le Crom, S., Casadó, V., Canela, E. I., et al. (2000). Dopamine D_1 and adenosine A_1 receptors form functionally interacting heteromeric complexes. *Proceedings of the National Academy of Sciences of the United States of America*, *97*(15), 8606–8611.

Goin, J. C., & Nathanson, N. M. (2006). Quantitative analysis of muscarinic acetylcholine receptor homo- and heterodimerization in live cells: Regulation of receptor down-regulation by heterodimerization. *Journal of Biological Chemistry*, *281*(9), 5416–5425.

Gomes, I., Ayoub, M. A., Fujita, W., Jaeger, W. C., Pfleger, K. D., & Devi, L. A. (2016). G protein-coupled receptor heteromers. *Annual Review of Pharmacology and Toxicology*, *56*, 403–425.

Gomes, I., Gupta, A., & Devi, L. A. (2013). G-protein-coupled heteromers: Regulation in disease. *Methods in Enzymology*, *521*, 219–238.

Gomes, I., Ijzerman, A. P., Ye, K., Maillet, E. L., & Devi, L. A. (2011). G protein-coupled receptor heteromerization: A role in allosteric modulation of ligand binding. *Molecular Pharmacology*, *79*(6), 1044–1052.

Gomes, I., Jordan, B. A., Gupta, A., Trapaidze, N., Nagy, V., & Devi, L. A. (2000). Heterodimerization of mu and delta opioid receptors: A role in opiate synergy. *Journal of Neuroscience*, *20*(22). RC110.

Gomes, I., Sierra, S., & Devi, L. A. (2016). Detection of receptor heteromerization using in situ proximity ligation assay. *Current Protocols in Pharmacology*, *75*, 2.16.1–2.16.31.

Gonzalez, A., Cordomí, A., Matsoukas, M., Zachmann, J., & Pardo, L. (2014). Modeling of G protein-coupled receptors using crystal structures: From monomers to signaling complexes. *Advances in Experimental Medicine and Biology*, *796*, 15–33.

González, S., Rangel-Barajas, C., Peper, M., Lorenzo, R., Moreno, E., Ciruela, F., et al. (2012). Dopamine D_4 receptor, but not the ADHD-associated $D_{4.7}$ variant, forms functional heteromers with the dopamine D_{2S} receptor in the brain. *Molecular Psychiatry*, *17*(6), 650–662.

Gracia, E., Moreno, E., Cortés, A., Lluís, C., Mallol, J., McCormick, P. J., et al. (2013). Homodimerization of adenosine A_1 receptors in brain cortex explains the biphasic effects of caffeine. *Neuropharmacology*, *71*, 56–69.

Gracia, E., Pérez-Capote, K., Moreno, E., Barkešová, J., Mallol, J., Lluís, C., et al. (2011). A_{2A} adenosine receptor ligand binding and signalling is allosterically modulated by adenosine deaminase. *Biochemical Journal*, *435*, 701–709.

Guitart, X., Navarro, G., Moreno, E., Yano, H., Cai, N. S., Sánchez-Soto, M., et al. (2014). Functional selectivity of allosteric interactions within G protein-coupled receptor oligomers: The dopamine D1-D3 receptor heterotetramer. *Molecular Pharmacology*, *86*(4), 417–429.

Gulyani, S., Earley, C. J., Camandola, S., Maudsley, S., Ferré, S., Mughal, M. R., et al. (2009). Diminished iron concentrations increase adenosine A(2A) receptor levels in mouse striatum and cultured human neuroblastoma cells. *Experimental Neurology*, *215*(2), 236–242.

Guo, C. N., Yang, W. J., Zhan, S. Q., Yang, X. F., Chen, M. C., Fuller, P. M., et al. (2017). Targeted disruption of supraspinal motor circuitry reveals a distributed network underlying restless legs syndrome (RLS)-like movements in the rat. *Scientific Reports*, 7(1), 9905.

Gupta, A., Mulder, J., Gomes, I., Rozenfeld, R., Bushlin, I., Ong, E., et al. (2010). Increased abundance of opioid receptor heteromers after chronic morphine administration. *Science Signaling*, *3*(131), ra54.

Gurevich, V. V., & Gurevich, E. V. (2017). Molecular mechanisms of GPCR signaling: A structural perspective. *International Journal of Molecular Sciences*, *18*(12). e2519.

Han, Y., Moreira, I. S., Urizar, E., Weinstein, H., & Javitch, J. A. (2009). Allosteric communication between protomers of dopamine class A GPCR dimers modulates activation. *Nature Chemical Biology*, *5*(9), 688–695.

Hanson, S. M., Gurevich, E. V., Vishnivetskiy, S. A., Ahmed, M. R., Song, X., & Gurevich, V. V. (2007). Each rhodopsin molecule binds its own arrestin. *Proceedings of the National Academy of Sciences of the United States of America*, *104*(9), 3125–3128.

Hare, D., Ayton, S., Bush, A., & Lei, P. (2013). A delicate balance: Iron metabolism and diseases of the brain. *Frontiers in Aging Neuroscience*, *5*, 34.

Harikumar, K. G., Lau, S., Sexton, P. M., Wootten, D., & Miller, L. J. (2017). Coexpressed class B G protein-coupled secretin and GLP-1 receptors self- and cross-associate: Impact on pancreatic islets. *Endocrinology*, *158*(6), 1685–1700.

Harikumar, K. G., Pinon, D. I., & Miller, L. J. (2007). Transmembrane segment IV contributes a functionally important interface for oligomerization of the class II G protein-coupled secretin receptor. *Journal of Biological Chemistry*, *282*(42), 30363–30372.

Hartmann, M., Pfister, R., & Pfadenhauer, K. (1999). Restless legs syndrome associated with spinal cord lesions. *Journal of Neurology, Neurosurgery, and Psychiatry*, *66*(5), 688–689.

Hauser, A. S., Attwood, M. M., Rask-Andersen, M., Schiöth, H. B., & Gloriam, D. E. (2017). Trends in GPCR drug discovery: New agents, targets and indications. *Nature Reviews Drug Discovery*, *16*(12), 829–842.

He, L., Fong, J., von Zastrow, M., & Whistler, J. L. (2002). Regulation of opioid receptor trafficking and morphine tolerance by receptor oligomerization. *Cell*, *108*, 271–282.

He, S. Q., Zhang, Z. N., Guan, J. S., Liu, H. R., Zhao, B., Wang, H. B., et al. (2011). Facilitation of μ-opioid receptor activity by preventing δ-opioid receptor-mediated codegradation. *Neuron*, *69*(1), 120–131.

Hening, W. A., Walters, A. S., Wagner, M., Rosen, R., Chen, V., Kim, S., et al. (1999). Circadian rhythm of motor restlessness and sensory symptoms in the idiopathic restless legs syndrome. *Sleep*, *22*(7), 901–912.

Herrick-Davis, K., Grinde, E., Cowan, A., & Mazurkiewicz, J. E. (2013). Fluorescence correlation spectroscopy analysis of serotonin, adrenergic, muscarinic, and dopamine receptor dimerization: The oligomer number puzzle. *Molecular Pharmacology*, *84*(4), 630–642.

Herrick-Davis, K., Grinde, E., Lindsley, T., Cowan, A., & Mazurkiewicz, J. E. (2012). Oligomer size of the serotonin 5-hydroxytryptamine 2C (5-HT2C) receptor revealed by fluorescence correlation spectroscopy with photon counting histogram analysis: Evidence for homodimers without monomers or tetramers. *Journal of Biological Chemistry*, *287*(28), 23604–23614.

Herrick-Davis, K., Grinde, E., Lindsley, T., Teitler, M., Mancia, F., Cowan, A., et al. (2015). Native serotonin 5-HT_{2C} receptors are expressed as homodimers on the apical surface of choroid plexus epithelial cells. *Molecular Pharmacology*, *87*(4), 660–673.

Herrick-Davis, K., Weaver, B. A., Grinde, E., & Mazurkiewicz, J. E. (2006). Serotonin 5-HT2C receptor homodimer biogenesis in the endoplasmic reticulum: Real-time visualization with confocal fluorescence resonance energy transfer. *Journal of Biological Chemistry*, *281*(37), 27109–27116.

Hillion, J., Canals, M., Torvinen, M., Casadó, V., Scott, R., Terasmaa, A., et al. (2002). Coaggregation, cointernalization, and codesensitization of adenosine A_{2A} receptors and dopamine D_2 receptors. *Journal of Biological Chemistry*, *277*(20), 18091–18097.

Hobson, B. D., O'Neill, C. E., Levis, S. C., Monteggia, L. M., Neve, R. L., Self, D. W., et al. (2013). Adenosine A_1 and dopamine D_1 receptor regulation of AMPA receptor phosphorylation and cocaine-seeking behavior. *Neuropsychopharmacology*, *38*(10), 1974–1983.

Hounsou, C., Margathe, J. F., Oueslati, N., Belhocine, A., Dupuis, E., & Thomas, C. (2015). Time-resolved FRET binding assay to investigate hetero-oligomer binding properties: Proof of concept with dopamine D_1/D_3 heterodimer. *ACS Chemical Biology*, *10*(2), 466–474.

Hurevich, M., Talhami, A., Shalev, D. E., & Gilon, C. (2014). Allosteric inhibition of g-protein coupled receptor oligomerization: Strategies and challenges for drug development. *Current Topics in Medicinal Chemistry*, *14*(15), 1842–1863.

Jacobs, B. A., Pando, M. M., Jennings, E., Chavera, T. A., Clarke, W. P., & Berg, K. A. (2018). Allosterism within δ opioid-κ opioid receptor heteromers in peripheral sensory neurons: Regulation of κ opioid agonist efficacy. *Molecular Pharmacology*, *93*(4), 376–386.

Jastrzebska, B., Comar, W. D., Kaliszewski, M. J., Skinner, K. C., Torcasio, M. H., Esway, A. S., et al. (2017). A G protein-coupled receptor dimerization interface in human cone opsins. *Biochemistry*, *56*(1), 61–72.

Jellen, L. C., Lu, L., Wang, X., Unger, E. L., Earley, C. J., Allen, R. P., et al. (2013). Iron deficiency alters expression of dopamine-related genes in the ventral midbrain in mice. *Neuroscience*, *252*, 13–23.

Jin, J., Momboisse, F., Boncompain, G., Koensgen, F., Zhou, Z., Cordeiro, N., et al. (2018). CCR5 adopts three homodimeric conformations that control cell surface delivery. *Science Signaling*, *11*(529), eaal2869.

Jonas, K. C., Chen, S., Virta, M., Mora, J., Franks, S., Huhtaniemi, I., et al. (2018). Temporal reprogramming of calcium signalling via crosstalk of gonadotrophin receptors that associate as functionally asymmetric heteromers. *Scientific Reports*, *8*(1), 2239.

Jonas, K. C., Fanelli, F., Huhtaniemi, I. T., & Hanyaloglu, A. C. (2015). Single molecule analysis of functionally asymmetric G protein-coupled receptor (GPCR) oligomers reveals diverse spatial and structural assemblies. *Journal of Biological Chemistry*, *290*(7), 3875–3892.

Jonas, K. C., & Hanyaloglu, A. C. (2017). Impact of G protein-coupled receptor heteromers in endocrine systems. *Molecular and Cellular Endocrinology*, *449*, 21–27.

Jonas, K. C., Huhtaniemi, I., & Hanyaloglu, A. C. (2016). Single-molecule resolution of G protein-coupled receptor (GPCR) complexes. *Methods in Cell Biology*, *132*, 55–72.

Jordan, B. A., & Devi, L. A. (1999). G-protein-coupled receptor heterodimerization modulates receptor function. *Nature*, *399*(6737), 697–700.

Katritch, V., Cherezov, V., & Stevens, R. C. (2012). Diversity and modularity of G protein-coupled receptor structures. *Trends in Pharmacological Sciences*, *33*(1), 17–27.

Keeler, B. E., Lallemand, P., Patel, M. M., de Castro Brás, L. E., & Clemens, S. (2016). Opposing aging-related shift of excitatory dopamine D_1 and inhibitory D_3 receptor protein expression in striatum and spinal cord. *Journal of Neurophysiology*, *115*(1), 363–369.

Kenakin, T., Agnati, L. F., Caron, M., Fredholm, B., Guidoli, D., Kobilka, B., et al. (2010). International workshop at the Nobel forum, Karolinska Institutet on G protein-coupled receptors: Finding the words to describe monomers, oligomers, and their molecular mechanisms and defining their meaning. Can a consensus be reached? *Journal of Receptors and Signal Transduction*, *30*(5), 284–286.

Kern, A., Albarran-Zeckler, R., Walsh, H. E., & Smith, R. G. (2012). Apo-ghrelin receptor forms heteromers with DRD2 in hypothalamic neurons and is essential for anorexigenic effects of DRD2 agonism. *Neuron*, *73*(2), 317–332.

Kim, E. S., & Deeks, E. D. (2016). Gabapentin enacarbil: A review in restless legs syndrome. *Drugs*, *76*(8), 879–887.

Kniazeff, J., Prézeau, L., Rondard, P., Pin, J. P., & Goudet, C. (2011). Dimers and beyond: The functional puzzles of class C GPCRs. *Pharmacology & Therapeutics*, *130*(1), 9–25.

Kuszak, A. J., Pitchiaya, S., Anand, J. P., Mosberg, H. I., Walter, N. G., & Sunahara, R. K. (2009). Purification and functional reconstitution of monomeric mu-opioid receptors: Allosteric modulation of agonist binding by Gi2. *Journal of Biological Chemistry*, *284*(39), 26732–26741.

Lao, J., He, H., Wang, X., Wang, Z., Song, Y., Yang, B., et al. (2017). Single-molecule imaging demonstrates ligand regulation of the oligomeric status of CXCR4 in living cells. *The Journal of Physical Chemistry B*, *121*(7), 1466–1474.

Le Crom, S., Prou, D., & Vernier, P. (2002). Autocrine activation of adenosine A1 receptors blocks D1A but not D1B dopamine receptor desensitization. *Journal of Neurochemistry*, *82*(6), 1549–1552.

Liste, M. J., Caltabiano, G., Ward, R. J., Alvarez-Curto, E., Marsango, S., & Milligan, G. (2015). The molecular basis of oligomeric organization of the human M3 muscarinic acetylcholine receptor. *Molecular Pharmacology*, *87*(6), 936–953.

Liu, J., Zhang, Z., Moreno-Delgado, D., Dalton, J. A., Rovira, X., Trapero, A., et al. (2017). Allosteric control of an asymmetric transduction in a G protein-coupled receptor heterodimer. *eLife*, *6*, e26985.

Lopez-Gimenez, J. F., Canals, M., Pediani, J. D., & Milligan, G. (2007). The alpha1b-adrenoceptor exists as a higher-order oligomer: Effective oligomerization is required for receptor maturation, surface delivery, and function. *Molecular Pharmacology*, *71*(4), 1015–1029.

Łukasiewicz, S., Błasiak, E., Faron-Górecka, A., Polit, A., Tworzydło, M., Górecki, A., et al. (2007). Fluorescence studies of homooligomerization of adenosine A_{2A} and serotonin 5-HT_{1A} receptors reveal the specificity of receptor interactions in the plasma membrane. *Pharmacological Reports*, *59*, 379–392.

Mandrika, I., Petrovska, R., & Klovins, J. (2010). Evidence for constitutive dimerization of niacin receptor subtypes. *Biochemical and Biophysical Research Communications*, *395*, 281–287.

Mango, D., Bonito-Oliva, A., Ledonne, A., Cappellacci, L., Petrelli, R., Nisticò, R., et al. (2014). Adenosine A_1 receptor stimulation reduces D_1 receptor-mediated GABAergic transmission from striato-nigral terminals and attenuates L-DOPA-induced dyskinesia in dopamine-denervated mice. *Experimental Neurology*, *261*, 733–743.

Matak, P., Matak, A., Moustafa, S., Aryal, D. K., Benner, E. J., Wetsel, W., et al. (2016). Disrupted iron homeostasis causes dopaminergic neurodegeneration in mice. *Proceedings of the National Academy of Sciences of the United States of America*, *113*(13), 3428–3435.

May, L. T., Bridge, L. J., Stoddart, L. A., Briddon, S. J., & Hill, S. J. (2011). Allosteric interactions across native adenosine-A3 receptor homodimers: Quantification using single-cell ligand-binding kinetics. *FASEB Journal*, *25*, 3465–3476.

Mercier, J. F., Salahpour, A., Angers, S., Breit, A., & Bouvier, M. (2002). Quantitative assessment of beta 1- and beta 2-adrenergic receptor homo- and heterodimerization by bioluminescence resonance energy transfer. *Journal of Biological Chemistry*, *277*, 44925–44931.

Mioranzza, S., Costa, M. S., Botton, P. H., Ardais, A. P., Matte, V. L., Espinosa, J., et al. (2011). Blockade of adenosine a(1) receptors prevents methylphenidate-induced impairment of object recognition task in adult mice. *Progress in Neuro-Psychopharmacology & Biological Psychiatry*, *35*(1), 169–176.

Mishra, A., Singh, S., & Shukla, S. (2018). Physiological and functional basis of dopamine receptors and their role in neurogenesis: Possible implication for Parkinson's disease. *Journal of Experimental Neuroscience*, *12*, 1179069518779829.

Molero, A., Vendrell, M., Bonaventura, J., Zachmann, J., López, L., Pardo, L., et al. (2015). A solid-phase combinatorial approach for indoloquinolizidine-peptides with high affinity at D(1) and D(2) dopamine receptors. *European Journal of Medicinal Chemistry*, *97*, 173–180.

Moller, T. C., Moreno-Delgado, D., Pin, J. P., & Kniazeff, J. (2017). Class C G protein-coupled receptors: Reviving old couples with new partners. *Biophysics Reports*, *3*(4), 57–63.

Moreira, I. S. (2014). Structural features of the G-protein/GPCR interactions. *Biochimica et Biophysica Acta*, *1840*(1), 16–33.

Moreno, E., Quiroz, C., Rea, W., Cai, N. S., Mallol, J., Cortés, A., et al. (2017). Functional μ-opioid-galanin receptor heteromers in the ventral tegmental area. *Journal of Neuroscience*, *37*(5), 1176–1186.

Moreno-Delgado, D., Møller, T. C., Ster, J., Giraldo, J., Maurel, D., Rovira, X., et al. (2017). Pharmacological evidence for a metabotropic glutamate receptor heterodimer in neuronal cells. *eLife*, *6*, e25233.

Mustafa, S., & Pfleger, K. D. (2011). G protein-coupled receptor heteromer identification technology: Identification and profiling of GPCR heteromers. *Journal of Laboratory Automation*, *16*, 285–291. https://doi.org/10.1016/j.jala.2011.03.002.

Navarro, G., Cordomí, A., Casadó-Anguera, V., Moreno, E., Cai, N. S., Cortés, A., et al. (2018). Evidence for functional pre-coupled complexes of receptor heteromers and adenylyl cyclase. *Nature Communications*, *9*(1), 1242.

Navarro, G., Cordomí, A., Zelman-Femiak, M., Brugarolas, M., Moreno, E., Aguinaga, D., et al. (2016). Quaternary structure of a G-protein-coupled receptor heterotetramer in complex with Gi and Gs. *BMC Biology*, *14*, 26.

Navarro, G., Quiroz, C., Moreno-Delgado, D., Sierakowiak, A., McDowell, K., Moreno, E., et al. (2015). Orexin-corticotropin-releasing factor receptor heteromers in the ventral tegmental area as targets for cocaine. *Journal of Neuroscience*, *35*(17), 6639–6653.

Nazario, L. R., da Silva, R. S., & Bonan, C. D. (2017). Targeting adenosine signaling in Parkinson's disease: From pharmacological to non-pharmacological approaches. *Frontiers in Neuroscience*, *11*, 658.

Nemoto, W., Yamanishi, Y., Limviphuvadh, V., Saito, A., & Toh, H. (2016). GGIP: Structure and sequence-based GPCR-GPCR interaction pair predictor. *Proteins*, *84*(9), 1224–1233.

Ng, H. K., & Chow, B. K. (2015). Oligomerization of family B GPCRs: Exploration in inter-family oligomer formation. *Frontiers in Endocrinology*, *6*, 10.

Ng, S. Y., Lee, L. T., & Chow, B. K. (2013). Receptor oligomerization: From early evidence to current understanding in class B GPCRs. *Frontiers in Endocrinology*, *3*, 175.

Nimczick, M., & Decker, M. (2015). New approaches in the design and development of cannabinoid receptor ligands: Multifunctional and bivalent compounds. *ChemMedChem*, *10*(5), 773–786.

Nunes, E. J., Randall, P. A., Podurgiel, S., Correa, M., & Salamone, J. D. (2013). Nucleus accumbens neurotransmission and effort-related choice behavior in food motivation: Effects of drugs acting on dopamine, adenosine, and muscarinic acetylcholine receptors. *Neuroscience & Biobehavioral Reviews*, *37*(9 Pt. A), 2015–2025.

Oboshi, Y., Ouchi, Y., Yagi, S., Kono, S., Nakai, N., Yoshikawa, E., et al. (2012). In vivo mesolimbic D2/3 receptor binding predicts posttherapeutic clinical responses in restless legs syndrome: A positron emission tomography study. *Journal of Cerebral Blood Flow & Metabolism*, *32*(4), 654–662.

Oliveira-Giacomelli, Á., Naaldijk, Y., Sardá-Arroyo, L., Gonçalves, M. C. B., Corrêa-Velloso, J., Pillat, M. M., et al. (2018). Purinergic receptors in neurological diseases with motor symptoms: Targets for therapy. *Frontiers in Pharmacology*, *9*, 325.

Palacios, N., Gao, X., McCullough, M. L., Schwarzschild, M. A., Shah, R., Gapstur, S., et al. (2012). Caffeine and risk of Parkinson's disease in a large cohort of men and women. *Movement Disorders*, *27*(10), 1276–1282.

Parmar, V. K., Grinde, E., Mazurkiewicz, J. E., & Herrick-Davis, K. (2017). $Beta_2$-adrenergic receptor homodimers: Role of transmembrane domain 1 and helix 8 in dimerization and cell surface expression. *Biochimica et Biophysica Acta, Biomembranes*, *1859*(9 Pt. A), 1445–1455.

Paulus, W., & Schomburg, E. D. (2006). Dopamine and the spinal cord in restless legs syndrome: Does spinal cord physiology reveal a basis for augmentation? *Sleep Medicine Reviews*, *10*(3), 185–196.

Pediani, J. D., Ward, R. J., Godin, A. G., Marsango, S., & Milligan, G. (2016). Dynamic regulation of quaternary organization of the M1 muscarinic receptor by subtype-selective antagonist drugs. *Journal of Biological Chemistry*, *291*(25), 13132–13146.

Peterson, C. D., Kitto, K. F., Akgün, E., Lunzer, M. M., Riedl, M. S., Vulchanova, L., et al. (2017). Bivalent ligand that activates mu opioid receptor and antagonizes mGluR5 receptor reduces neuropathic pain in mice. *Pain*, *158*(12), 2431–2441.

Pioszak, A. A., Harikumar, K. G., Parker, N. R., Miller, L. J., & Xu, H. E. (2010). Dimeric arrangement of the parathyroid hormone receptor and a structural mechanism for ligand-induced dissociation. *Journal of Biological Chemistry*, *285*(16), 12435–12444.

Pitarokoili, K., Fels, M., Kerasnoudis, A., Tönges, L., Gold, R., & Yoon, M. S. (2018). High-resolution nerve ultrasound and electrophysiological findings in restless legs syndrome. *Journal of Neuroimaging*, *28*(5), 506–514.

Pou, C., Mannoury la Cour, C., Stoddart, L. A., Millan, M. J., & Milligan, G. (2012). Functional homomers and heteromers of dopamine D_{2L} and D_3 receptors co-exist at the cell surface. *Journal of Biological Chemistry*, *287*, 8864–8878.

Provasi, D., Boz, M. B., Johnston, J. M., & Filizola, M. (2015). Preferred supramolecular organization and dimer interfaces of opioid receptors from simulated self-association. *PLoS Computational Biology*, *11*(3), e1004148.

Puig, M. V., Rose, J., Schmidt, R., & Freund, N. (2014). Dopamine modulation of learning and memory in the prefrontal cortex: Insights from studies in primates, rodents, and birds. *Frontiers in Neural Circuits*, *8*, 93.

Pulido, D., Casadó-Anguera, V., Pérez-Benito, L., Moreno, E., Cordomí, A., López, L., et al. (2018). Design of a true bivalent ligand with picomolar binding affinity for a G protein-coupled receptor homodimer. *Journal of Medicinal Chemistry*, *61*(20), 9335–9346.

Qian, M., Vasudevan, L., Huysentruyt, J., Risseeuw, M. D. P., Stove, C., Vanderheyden, P. M. L., et al. (2018). Design, synthesis, and biological evaluation of bivalent ligands targeting dopamine D2-like receptors and the μ-opioid receptor. *ChemMedChem*, *13*, 944–956. https://doi.org/10.1002/cmdc.201700787.

Qian, M., Wouters, E., Dalton, J. A. R., Risseeuw, M. D. P., Crans, R. A. J., Stove, C., et al. (2018). Synthesis toward bivalent ligands for the dopamine D2 and metabotropic glutamate 5 receptors. *Journal of Medicinal Chemistry*, *61*, 8212–8225. https://doi.org/10.1021/acs.jmedchem.8b00671.

Quiroz, C., Gulyani, S., Ruiqian, W., Bonaventura, J., Cutler, R., Pearson, V., et al. (2016). Adenosine receptors as markers of brain iron deficiency: Implications for restless legs syndrome. *Neuropharmacology*, *111*, 160–168.

Quiroz, C., Pearson, V., Gulyani, S., Allen, R., Earley, C., & Ferré, S. (2010). Up-regulation of striatal adenosine A(2A) receptors with iron deficiency in rats: Effects on locomotion and cortico-striatal neurotransmission. *Experimental Neurology*, *224*(1), 292–298.

Rivera-Oliver, M., & Díaz-Ríos, M. (2014). Using caffeine and other adenosine receptor antagonists and agonists as therapeutic tools against neurodegenerative diseases: A review. *Life Sciences*, *101*(1–2), 1–9.

Rivera-Oliver, M., Moreno, E., Álvarez-Bagnarol, Y., Ayala-Santiago, C., Cruz-Reyes, N., Molina-Castro, G. C., et al. (2018). Adenosine A_1-dopamine D_1 receptor heteromers control the excitability of the spinal motoneuron. *Molecular Neurobiology*. https://doi.org/10.1007/s12035-018-1120-y. Epub ahead of print.

Rizzo, G., Li, X., Galantucci, S., Filippi, M., & Cho, Y. W. (2017). Brain imaging and networks in restless legs syndrome. *Sleep Medicine*, *31*, 39–48.

Roberts, K. M., & Fitzpatrick, P. F. (2013). Mechanisms of tryptophan and tyrosine hydroxylase. *IUBMB Life*, *65*(4), 350–357.

Rubí, B., & Maechler, P. (2010). Minireview: New roles for peripheral dopamine on metabolic control and tumor growth: Let's seek the balance. *Endocrinology*, *151*(12), 5570–5581.

Sales, S., Sanghera, M. K., Klocko, D. J., & Stewart, R. M. (2016). Diagnosis and treatment of restless legs syndrome. *Journal of the American Academy of Physician Assistants*, *29*(7), 15–20.

Salvemini, D., Kim, S. F., & Mollace, V. (2013). Reciprocal regulation of the nitric oxide and cyclooxygenase pathway in pathophysiology: Relevance and clinical implications. *American Journal of Physiology-Regulatory, Integrative and Comparative*, *304*(7), R473–R487.

Scarselli, M., Annibale, P., McCormick, P. J., Kolachalam, S., Aringhieri, S., Radenovic, A., et al. (2016). Revealing G-protein-coupled receptor oligomerization at the single-molecule level through a nanoscopic lens: Methods, dynamics and biological function. *The FEBS Journal*, *283*(7), 1197–1217.

Scholz, S. W. (2017). Restless legs syndrome: Is it all in the genes? *Lancet Neurology*, *16*, 859–860.

Schormair, B., Zhao, C., Bell, S., Tilch, E., Salminen, A. V., Pütz, B., et al. (2017). Identification of novel risk loci for restless legs syndrome in genome-wide association studies in individuals of European ancestry: A meta-analysis. *Lancet Neurology*, *16*(11), 898–907.

Sharples, S. A., Koblinger, K., Humphreys, J. M., & Whelan, P. J. (2014). Dopamine: A parallel pathway for the modulation of spinal locomotor networks. *Frontiers in Neural Circuits*, *8*, 55.

Shen, J., Zhang, L., Song, W. L., Meng, T., Wang, X., Chen, L., et al. (2013). Design, synthesis and biological evaluation of bivalent ligands against A(1)-D(1) receptor heteromers. *Acta Pharmacologica Sinica*, *34*(3), 441–452.

Silber, M. H., Becker, P. M., Buchfuhrer, M. J., Earley, C. J., Ondo, W. G., Walters, A. S., et al. (2018). The appropriate use of opioids in the treatment of refractory restless legs syndrome. *Mayo Clinic Proceedings*, *93*(1), 59–67.

Smith, N. J., & Milligan, G. (2010). Allostery at G protein-coupled receptor homo- and heteromers: Uncharted pharmacological landscapes. *Pharmacological Reviews*, *62*(4), 701–725.

Soares, P. M., Patrocínio, M. C., Assreuy, A. M., Siqueira, R. C., Lima, N. M., Arruda, M. d. O., et al. (2009). Aminophylline (a theophylline-ethylenediamine complex) blocks ethanol behavioral effects in mice. *Behavioural Pharmacology*, *20*(4), 297–302.

Söderberg, O., Leuchowius, K. J., Gullberg, M., Jarvius, M., Weibrecht, I., Larsson, L. G., et al. (2008). Characterizing proteins and their interactions in cells and tissues using the in situ proximity ligation assay. *Methods*, *45*, 227–232. https://doi.org/10.1016/j.ymeth.2008.06.014.

Sohy, D., Parmentier, M., & Springael, J. Y. (2007). Allosteric transinhibition by specific antagonists in CCR2/CXCR4 heterodimers. *Journal of Biological Chemistry*, *282*(41), 30062–30069.

Stone, T. W., Ceruti, S., & Abbracchio, M. P. (2009). Adenosine receptors and neurological disease: Neuroprotection and neurodegeneration. *Handbook of Experimental Pharmacology*, *193*, 535–587.

Szalai, B., Barkai, L., Turu, G., Szidonya, L., Várnai, P., & Hunyady, L. (2012). Allosteric interactions within the AT1 angiotensin receptor homodimer: Role of the conserved DRY motif. *Biochemical Pharmacology*, *84*, 477–485.

Tabor, A., Weisenburger, S., Banerjee, A., Purkayastha, N., Kaindl, J. M., Hübner, H., et al. (2016). Visualization and ligand-induced modulation of dopamine receptor dimerization at the single molecule level. *Scientific Reports*, *6*, 33233.

Taura, J., Fernández-Dueñas, V., & Ciruela, F. (2015). Visualizing G protein-coupled receptor-receptor interactions in brain using proximity ligation in situ assay. *Current Protocols in Cell Biology*, *67*, 17.17.1–16. https://doi.org/10.1002/0471143030.cb1717s67.

Teichmann, A., Gibert, A., Lampe, A., Grzesik, P., Rutz, C., Furkert, J., et al. (2014). The specific monomer/dimer equilibrium of the corticotropin-releasing factor receptor type 1 is established in the endoplasmic reticulum. *Journal of Biological Chemistry*, *289*(35), 24250–24262.

Teitler, M., Toohey, N., Knight, J. A., Klein, M. T., & Smith, C. (2010). Clozapine and other competitive antagonists reactivate risperidone-inactivated h5-HT7 receptors: Radioligand binding and functional evidence for GPCR homodimer protomer interactions. *Psychopharmacology (Berlin)*, *212*, 687–697.

Terrillon, S., Barberis, C., & Bouvier, M. (2004). Heterodimerization of V1a and V2 vasopressin receptors determines the interaction with beta-arrestin and their trafficking patterns. *Proceedings of the National Academy of Sciences of the United States of America*, *101*(6), 1548–1553.

Tian, H., Fürstenberg, A., & Huber, T. (2017). Labeling and single-molecule methods to monitor G protein-coupled receptor dynamics. *Chemical Reviews*, *117*(1), 186–245.

Toda, S., Alguacil, L. F., & Kalivas, P. W. (2003). Repeated cocaine administration changes the function and subcellular distribution of adenosine A_1 receptor in the rat nucleus accumbens. *Journal of Neurochemistry*, *87*(6), 1478–1484.

Torvinen, M., Gines, S., Hillion, J., Latini, S., Canals, M., Ciruela, F., et al. (2002). Interactions among adenosine deaminase, adenosine A(1) receptors and dopamine D(1) receptors in stably cotransfected fibroblast cells and neurons. *Neuroscience*, *113*, 709–719.

Trenkwalder, C., Allen, R., Högl, B., Paulus, W., & Winkelmann, J. (2016). Restless legs syndrome associated with major diseases: A systematic review and new concept. *Neurology*, *86*(14), 1336–1343.

Trenkwalder, C., & Paulus, W. (2010). Restless legs syndrome: Pathophysiology, clinical presentation and management. *Nature Reviews Neurology*, *6*(6), 337–346.

Trenkwalder, C., Winkelmann, J., Inoue, Y., & Paulus, W. (2015). Restless legs syndrome—Current therapies and management of augmentation. *Nature Reviews Neurology*, *11*(8), 434–445.

Trenkwalder, C., Zieglgänsberger, W., Ahmedzai, S. H., & Högl, B. (2017). Pain, opioids, and sleep: Implications for restless legs syndrome treatment. *Sleep Medicine*, *31*, 78–85.

Trifilieff, P., Rives, M. L., Urizar, E., Piskorowski, R. A., Vishwasrao, H. D., Castrillon, J., et al. (2011). Detection of antigen interactions ex vivo by proximity ligation assay: Endogenous dopamine D_2-adenosine A_{2A} receptor complexes in the striatum. *BioTechniques*, *51*(2), 111–118.

Trincavelli, M. L., Daniele, S., Orlandini, E., Navarro, G., Casadó, V., Giacomelli, C., et al. (2012). A new D_2 dopamine receptor agonist allosterically modulates A(2A) adenosine receptor signalling by interacting with the A(2A)/D_2 receptor heteromer. *Cellular Signalling*, *24*, 951–960. https://doi.org/10.1016/j.cellsig.2011.12.018.

Varani, K., Vincenzi, F., Merighi, S., Gessi, S., & Borea, P. A. (2017). Biochemical and pharmacological role of A_1 adenosine receptors and their modulation as novel therapeutic strategy. *Advances in Experimental Medicine and Biology*, *1051*, 193–232.

Vilardaga, J. P., Agnati, L. F., Fuxe, K., & Ciruela, F. (2010). G-protein-coupled receptor heteromer dynamics. *Journal of Cell Science*, *123*(24), 4215–4220.

Viñals, X., Moreno, E., Lanfumey, L., Cordomí, A., Pastor, A., de La Torre, R., et al. (2015). Cognitive impairment induced by delta9-tetrahydrocannabinol occurs through heteromers between cannabinoid CB_1 and serotonin 5-HT_{2A} receptors. *PLoS Biology*, *13*(7), e1002194.

Vischer, H. F., Castro, M., & Pin, J. P. (2015). G protein-coupled receptor multimers: A question still open despite the use of novel approaches. *Molecular Pharmacology*, *88*(3), 561–571.

Volkow, N. D., Wang, G. J., Logan, J., Alexoff, D., Fowler, J. S., Thanos, P. K., et al. (2015). Caffeine increases striatal dopamine D_2/D_3 receptor availability in the human brain. *Translational Psychiatry*, *5*, e549.

Wade, F., Espagne, A., Persuy, M. A., Vidic, J., Monnerie, R., Merola, F., et al. (2011). Relationship between homo-oligomerization of a mammalian olfactory receptor and its activation state demonstrated by bioluminescence resonance energy transfer. *Journal of Biological Chemistry*, *286*(17), 15252–15259.

Wang, D., Yu, H., Liu, X., Liu, J., & Song, C. (2017). The orientation and stability of the GPCR-Arrestin complex in a lipid bilayer. *Scientific Reports*, 7(1), 16985.

Ward, R. J., Pediani, J. D., Harikumar, K. G., Miller, L. J., & Milligan, G. (2017). Spatial intensity distribution analysis quantifies the extent and regulation of homodimerization of the secretin receptor. *Biochemical Journal*, *474*(11), 1879–1895.

Weber, K. A., Sentis, A. I., Bernadel-Huey, O. N., Chen, Y., Wang, X., Parrish, T. B., et al. (2018). Thermal stimulation alters cervical spinal cord functional connectivity in humans. *Neuroscience*, *369*, 40–50.

Whorton, M. R., Bokoch, M. P., Rasmussen, S. G., Huang, B., Zare, R. N., Kobilka, B., et al. (2007). A monomeric G protein-coupled receptor isolated in a high-density lipoprotein particle efficiently activates its G protein. *Proceedings of the National Academy of Sciences of the United States of America*, *104*(18), 7682–7687.

Wijemanne, S., & Ondo, W. (2017). Restless legs syndrome: Clinical features, diagnosis and a practical approach to management. *Practical Neurology*, *17*(6), 444–452.

Winkelman, J. (2008). Genetics of restless legs syndrome. *Current Neurology and Neuroscience Reports*, *8*(3), 211–216.
Winkelman, J. W., Armstrong, M. J., Allen, R. P., Chaudhuri, K. R., Ondo, W., Trenkwalder, C., et al. (2016). Practice guideline summary: Treatment of restless legs syndrome in adults. *Neurology*, *87*(24), 2585–2593.
Winkelman, J., Czamara, D., Schormair, B., Knauf, F., Schulte, E. C., Trenkwalder, C., et al. (2011). Genome-wide association study identifies novel restless legs syndrome susceptibility loci on 2p14 and 16q12.1. *PLoS Genetics*, 7(7), e1002171.
Winkelman, J., Schormair, B., Lichtner, P., Ripke, S., Xiong, L., Jalilzadeh, S., et al. (2007). Genome-wide association study of restless legs syndrome identifies common variants in three genomic regions. *Nature Genetics*, *39*(8), 1000–1006.
Witts, E. C., Nascimento, F., & Miles, G. B. (2015). Adenosine-mediated modulation of ventral horn interneurons and spinal motoneurons in neonatal mice. *Journal of Neurophysiology*, *114*(4), 2305–2315.
Xue, L., Rovira, X., Scholler, P., Zhao, H., Liu, J., Pin, J. P., et al. (2015). Major ligand-induced rearrangement of the heptahelical domain interface in a GPCR dimer. *Nature Chemical Biology*, *11*(2), 134–140.
Yepes, G., Guitart, X., Rea, W., Newman, A. H., Allen, R. P., Earley, C. J., et al. (2017). Targeting hypersensitive corticostriatal terminals in restless legs syndrome. *Annals of Neurology*, *82*(6), 951–960.
Yin, S., Noetzel, M. J., Johnson, K. A., Zamorano, R., Jalan-Sakrikar, N., Gregory, K. J., et al. (2014). Selective actions of novel allosteric modulators reveal functional heteromers of metabotropic glutamate receptors in the CNS. *Journal of Neuroscience*, *34*(1), 79–94.
Zhang, Q., Yu, Y. P., Ye, Y. L., Zhang, J. T., Zhang, W. P., & Wei, E. Q. (2011). Spatiotemporal properties of locomotor activity after administration of central nervous stimulants and sedatives in mice. *Pharmacology Biochemistry and Behavior*, *97*(3), 577–585.

CHAPTER FOUR

D3 and D1 receptors: The Yin and Yang in the treatment of restless legs syndrome with dopaminergics

Stefan Clemens[a,*], Imad Ghorayeb[b,c,d]
[a]Brody School of Medicine, Department of Physiology, East Carolina University, Greenville, NC, United States
[b]Clinical Neurophysiology Department, Clinical Neurosciences Pole, Bordeaux Teaching Hospital, Bordeaux, France
[c]Aquitaine Institute for Cognitive and Integrative Neuroscience, Bordeaux University, CNRS-UMR 5287, Bordeaux, France
[d]CNRS, Aquitaine Institute of Cognitive and Integrative Neurosciences, UMR, Bordeaux, France
*Corresponding author: e-mail address: clemenss@ecu.edu

Contents

Abstract

Dopaminergic treatments targeting the D3 receptor subtype to reduce the symptoms of RLS show substantial initial clinical benefits but fail to maintain their efficacy over time. Sensorimotor circuits in the spinal cord are the gateway for the sensory processing of the symptoms and critical for the associated leg movements that relieve the symptoms and the periodic limb movements that often develop during sleep. There is a high preponderance of the inhibitory D3 receptor in the sensory-processing areas of the spinal cord (dorsal horn), whereas the motor areas in the ventral horn more strongly express the excitatory D1 receptor subtype. D3 and D1 receptors can form functional heteromeric ensembles that influence each other. In the spinal cord, long-term treatment with D3 receptor agonists is associated with the upregulation of the D1 receptor subtype and block of D1 receptor function at this stage can restore the D3 receptor

Advances in Pharmacology, Volume 84
ISSN 1054-3589
https://doi.org/10.1016/bs.apha.2019.01.002
© 2019 Elsevier Inc.
All rights reserved.

effect. Alternate scenarios for a role of dopamine involve a role for the D5 receptor in regulating motor excitability and for the D4 receptor subtype in controlling D3-like effects. A model emerges that proposes that the behavioral changes in RLS, while responsive to D3 receptor agonists, may be ultimately be the result of unmasked increased D1-like receptor activities.

Abbreviations

6-OHDA 6-hydroxydopamine
AMP adenosine-mono-phosphate
cAMP cyclic AMP
D1 dopamine D1 receptor
D2 dopamine D2 receptor
D3 dopamine D3 receptor
D4 dopamine D4 receptor
D5 dopamine D5 receptor
GPCR G protein-coupled receptor
ID iron deficient
K_i inhibitory binding constant
L-dopa levodopa
LTP long-term potentiation
PD Parkinson's disease
PLMS periodic limb movements during sleep
QoL quality of life
RLS restless legs syndrome
rt-PCR real-time polymerase chain reaction
SDH superficial dorsal horn
SN substantia nigra
VTA ventral tegmental area

1. Introduction

Restless Legs Syndrome (RLS) has the reputation of a "modern" neurological disorder, despite the fact that it was first described as disorder of the nervous system in the 17th century (Willis, 1685). Moreover, following this first description in a clinical textbook, there is a long trail of medical literature over the centuries that reports "anxietas tibiarum," "fidgeting and nervousness," and "the inability to keep still" (reviewed in Langebner & Lampl, 2018). RLS was clinically re-defined in the mid-20th century (Ekbom, 1945, 1960) and it is now considered a common sensorimotor disorder with symptoms that primarily and predominantly affects the legs in a circadian manner. Restless legs syndrome is now defined by the following five essential criteria: (1) An urge to move the legs usually but not always accompanied by, or felt to be caused by, uncomfortable and unpleasant sensations in the legs; (2) The urge to move the legs and any accompanying unpleasant sensations begin or worsen during periods of rest or inactivity such as lying down or sitting; (3) The urge to move the legs and any accompanying unpleasant sensations are partially or totally relieved by movement, such as walking or stretching, at least as long as the activity continues; (4) The urge to move the legs and any accompanying unpleasant sensations during rest or inactivity only occur or are worse in the evening or night than during the day; (5) The occurrence of the above features is not solely accounted for as symptoms primary to another medical or a behavioral condition (e.g., myalgia, venous stasis, leg edema, arthritis, leg cramps, positional discomfort, habitual foot tapping) (Allen et al., 2014).

The sensorimotor symptoms of RLS impede the quality of life (QoL) and sleep of the patients affected (Allen et al., 2005; Earley & Silber, 2010; Trenkwalder et al., 2018; Winkelman et al., 2009), and RLS is considered by many as "The most important sleep disorder you've never heard of" (Owens, 2016). In addition to the sensory symptoms, RLS patients often also manifest with periodic limb movements during sleep (PLMS) (Ferri et al., 2015; Zucconi et al., 2006), which contributes to reduced QoL of the patients.

The cause of RLS remains unclear (Chokroverty, 2014). While there is substantial evidence from genome-wide association studies in humans indicating an association of several distinct key genes with the disorder (Schormair et al., 2011, 2017; Stefansson et al., 2007; Trotti, Bhadriraju, & Rye, 2008; Winkelmann & Ferini-Strambi, 2006; Winkelmann et al., 2007, 2017), none of these genes alone can explain the pathophysiology of the symptoms on its own. Central to the pathophysiology of RLS, brain iron insufficiency could be the primary event that triggers an altered dopaminergic state in the nervous system, as well as dysfunctions of other neurotransmitter systems, including serotonin and adenosine (Hyacinthe et al., 2015; Quiroz et al., 2016). Further, the success of clinical trials suggests a role for dopamine in the pathophysiology of RLS, although it remains unclear whether the dopamine effect is due to an hyper- or hypodopaminergic state of the nervous system and if this dopamine dysfunction originates in the basal ganglia or the spinal cord, which is the first site of sensory integration and the final common output for all locomotor function (Chokroverty, 2014; Mrowka, Chaudhuri, & Odin, 2004).

With an incidence rate of 4.5–11% in otherwise healthy populations (Didriksen et al., 2017; Phillips, Hening, Britz, & Mannino, 2006), RLS is, adjusted to age, as common as dementia and more prevalent than the next most widespread neurological disorders combined (Tourette's, <1%; Epilepsy, 0.6%; Parkinson's disease, 0.3%; and Cerebral palsy, 0.2%) (Pringsheim, Fiest, & Jette, 2014). Against this background, it is surprising that no pharmacological treatments have been developed with RLS as a primary target.

2. L-dopa, the first dopaminergic drug approach to treat RLS

Early reports suggested a relationship between anemia and the emergence of the symptoms, thus supporting the concept of a role of the iron system in RLS, and initial attempts to treat RLS symptoms pharmacologically focused with varying effects on vasodilating drugs, blood transfusions, or iron therapy (Murray, 1967). The high prevalence of PLMS in RLS patients suggests that the descending motor system might play an important role in the overall symptomatology. Intriguingly, while there is no evidence of a direct link between Parkinson's disease (PD) and RLS (Ondo, Vuong, & Jankovic, 2002) or suggesting that RLS patients may have a higher predisposition to PD (Walters et al., 2003), recent studies indicate high similarities between RLS and PD in regard to iron homeostasis and dopamine function (Ferini-Strambi, Carli, Casoni, & Galbiati, 2018; Piao et al., 2017). Initially, PD was associated with low DA metabolite levels in the brain (Bernheimer, Birkmayer, Hornykiewicz, Jellinger, & Seitelberger, 1973; Price, Farley, & Hornykiewicz, 1978), and treatment of PD was successful with L-dopa medication or a combination of L-dopa plus benserazide (inhibitor of the peripheral decarboxylase) (Birkmayer & Hornykiewicz, 1962). In a subsequent study, the first of its kind in RLS patients, this combination of L-dopa/benserazide also showed beneficial responses in treating the symptoms of RLS (Akpinar, 1982). In that proof-of-concept trial with five patients enrolled, L-dopa/benserazide completely resolved the symptoms in all patients and these effects were mimicked by the D2 receptor agonist bromocriptine, but worsened by pimozide, a dopamine receptor antagonist with high binding affinities to D2, D3, and D4 receptor subtypes (Pearlstein, Vaz, & Rampe, 2003; Silvestre & Prous, 2005). The efficacy of L-dopa and D2-like receptor agonists to significantly improve the primary symptom of RLS has been confirmed since (Garcia-Borreguero et al., 2013; Hening, Allen, Earley, Picchietti, & Silber, 2004), but while these data suggest a role for the DA system, and in particular the D2-like receptor system, in RLS, it remains unclear if the underlying pathology is based on a hypo- (Akpinar, 1987; Connor et al., 2009; Montplaisir, Godbout, Poirier, & Bedard, 1986; Montplaisir, Lorrain, & Godbout, 1991) or hyper-dopaminergic state (Earley et al., 2014, 2013; Earley, Uhl, Clemens, & Ferre, 2017; Khan, Ahlberg, Chow, Shah, & Koo, 2017).

The answer to this ongoing controversy may come from experiments that manipulated iron levels in non-human primates and in rodents and that highlighted the pivotal role of iron in the modulation of the dopaminergic system. In RLS patients, dopaminergic abnormalities were characterized as an overly active dopaminergic system at the presynaptic level (Earley, Allen, & Hening, 2011), and changes in iron levels reproduced these key features in macaques, where an increase in nigrostriatal dopaminergic function together with a specific alteration of the serotonin/dopamine interaction in the central nervous system was documented after serum depletion of iron (Hyacinthe et al., 2015). In rats with nutritional iron deficiency, a significant reduction in density and functioning of DAT was observed (Erikson, Jones, & Beard, 2000), and, in addition, iron deficiency can alter dopamine extracellular levels in the caudate-putamen at different biological times of the day and night and decrease D1 and D2 receptor density in the caudate-putamen of rat brains (Ashkenazi, Ben-Shachar, & Youdim, 1982; Erikson, Jones, Hess, Zhang, & Beard, 2001).

3. Dopamine and its receptors

DA cannot pass through the blood-brain barrier, but L-dopa is converted in the nervous system to DA, where it then exerts its modulatory actions through five identified trans-membrane G protein-coupled receptor (GPCR) subtypes (D1–D5) that activate (D1-like) or inhibit (D2-like) cyclic AMP-mediated second messenger pathways. The D1-like group of receptors consists of the D1 and the D5 receptor subtypes, while the D2-like group consists of the D2, D3, and D4 receptors. All receptors express different binding K_i-binding affinities to dopamine (compiled from public database available at: https://pdsp.unc.edu/databases/kidb.php, see Table 1 and Fig. 1).

Together, these data suggest that D3 and D4 receptor subtypes have the highest affinities to dopamine and that the D2 receptor has a nearly ~20-fold reduced affinity to dopamine compared to D3 or D4, and a ~twofold reduced affinity when compared to the D5 receptor subtype. Note that the K_i value for the D5 receptor subtype stems from only a single study

Table 1 Synopsis of all dopamine receptors and their different binding Ki-binding affinities to the monoamine.

	D1	D2	D3	D4	D5
# Of studies	**17**	**36**	**13**	**6**	**1**
Range K_i	11.7–10,000	2.8–10,000	1.4–266	6.2–407	228
Avg K_i	3580	519	69	39	228
Std dev K_i	4222	2154	86	158	–
Median K_i	1450	544	29	35	228

Data were compiled from the Psychoactive Drug Screening Program (PDSP) K_i Database available at https://pdsp.unc.edu/databases/kidb.php.

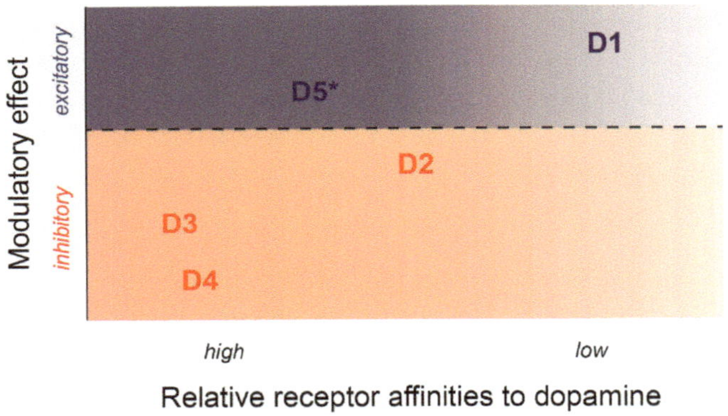

Fig. 1 Summary of the relative dopamine receptor affinities to their substrate. Shown are the approximate affinities based on their median K_i values. Based on data obtained from the K_i-database, https://pdsp.unc.edu/databases/kidb.php.

and that its position on this model may change as more data come in. Evidence suggests that D1-like and D2-like receptors can be found on the same neurons (Zhu, Clemens, Sawchuk, & Hochman, 2007b), and that dopamine can up- or downregulate cellular and network functions in a dose-dependent manner (Clemens, Belin-Rauscent, Simmers, & Combes, 2012; Missale, Nash, Robinson, Jaber, & Caron, 1998; Thirumalai & Cline, 2008). Additionally, the rate of dopamine neuron firing can dictate the outcome of how the different receptor subtypes are activated (Dreyer, Herrik, Berg, & Hounsgaard, 2010; Kishore & McLean, 2015). Therefore, based on the concept that dopamine receptors form individual entities in the cell membrane, the high affinities of the D3 and the D4 receptors to DA suggest that these receptor subtypes may be activated in the presence of relatively low levels of the compound that are based on a tonic background release of dopamine, while activation of the low-affinity D1 receptor might require relatively larger amounts of dopamine in the synaptic cleft that may be present after increased dopamine neuron bursting activity.

4. Dopamine, where does it act?

Dopamine receptors can be found both presynaptically (Barrett & Lokhandwala, 1982; Bonaventura et al., 2017; Gajendiran, Seth, & Ganguly, 1996; Jackisch, Hotz, Allgaier, & Hertting, 1994; Kondo, Fujiwara, & Tanaka, 1986; Lindgren et al., 2003; Wu, Dougherty, & Nichols, 2006) and postsynaptically (Centonze et al., 2003; Huang et al., 1992; Navarro et al., 1992; Olianas, Dedoni, & Onali, 2012; Shin et al., 2003; Swant, Stramiello, & Wagner, 2008; Waters, Svensson, Haadsma-Svensson, Smith, & Carlsson, 1993; Yang, 2000). The presence of these receptors on both sides of the synapse provides a wealth of opportunity for the nervous system to fine-tune dopamine-mediated responses, but it also makes it difficult to ascribe specific modulatory actions to any given receptor subtype and location.

There are several dopamine pathways intrinsic to the brain that are receptive to increasing dopamine levels: the mesocortical pathway, ascending from the ventral tegmental area (VTA); the mesolimbic pathway, also originating from the VTA; the tuberofundibular pathway, originating from the hypothalamus, and the nigrostriatal pathway, which originates from the substantia nigra (SN) (Chakravarthy, Balasubramani, Mandali, Jahanshahi, & Moustafa, 2018). As the symptoms of RLS are sensory in nature, as described by the "urge to move", and as these aforementioned projections do not directly modulate sensory circuits in the brain, it is unlikely that the symptomatic relief of L-dopa can be attributed to any of these four pathways. However, as the basal ganglia provide pre-motor information to the spinal cord, the nigrostriatal projections may play an instrumental role in setting the tone for the descending motor commands and the emergence of PLMS movements, and this modulation can occur via D1-like (predominantly located on the direct pathway) and D2-like receptors (mainly on the indirect pathway).

There exists a fifth group of dopamine neurons in the brain, located in the dorso-posterior aspect of the hypothalamus (A11), that has projections not only to the frontal cortex but is also the only one with descending projections throughout the entire length of the spinal cord, the primary site for sensory integration (Barraud et al., 2010; Bjorklund & Skagerberg, 1979; Holstege et al., 1996; Skagerberg, Bjorklund, Lindvall, & Schmidt, 1982). With its widespread projections notably to the dorsal horn and the intermediate and ventral laminae (Holstege et al., 1996), these dopamine fibers are ideally situated to modulate sensory signals at the site of entry from the periphery to the CNS and the motoneurons and central pattern generating (CPG) networks that coordinate locomotion and leg movements (Clemens, Rye, & Hochman, 2006; Trenkwalder et al., 2018). Intriguingly, partial deletion of A11 neurons with 6-OHDA was associated with an increase in locomotor activity that could be brought back by treating animals with a D3 agonist (Ondo, He, Rajasekaran, & Le, 2000), and iron deprivation further increased locomotor activities (Qu et al., 2007). Together with data showing that D3 receptor dysfunction increased the sensitivity of spinal reflex pathways (Clemens & Hochman, 2004; Keeler, Baran, Brewer, & Clemens, 2012) and that iron-deficiency in D3 receptor knockout animals further increased the already elevated responses in these animals to acute and persistent pain stimuli and also changed circadian activity (Dowling et al., 2011), these findings further support the aforementioned link between dopamine and iron and indicate a potential role of the spinal dopamine system in modulating both sensory and motor symptoms as observed in RLS.

In situ hybridization and rt-PCR studies have reported the presence of all DA receptor mRNAs in the rodent spinal cord (Zhu, Clemens, Sawchuk, & Hochman, 2007a, 2008), independent of the iron status of the animals (Zhao et al., 2007). While in rodents all receptors are present throughout the gray matter, the ratio of labeling was Lamina-specific for each receptor subtype (Zhu et al., 2007a). Additionally, across all Laminae, D2 and D5 receptors had the highest abundance and were expressed in about 50% of all identified neurons, D4 receptors in ~30% of the neurons, and D1 and D3 receptors in only 15–20%. However, the spatial distribution of the receptors was more diverse: in Laminae 1–3, D1 expression was low and similar to D3 (each in ~10% of the neurons), D4 was expressed in ~20% of the neurons, while D2 and D5 were found in ~40% of the cells. In contrast, in Lamina IX, D1, D2, and D5 receptors were found in >80% of the neurons (including motoneurons), while D3 and D4 receptors were present in less than half of the cells. Together with the different affinities of the dopamine receptor subtypes to their substrate (cf. Table 1, Fig. 1), these spatial characteristics suggest a preferential inhibitory role for dopamine in the dorsal (sensory) horn of the spinal cord and a preferential excitatory role of the monoamine in the ventral (motor) horn. A subsequent neuro-anatomical study, performed in non-human primates, detected only four receptor subtypes in the monkey spinal cord (D2, D3, D4, and D5) (Barraud et al., 2010), however the functional analogy of D1 and D5 receptors would still allow for a co-modulation of dopamine signals through inhibitory and excitatory pathways.

In addition to these mRNA studies, quantitative autoradiography assessed D1 and D3 receptor expression across the spinal gray matter in rodents and identified a two- to fourfold higher expression of the D3 receptor subtype in the superficial dorsal horn (SDH) over dorsal horn, ventral horn, and pars centralis in all areas of the cord (cervical, thoracic, lumbar, and sacral), while D1-like receptor expression was generally similar across all laminae and only slightly increased in the SDH of the lumbar cord (Levant & McCarson, 2001). As dopamine directly inhibits neurons in the pain-encoding SDH (Tamae et al., 2005), it is conceivable that the beneficial actions of L-dopa initially target this particular cell population to relieve RLS symptoms, and that a blocking action of the nociceptive pathway in the dorsal horn by D3 receptor agonists could also explain the high symptomatic relief these drugs are achieving in the clinical setting (Manconi et al., 2011, 2007). At the same time, dopamine and D3 receptor agonists will also act on receptors in other areas of the brain and the spinal cord, additionally camouflaging the mechanistic pathways that provide the symptomatic relief for RLS symptoms.

For example, excitatory D1-like receptors are not only implicated in the induction of LTP phenomena in C-fibers in the dorsal horn (Yang, Zhou, Hu, Xin, & Liu, 2005) and the activation of leg movements in the ventral horn (Barriere, Mellen, & Cazalets, 2004), D3 receptor activation can even potentiate the recruitment of D1 receptors in a heterodimer configuration (Marcellino et al., 2008). The possible interplay of D3 and D1 receptors with regard to their location with the sensorimotor circuitry of the spinal cord is illustrated in Fig. 2.

5. Dopamine receptor heteromers and D3–D1 receptor interactions

The concept that G protein-coupled receptors (GPCRs) such as dopamine receptors form independent entities in the cell membrane that act independently of each other has undergone a major revision in the last two decades. There is growing evidence that the classical view of GPCR function and signaling, i.e., of individual receptors in the membrane that

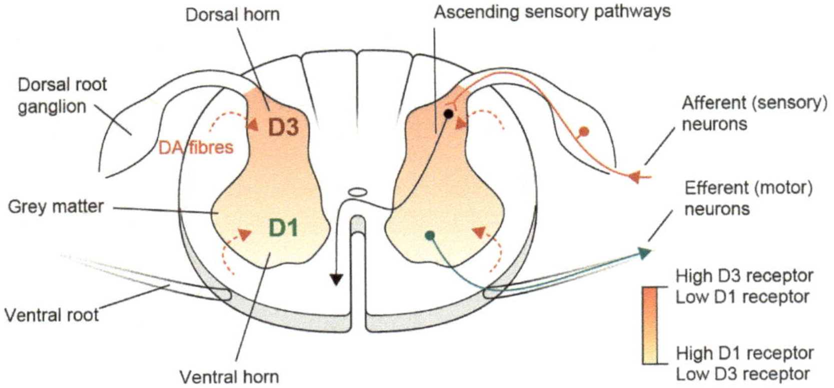

Fig. 2 Model of D1 and D3 and receptor expression in the spinal cord, the site of sensorimotor integration for ascending sensory signals and descending pre-motor signals. D3 receptors are predominantly expressed in the dorsal horn where they are well placed to modulate the sensory symptoms that define RLS. In contrast, D1 receptors are more prominent in the ventral areas of the cord where they are in a prime location to modulate the interneurons of the CPG for locomotion and the motoneurons that ultimately drive leg movements. *Adapted from, and used with permission: Trenkwalder, C., Allen, R., Hogl, B., Clemens, S., Patton, S., Schormair, B., et al. (2018). Comorbidities, treatment, and pathophysiology in restless legs syndrome.* Lancet Neurol, 17*(11), 994–1005. doi:10.1016/S1474-4422(18)30311-9.*

float in the plasma membrane where they can couple to their ligand, is outdated and that GPCRs can form heteromers (both heterodimers and heterotetramers) that provide the basis for the interactions of the GPCRs with adenylate-cyclase (Ferre, 2015; Ferre et al., 2007; Fuxe, Ferre, Genedani, Franco, & Agnati, 2007). For example, evidence suggests that there is an anatomical basis for the existence of functional interactions between adenosine A(1) and dopamine D1 and between adenosine A(2A) and dopamine D2 receptors in the same neurons, and that selective A(1) agonists affect negatively the affinity binding of D1 receptors (Franco et al., 2000). Dopamine D1 and D2 receptors can also form functional heteromers with the histamine (H3) receptor and provide a link between the MAPK pathway and the GABA-ergic neurons in the direct striatal efferent pathway (Moreno et al., 2011). Such heteromers may even alter the affinity of the neurotransmitter to either receptor subunit and thus they might provide an additional layer of complexity in modulating second messenger signaling in the target neuron (Earley et al., 2017).

Further, besides functionally coupling to other receptor classes, dopamine receptors themselves can also form both homomers and heteromers with each other, thereby modifying the dopamine-evoked response at the level of the GPCRs (Earley et al., 2017; Fuxe, Guidolin, Agnati, & Borroto-Escuela, 2015; Rashid et al., 2007; Verma, Hasbi, O'Dowd, & George, 2010). Dopamine receptor heteromers, apart from their canonical action on cAMP-mediated signaling, can therefore regulate a wide range of cellular responses to fine-tune the expression of dopamine-associated behaviors and functions, and it has been proposed that such pathways may be involved in the desensitization of GPCR activity (Beaulieu, Espinoza, & Gainetdinov, 2015).

With regard to RLS, D1–D3 receptor heteromers are a particularly promising target. First, these receptors can display functional interactions in both hetero-dimer (Cruz-Trujillo et al., 2013; Fiorentini et al., 2008; Marcellino et al., 2008) or hetero-tetramer configurations (Guitart et al., 2014). Second, the D1 receptor coimmunoprecipitates with the D3 receptor in striatal protein preparations, and as a result of this dimerization, the D3R is switched to the desensitization mechanisms typical of the D1R (Fiorentini et al., 2008). Third, a unique characteristic of this receptor complex in the striatum is a synergistic interaction by which D3 receptor stimulation increases D1 receptor agonist affinity, which in turn allows a stronger stimulatory coupling of the D1R to the cAMP system and potentiates D1 receptor-mediated behavior (Fiorentini, Busi, Spano, & Missale, 2010). Lastly, the reciprocal regulation of D3 and D1 receptor function in the striatum points to a role of this mechanism in the development of motor dysfunctions and may possibly be a key feature in the emergence of PLMS in RLS patients.

In addition to these potential supraspinal actions of the D1–D3 receptor system, the distinct distribution patterns of dopamine D1 and D3 receptors in the spinal cord indicate specific tasks in those neural circuits they modulate, with D3 receptors preferentially modulating sensory afferences and D1 receptors controlling locomotor output (cf. Fig. 2). However, despite the spatial differences, there is also substantial overlap between D1 and D3 receptors (Zhu et al., 2007a), which would allow for D1–D3 receptors to form and be functionally active. Externally applied drug effects appear to be contiguous across spinal cord neurons in be present in sensory and motor laminae alike. Activation of the D3 pathway reduces both overall sensory (Keeler et al., 2012) and motor excitability in the isolated spinal cord (Sharples et al., 2015), while activation of the D1 receptor pathways tends to increase the excitability or the performance of neural networks that underlie or control fictive locomotion in different animal models (Clemens et al., 2012; Han & Whelan, 2009).

The interplay between D3 and D1 receptors in the spinal cord has recently garnered more interest, as a dysfunction of the D3 receptor system was associated with an increase of D1 receptor protein expression in the spinal cord (Brewer, Baran, Whitfield, Jensen, & Clemens, 2014). Moreover D1R expression levels increased in both striatum and spinal cord, while D3R expression levels remained stable in the striatum or slightly decreased in the spinal cord. The resulting D1-to-D3 ratio indicated a strong upregulation of D1R-mediated pathways in old animals, which was particularly pronounced in the lumbar spinal cord. These data suggest that aging may be associated with a shift in D1 and D3 receptor-mediated pathways in striatum and spinal cord, which in turn could be an underlying factor in the emergence of RLS and its increased prevalence in the elderly (Keeler, Patel, Lallemand, de Castro Brás, & Clemens, 2016).

An important argument against the use of D3 receptor agonists to treat RLS symptoms is the emergence of augmentation over time, which has become the single-most important side-effect (e.g., Allen & Earley, 1996; Trenkwalder et al., 2017; Williams & Garcia-Borreguero, 2009; Winkelman & Johnston, 2004). The presence of D1–D3 receptor heterodimers in the key nervous system tissues that regulate sensory and motor functions with regard to RLS provides a tempting background to speculate if the prolonged activation of the D3 receptor pathway during treatment may inadvertently recruit and strengthen D1 receptor-mediated excitatory pathways, as also reported from other tissues (Fiorentini et al., 2010; Zeng et al., 2004) and thus induce the opposite of the desired clinical outcome. As block of D1 receptor function has recently been reported to improve the motor outcome in Tourette's syndrome (Chipkin, 2014; Gilbert, Budman, Singer, Kurlan, & Chipkin, 2014), it is conceivable that this receptor may be a potential target to control increased motor outputs in RLS and in general.

In support of the hypothetical model that an upregulation of the D1 receptor subtype may play a role in the augmentation phenotype of RLS, a preclinical study recently showed that the gradual decline in responsiveness to long-term treatment with D3 receptor agonists in a rodent model could be reversed or rescued by adjuvant block of D1 receptors in animals that were no longer responsive to the D3 receptor agonist alone (Dinkins, Lallemand, & Clemens, 2017). If repeatable in the clinic, the mechanisms leading to augmentation in RLS patients after long-term use of D3R drugs might then be related to a parallel stimulation of the D1R system that is based on D1–D3 receptor heteromers (Dinkins et al., 2017). Such a transition

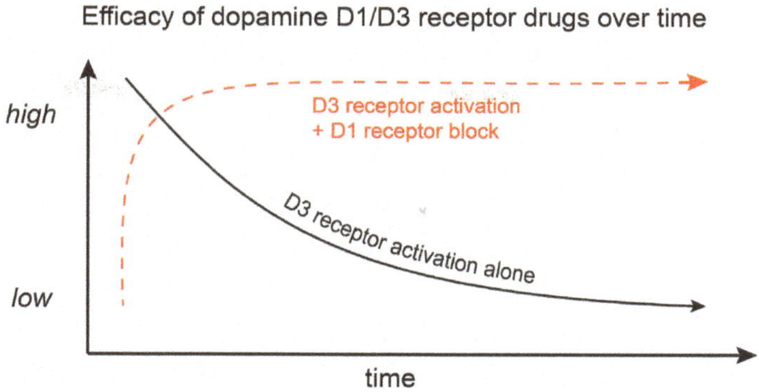

Fig. 3 Model of the efficacy of D3 and D1 receptor compounds over time. Clinical and pre-clinical data report a decline of efficacy of D3 receptor compounds in the treatment of RLS over time that, in humans, is acted on by increasing dosages and eventually leads to augmentation. Pre-clinical data indicate that prolonged D3 receptor activation is associated with an increase of D1 receptor expression, and that adjuvant administration of a D1 receptor blocker under such conditions can maintain or rescue the D3 receptor agonist effect. *Adapted from, and used with permission: Dinkins, M. -L., Lallemand, P., & Clemens, S. (2017). Long-term treatment with dopamine D3 receptor agonists induces a behavioral switch that can be rescued by blocking the dopamine D1 receptor.* Sleep Medicine, 40, *47–52. https://doi.org/10.1016/j.sleep.2017.10.001.*

from D3R to D1R-mediated actions over time would point to a synergistic role of the D1 and D3 receptor system in RLS, and it could provide a new D1 receptor-based avenue to explore as a potential pharmacological target in RLS (Fig. 3).

6. Beyond dopamine D1 and D3 receptors

Dopamine receptors can form multiple versions of heterodimers and heterotetramers (Fuxe et al., 2015), and the aforementioned D1–D3 receptor model is just one of several possible scenarios that may explain the efficacy of D3 receptor-preferring agonists in treating the initial RLS symptoms and the augmentation that usually occurs after long-lasting treatment. Other configurations might occur that may lead to similar functional and behavioral outcomes as in the postulated D1–D3 heteromer model. First and foremost, there is no evidence to date that all five dopamine receptors are expressed in the human spinal cord. The rodent data suggest that all 5 DA receptor are expressed in the spinal cord (Zhu et al., 2007a), however a non-human primate study found no evidence of the D1R subtype, only a presence of D2R-D5R subtypes (Barraud et al., 2010). Thus, while the projections from the animal models indicate a likely role of DA that is also present in the human spinal cord, it is possible that, in man, DA receptor distribution may differ from those reported in rodents or the non-human primate. Immunohistochemical studies assessing receptor distributions in human spinal cord and comparing them to animal models are rare, but evidence indicates that in those studies human and animal data diverge slightly (Gillberg, d'Argy, & Aquilonius, 1988). If, as in the macaque, the human spinal cord does not express the D1 receptor, the D5 subtype might functionally take over its role and emerging receptor heterodimer could be of the D3–D5 type. This putative heteromer would be functional similar to the D1–D3 subtype, and, due to the higher affinity of the D5 over the D1 subtype to dopamine (cf. Fig. 1), may even have a stronger impact on inhibitory and excitatory homeostasis. Alternatively, but not mutually exclusive from the previous scenario, the D4 receptor subtype may also play a more prominent role than previously thought. Both D4 and D3 receptors have the highest affinities to dopamine, and the D4 subtype has begun to emerge as a potential new target in controlling dopamine-mediated inhibitory tone (Bonaventura et al., 2017), and selective D4 receptor agonists, by specifically targeting these terminals, may provide a new efficient treatment for RLS (Yepes et al., 2017).

7. Conclusion

Dopaminergic treatments targeting the D3 receptor subtype to reduce the symptoms of RLS show high initial clinical benefits but fail to maintain their efficacy over time.

Dopamine receptors show a high variability in their substrate affinity, and the higher-affinity D3 and D4 subtypes promote inhibitory effects, suggesting that an increase in inhibitory DA tone underlies the initial symptomatic relief in the clinical setting. Sensorimotor circuits in the spinal cord are the gateway for the sensory processing of the symptoms and critical for the associated leg movements that relieve the symptoms and the periodic limb movements that often develop during sleep. There is a high preponderance of the inhibitory D3 receptor in the sensory-processing areas of the spinal cord (dorsal horn), whereas the motor areas in the ventral horn more strongly express the excitatory D1 receptor subtype. D3 and D1 receptors can form functional heteromeric ensembles that influence each other. In the spinal cord, long-term treatment with D3 receptor agonists is associated with the upregulation of the D1 receptor subtype and block of D1 receptor function at this stage can restore the D3 receptor effect. These findings suggest that the D3 receptor agonist mediated sensory excitability and D3 receptor treatment triggered-augmentation may be ultimately the result of unmasked increased D1 receptor activities, and that D1-like receptors may be the underlying target in the treatment of RLS.

Conflict of interest statement

No conflict of interest to declare.

Acknowledgments

We would like to thank Walter Paulus for his input and suggestions into an earlier version of the ideas presented in this chapter.

References

Akpinar, S. (1982). Treatment of restless legs syndrome with levodopa plus benserazide. *Archives of Neurology*, *39*(11), 739.

Akpinar, S. (1987). Restless legs syndrome treatment with dopaminergic drugs. *Clinical Neuropharmacology*, *10*(1), 69–79.

Allen, R. P., & Earley, C. J. (1996). Augmentation of the restless legs syndrome with carbidopa/levodopa. *Sleep*, *19*(3), 205–213.

Allen, R. P., Picchietti, D. L., Garcia-Borreguero, D., Ondo, W. G., Walters, A. S., Winkelman, J. W., et al. (2014). Restless legs syndrome/Willis-Ekbom disease diagnostic criteria: Updated International Restless Legs Syndrome Study Group (IRLSSG) consensus criteria–history, rationale, description, and significance. *Sleep Medicine*, *15*(8), 860–873. https://doi.org/10.1016/j.sleep.2014.03.025.

Allen, R. P., Walters, A. S., Montplaisir, J., Hening, W., Myers, A., Bell, T. J., et al. (2005). Restless legs syndrome prevalence and impact: REST general population study. *Archives of Internal Medicine*, *165*(11), 1286–1292. https://doi.org/10.1001/archinte.165.11.1286.

Ashkenazi, R., Ben-Shachar, D., & Youdim, M. B. (1982). Nutritional iron and dopamine binding sites in the rat brain. *Pharmacology, Biochemistry, and Behavior*, *17*(Suppl 1), 43–47.

Barraud, Q., Obeid, I., Aubert, I., Barriere, G., Contamin, H., McGuire, S., et al. (2010). Neuroanatomical study of the A11 diencephalospinal pathway in the non-human primate. *PLoS One*, *5*(10), e13306. doi:e13306 [pii]. https://doi.org/10.1371/journal.pone.0013306.

Barrett, R. J., & Lokhandwala, M. F. (1982). Presynaptic dopamine receptor stimulation and the antihypertensive action of pergolide in experimental neurogenic hypertension. *Proceedings of the Western Pharmacology Society*, *25*, 39–42.

Barriere, G., Mellen, N., & Cazalets, J. R. (2004). Neuromodulation of the locomotor network by dopamine in the isolated spinal cord of newborn rat. *The European Journal of Neuroscience*, *19*(5), 1325–1335.

Beaulieu, J. M., Espinoza, S., & Gainetdinov, R. R. (2015). Dopamine receptors–IUPHAR Review 13. *British Journal of Pharmacology*, *172*(1), 1–23. https://doi.org/10.1111/bph.12906.

Bernheimer, H., Birkmayer, W., Hornykiewicz, O., Jellinger, K., & Seitelberger, F. (1973). Brain dopamine and the syndromes of Parkinson and Huntington. Clinical, morphological and neurochemical correlations. *Journal of the Neurological Sciences*, *20*(4), 415–455.

Birkmayer, W., & Hornykiewicz, O. (1962). The L-dihydroxyphenylalanine (L-DOPA) effect in Parkinson's syndrome in man: On the pathogenesis and treatment of Parkinson akinesis. *Arch Psychiatr Nervenkr Z Gesamte Neurol Psychiatr*, *203*, 560–574.

Bjorklund, A., & Skagerberg, G. (1979). Evidence for a major spinal cord projection from the diencephalic A11 dopamine cell group in the rat using transmitter-specific fluorescent retrograde tracing. *Brain Research*, *177*(1), 170–175.

Bonaventura, J., Quiroz, C., Cai, N. S., Rubinstein, M., Tanda, G., & Ferre, S. (2017). Key role of the dopamine D4 receptor in the modulation of corticostriatal glutamatergic neurotransmission. *Science Advances*, *3*(1), e1601631. https://doi.org/10.1126/sciadv.1601631.

Brewer, K. L., Baran, C. A., Whitfield, B. R., Jensen, A. M., & Clemens, S. (2014). Dopamine D3 receptor dysfunction prevents anti-nociceptive effects of morphine in the spinal cord. *Frontiers in Neural Circuits*, *8*. https://doi.org/10.3389/fncir.2014.00062. 62-01–62-10.

Centonze, D., Grande, C., Usiello, A., Gubellini, P., Erbs, E., Martin, A. B., et al. (2003). Receptor subtypes involved in the presynaptic and postsynaptic actions of dopamine on striatal interneurons. *The Journal of Neuroscience*, *23*(15), 6245–6254. doi:23/15/6245 [pii].

Chakravarthy, S., Balasubramani, P. P., Mandali, A., Jahanshahi, M., & Moustafa, A. A. (2018). The many facets of dopamine: Toward an integrative theory of the role of dopamine in managing the body's energy resources. *Physiology & Behavior*, *195*, 128–141. https://doi.org/10.1016/j.physbeh.2018.06.032.

Chipkin, R. E. (2014). *Ecopipam treatment of Tourette's syndrome in subjects 7–17 years*. from ClinicalTrials.gov. https://clinicaltrials.gov/ct2/show/NCT02102698.

Chokroverty, S. (2014). Therapeutic dilemma for restless legs syndrome. *The New England Journal of Medicine*, *370*(7), 667–668. https://doi.org/10.1056/NEJMe1313155.

Clemens, S., Belin-Rauscent, A., Simmers, J., & Combes, D. (2012). Opposing modulatory effects of D1- and D2-like receptor activation on a spinal central pattern generator. *Journal of Neurophysiology*, *107*, 2250–2259. https://doi.org/10.1152/jn.00366.2011.

Clemens, S., & Hochman, S. (2004). Conversion of the modulatory actions of dopamine on spinal reflexes from depression to facilitation in D3 receptor knock-out mice. *The Journal of Neuroscience*, *24*(50), 11337–11345. doi:24/50/11337 [pii]. https://doi.org/10.1523/JNEUROSCI.3698-04.2004.

Clemens, S., Rye, D., & Hochman, S. (2006). Restless legs syndrome: Revisiting the dopamine hypothesis from the spinal cord perspective. *Neurology*, *67*(1), 125–130. doi:67/1/125 [pii]. https://doi.org/10.1212/01.wnl.0000223316.53428.c9.

Connor, J. R., Wang, X. S., Allen, R. P., Beard, J. L., Wiesinger, J. A., Felt, B. T., et al. (2009). Altered dopaminergic profile in the putamen and substantia nigra in restless leg syndrome. *Brain*, *132*(Sep), 2403–2412.

Cruz-Trujillo, R., Avalos-Fuentes, A., Rangel-Barajas, C., Paz-Bermudez, F., Sierra, A., Escartin-Perez, E., et al. (2013). D3 dopamine receptors interact with dopamine D1 but not D4 receptors in the GABAergic terminals of the SNr of the rat. *Neuropharmacology*, *67*, 370–378. https://doi.org/10.1016/j.neuropharm.2012.11.032.

Didriksen, M., Rigas, A. S., Allen, R. P., Burchell, B. J., Di Angelantonio, E., Nielsen, M. H., et al. (2017). Prevalence of restless legs syndrome and associated factors in an otherwise healthy population: Results from the Danish Blood Donor Study. *Sleep Medicine*, *36*, 55–61. https://doi.org/10.1016/j.sleep.2017.04.014.

Dinkins, M.-L., Lallemand, P., & Clemens, S. (2017). Long-term treatment with dopamine D3 receptor agonists induces a behavioral switch that can be rescued by blocking the dopamine D1 receptor. *Sleep Medicine*, *40*, 47–52. https://doi.org/10.1016/j.sleep.2017.10.001.

Dowling, P., Klinker, F., Stadelmann, C., Hasan, K., Paulus, W., & Liebetanz, D. (2011). Dopamine D3 receptor specifically modulates motor and sensory symptoms in iron-deficient mice. *The Journal of Neuroscience*, *31*(1), 70–77. https://doi.org/10.1523/JNEUROSCI.0959-10.2011.

Dreyer, J. K., Herrik, K. F., Berg, R. W., & Hounsgaard, J. D. (2010). Influence of phasic and tonic dopamine release on receptor activation. *The Journal of Neuroscience, 30*(42), 14273–14283. https://doi.org/10.1523/JNEUROSCI.1894-10.2010.

Earley, C. J., Allen, R. P., & Hening, W. (2011). Restless legs syndrome and periodic leg movements in sleep. *Handbook of Clinical Neurology, 99*, 913–948. B978-0-444-52007-4.00015-1 [pii]. https://doi.org/10.1016/B978-0-444-52007-4.00015-1.

Earley, C. J., Connor, J., Garcia-Borreguero, D., Jenner, P., Winkelman, J., Zee, P. C., et al. (2014). Altered brain iron homeostasis and dopaminergic function in restless legs syndrome (Willis–Ekbom Disease). *Sleep Medicine, 15*(11), 1288–1301. https://doi.org/10.1016/j.sleep.2014.05.009.

Earley, C. J., Kuwabara, H., Wong, D. F., Gamaldo, C., Salas, R. E., Brasic, J. R., et al. (2013). Increased synaptic dopamine in the putamen in restless legs syndrome. *Sleep, 36*(1), 51–57. https://doi.org/10.5665/sleep.2300.

Earley, C. J., & Silber, M. H. (2010). Restless legs syndrome: Understanding its consequences and the need for better treatment. *Sleep Medicine, 11*(9), 807–815. https://doi.org/10.1016/j.sleep.2010.07.007.

Earley, C. J., Uhl, G. R., Clemens, S., & Ferre, S. (2017). Connectome and molecular pharmacological differences in the dopaminergic system in restless legs syndrome (RLS): Plastic changes and neuroadaptations that may contribute to augmentation. *Sleep Medicine, 31*, 71–77. https://doi.org/10.1016/j.sleep.2016.06.003.

Ekbom, K. A. (1945). Restless legs syndrome. *Acta Medica Scandinavica, 158*, 4–122. (Suppl).

Ekbom, K. A. (1960). Restless legs syndrome. *Neurology, 10*, 868–873.

Erikson, K. M., Jones, B. C., & Beard, J. L. (2000). Iron deficiency alters dopamine transporter functioning in rat striatum. *The Journal of Nutrition, 130*(11), 2831–2837. https://doi.org/10.1093/jn/130.11.2831.

Erikson, K. M., Jones, B. C., Hess, E. J., Zhang, Q., & Beard, J. L. (2001). Iron deficiency decreases dopamine D1 and D2 receptors in rat brain. *Pharmacology, Biochemistry, and Behavior, 69*(3-4), 409–418.

Ferini-Strambi, L., Carli, G., Casoni, F., & Galbiati, A. (2018). Restless legs syndrome and Parkinson disease: A causal relationship between the two disorders? *Frontiers in Neurology. 9, 551*. https://doi.org/10.3389/fneur.2018.00551.

Ferre, S. (2015). The GPCR heterotetramer: Challenging classical pharmacology. *Trends in Pharmacological Sciences, 36*(3), 145–152. https://doi.org/10.1016/j.tips.2015.01.002.

Ferre, S., Agnati, L. F., Ciruela, F., Lluis, C., Woods, A. S., Fuxe, K., et al. (2007). Neurotransmitter receptor heteromers and their integrative role in 'local modules': The striatal spine module. *Brain Research Reviews, 55*(1), 55–67. https://doi.org/10.1016/j.brainresrev.2007.01.007.

Ferri, R., Rundo, F., Zucconi, M., Manconi, M., Bruni, O., Ferini-Strambi, L., et al. (2015). An evidence-based analysis of the association between periodic leg movements during sleep and arousals in restless legs syndrome. *Sleep, 38*(6), 919–924. https://doi.org/10.5665/sleep.4740.

Fiorentini, C., Busi, C., Gorruso, E., Gotti, C., Spano, P., & Missale, C. (2008). Reciprocal regulation of dopamine D1 and D3 receptor function and trafficking by heterodimerization. *Molecular Pharmacology, 74*(1), 59–69. doi:mol.107.043885 [pii]. https://doi.org/10.1124/mol.107.043885.

Fiorentini, C., Busi, C., Spano, P., & Missale, C. (2010). Dimerization of dopamine D1 and D3 receptors in the regulation of striatal function. *Current Opinion in Pharmacology, 10*(1), 87–92. https://doi.org/10.1016/j.coph.2009.09.008.

Franco, R., Ferre, S., Agnati, L., Torvinen, M., Gines, S., Hillion, J., et al. (2000). Evidence for adenosine/dopamine receptor interactions: Indications for heteromerization. *Neuropsychopharmacology, 23*(4 Suppl), S50–S59. https://doi.org/10.1016/S0893-133X(00)00144-5.

Fuxe, K., Ferre, S., Genedani, S., Franco, R., & Agnati, L. F. (2007). Adenosine receptor-dopamine receptor interactions in the basal ganglia and their relevance for brain function. *Physiology & Behavior*, *92*(1-2), 210–217. https://doi.org/10.1016/j.physbeh.2007.05.034.
Fuxe, K., Guidolin, D., Agnati, L. F., & Borroto-Escuela, D. O. (2015). Dopamine heteroreceptor complexes as therapeutic targets in Parkinson's disease. *Expert Opinion on Therapeutic Targets*, *19*(3), 377–398. https://doi.org/10.1517/14728222.2014.981529.
Gajendiran, M., Seth, P., & Ganguly, D. K. (1996). Involvement of the presynaptic dopamine D2 receptor in the depression of spinal reflex by apomorphine. *Neuroreport*, 7(2), 513–516.
Garcia-Borreguero, D., Kohnen, R., Silber, M. H., Winkelman, J. W., Earley, C. J., Högl, B., et al. (2013). The long-term treatment of restless legs syndrome/Willis–Ekbom disease: Evidence-based guidelines and clinical consensus best practice guidance: A report from the International Restless Legs Syndrome Study Group. *Sleep Medicine*, *14*(7), 675–684. https://doi.org/10.1016/j.sleep.2013.05.016.
Gilbert, D. L., Budman, C. L., Singer, H. S., Kurlan, R., & Chipkin, R. E. (2014). A D1 receptor antagonist, ecopipam, for treatment of tics in Tourette syndrome. *Clinical Neuropharmacology*, *37*(1), 26–30. https://doi.org/10.1097/WNF.0000000000000017.
Gillberg, P. G., d'Argy, R., & Aquilonius, S. M. (1988). Autoradiographic distribution of [3H]acetylcholine binding sites in the cervical spinal cord of man and some other species. *Neuroscience Letters*, *90*(1-2), 197–202.
Guitart, X., Navarro, G., Moreno, E., Yano, H., Cai, N. S., Sanchez-Soto, M., et al. (2014). Functional selectivity of allosteric interactions within G protein-coupled receptor oligomers: The dopamine D1–D3 receptor heterotetramer. *Molecular Pharmacology*, *86*(4), 417–429. https://doi.org/10.1124/mol.114.093096.
Han, P., & Whelan, P. J. (2009). Modulation of AMPA currents by D(1)-like but not D(2)-like receptors in spinal motoneurons. *Neuroscience*, *158*(4), 1699–1707.
Hening, W. A., Allen, R. P., Earley, C. J., Picchietti, D. L., & Silber, M. H. (2004). An update on the dopaminergic treatment of restless legs syndrome and periodic limb movement disorder. *Sleep*, *27*(3), 560–583.
Holstege, J. C., Dijken, H. v., Buijs, R. M., Goedkengt, H., Gosens, T., & Bongers, C. M. (1996). Distribution of dopamine immunoreactivity in the rat, cat, and monkey spinal cord. *The Journal of Comparative Neurology*, *376*, 631–652.
Huang, Q., Zhou, D., Chase, K., Gusella, J. F., Aronin, N., & DiFiglia, M. (1992). Immunohistochemical localization of the D1 dopamine receptor in rat brain reveals its axonal transport, pre- and postsynaptic localization, and prevalence in the basal ganglia, limbic system, and thalamic reticular nucleus. *Proceedings of the National Academy of Sciences of the United States of America*, *89*(24), 11988–11992.
Hyacinthe, C., De Deurwaerdere, P., Thiollier, T., Li, Q., Bezard, E., & Ghorayeb, I. (2015). Blood withdrawal affects iron store dynamics in primates with consequences on monoaminergic system function. *Neuroscience*, *290*, 621–635. https://doi.org/10.1016/j.neuroscience.2015.01.057.
Jackisch, R., Hotz, H., Allgaier, C., & Hertting, G. (1994). Presynaptic opioid receptors on dopaminergic nerves in the rabbit caudate nucleus: Coupling to pertussis toxin-sensitive G-proteins and interaction with D2 autoreceptors? *Naunyn-Schmiedeberg's Archives of Pharmacology*, *349*(3), 250–258.
Keeler, B. E., Baran, C. A., Brewer, K. L., & Clemens, S. (2012). Increased excitability of spinal pain reflexes and altered frequency-dependent modulation in the dopamine D3-receptor knockout mouse. *Experimental Neurology*, *238*(2), 273–283.
Keeler, B. E., Patel, M. M., Lallemand, P., de Castro Brás, L. E., & Clemens, S. (2016). Opposing aging-related shift of excitatory dopamine D1and inhibitory D3 receptor protein expression in striatum and spinal cord. *Journal of Neurophysiology*, *115*(1), 363–369. https://doi.org/10.1152/jn.00390.2015.

Khan, F. H., Ahlberg, C. D., Chow, C. A., Shah, D. R., & Koo, B. B. (2017). Iron, dopamine, genetics, and hormones in the pathophysiology of restless legs syndrome. *Journal of Neurology, 264*(8), 1634–1641. https://doi.org/10.1007/s00415-017-8431-1.

Kishore, S., & McLean, D. L. (2015). Neuromodulation: Letting sources of spinal dopamine speak for themselves. *Current Biology, 25*(4), R146–R148. https://doi.org/10.1016/j.cub.2015.01.001.

Kondo, M., Fujiwara, H., & Tanaka, C. (1986). Dopamine release and presynaptic dopaminergic regulation in guinea pig spinal cord. *Japanese Journal of Pharmacology, 41*(1), 39–46.

Langebner, T., & Lampl, C. (2018). Two early descriptions of restless legs syndrome by J. Astruc (1736) and M.A. Weikard (1796). *Neurology, 91*(17), 786–789. https://doi.org/10.1212/WNL.0000000000006393.

Levant, B., & McCarson, K. E. (2001). D(3) dopamine receptors in rat spinal cord: Implications for sensory and motor function. *Neuroscience Letters, 303*(1), 9–12.

Lindgren, N., Usiello, A., Goiny, M., Haycock, J., Erbs, E., Greengard, P., et al. (2003). Distinct roles of dopamine D2L and D2S receptor isoforms in the regulation of protein phosphorylation at presynaptic and postsynaptic sites. *Proceedings of the National Academy of Sciences of the United States of America, 100*(7), 4305–4309. https://doi.org/10.1073/pnas.0730708100. 0730708100 [pii].

Manconi, M., Ferri, R., Zucconi, M., Clemens, S., Giarolli, L., Bottasini, V., et al. (2011). Preferential D2 or preferential D3 dopamine agonists in restless legs syndrome. *Neurology, 77*(2), 110–117. https://doi.org/10.1212/WNL.0b013e3182242d91.

Manconi, M., Ferri, R., Zucconi, M., Oldani, A., Fantini, M. L., Castronovo, V., et al. (2007). First night efficacy of pramipexole in restless legs syndrome and periodic leg movements. *Sleep Medicine, 8*(5), 491–497. https://doi.org/10.1016/j.sleep.2006.10.008.

Marcellino, D., Ferre, S., Casado, V., Cortes, A., Le Foll, B., Mazzola, C., et al. (2008). Identification of dopamine D1–D3 receptor heteromers. Indications for a role of synergistic D1–D3 receptor interactions in the striatum. *The Journal of Biological Chemistry, 283*(38), 26016–26025. https://doi.org/10.1074/jbc.M710349200.

Missale, C., Nash, S. R., Robinson, S. W., Jaber, M., & Caron, M. G. (1998). Dopamine receptors: From structure to function. *Physiological Reviews, 78*(1), 189–225.

Montplaisir, J., Godbout, R., Poirier, G., & Bedard, M. A. (1986). Restless legs syndrome and periodic movements in sleep: Physiopathology and treatment with L-dopa. *Clinical Neuropharmacology, 9*(5), 456–463.

Montplaisir, J., Lorrain, D., & Godbout, R. (1991). Restless legs syndrome and periodic leg movements in sleep: The primary role of dopaminergic mechanism. *European Neurology, 31*(1), 41–43.

Moreno, E., Hoffmann, H., Gonzalez-Sepulveda, M., Navarro, G., Casado, V., Cortes, A., et al. (2011). Dopamine D1-histamine H3 receptor heteromers provide a selective link to MAPK signaling in GABAergic neurons of the direct striatal pathway. *The Journal of Biological Chemistry, 286*(7), 5846–5854. https://doi.org/10.1074/jbc.M110.161489.

Mrowka, M., Chaudhuri, K. R., & Odin, P. (2004). Pathophysiology of restless legs syndrome. In K. R. Chaudhuri, P. Odin, & C. W. Olanow (Eds.), *Restless legs syndrome* (pp. 37–48). Taylor & Francis.

Murray, T. J. (1967). The restless leg syndrome. *Canadian Medical Association Journal, 96*(24), 1571–1574.

Navarro, M., Fernandez-Ruiz, J. J., Rodriguez de Fonseca, F., Hernandez, M. L., Cebeira, M., & Ramos, J. A. (1992). Modifications of striatal D2 dopaminergic postsynaptic sensitivity during development of morphine tolerance-dependence in mice. *Pharmacology, Biochemistry, and Behavior, 43*(2), 603–608.

Olianas, M. C., Dedoni, S., & Onali, P. (2012). Potentiation of dopamine D1-like receptor signaling by concomitant activation of delta- and mu-opioid receptors in mouse medial prefrontal cortex. *Neurochemistry International, 61*(8), 1404–1416. https://doi.org/10.1016/j.neuint.2012.10.005.

Ondo, W. G., He, Y., Rajasekaran, S., & Le, W. D. (2000). Clinical correlates of 6-hydroxydopamine injections into A11 dopaminergic neurons in rats: A possible model for restless legs syndrome. *Movement Disorders*, *15*(1), 154–158.

Ondo, W. G., Vuong, K. D., & Jankovic, J. (2002). Exploring the relationship between Parkinson disease and restless legs syndrome. *Archives of Neurology*, *59*(3), 421–424.

Owens, J. (2016). *Restless legs syndrome: The most important sleep disorder you've never heard of [Press release]*. Retrieved from https://notes.childrenshospital.org/restless-legs-syndrome-the-most-important-sleep-disorder-youve-never-heard-of/.

Pearlstein, R., Vaz, R., & Rampe, D. (2003). Understanding the structure-activity relationship of the human ether-a-go-go-related gene cardiac K+ channel. A model for bad behavior. *Journal of Medicinal Chemistry*, *46*(11), 2017–2022. https://doi.org/10.1021/jm0205651.

Phillips, B., Hening, W., Britz, P., & Mannino, D. (2006). Prevalence and correlates of restless legs syndrome: Results from the 2005 National Sleep Foundation Poll. *Chest*, *129*(1), 76–80. doi:129/1/76 [pii]. https://doi.org/10.1378/chest.129.1.76.

Piao, Y. S., Lian, T. H., Hu, Y., Zuo, L. J., Guo, P., Yu, S. Y., et al. (2017). Restless legs syndrome in Parkinson disease: Clinical characteristics, abnormal iron metabolism and altered neurotransmitters. *Scientific Reports*, 7(1), 10547. https://doi.org/10.1038/s41598-017-10593-7.

Price, K. S., Farley, I. J., & Hornykiewicz, O. (1978). Neurochemistry of Parkinson's disease: Relation between striatal and limbic dopamine. *Advances in Biochemical Psychopharmacology*, *19*, 293–300.

Pringsheim, T., Fiest, K., & Jette, N. (2014). The international incidence and prevalence of neurologic conditions: How common are they? *Neurology*, *83*(18), 1661–1664. https://doi.org/10.1212/WNL.0000000000000929.

Qu, S., Le, W., Zhang, X., Xie, W., Zhang, A., & Ondo, W. G. (2007). Locomotion is increased in a11-lesioned mice with iron deprivation: A possible animal model for restless legs syndrome. *Journal of Neuropathology and Experimental Neurology*, *66*(5), 383–388. https://doi.org/10.1097/nen.0b013e3180517b5f.

Quiroz, C., Gulyani, S., Ruiqian, W., Bonaventura, J., Cutler, R., Pearson, V., et al. (2016). Adenosine receptors as markers of brain iron deficiency: Implications for restless legs syndrome. *Neuropharmacology*, *111*, 160–168. https://doi.org/10.1016/j.neuropharm.2016.09.002.

Rashid, A. J., So, C. H., Kong, M. M., Furtak, T., El-Ghundi, M., Cheng, R., et al. (2007). D1–D2 dopamine receptor heterooligomers with unique pharmacology are coupled to rapid activation of Gq/11 in the striatum. *Proceedings of the National Academy of Sciences of the United States of America*, *104*(2), 654–659.

Schormair, B., Plag, J., Kaffe, M., Gross, N., Czamara, D., Samtleben, W., et al. (2011). MEIS1 and BTBD9: Genetic association with restless leg syndrome in end stage renal disease. *Journal of Medical Genetics*, *48*(7), 462–466. https://doi.org/10.1136/jmg.2010.087858.

Schormair, B., Zhao, C., Bell, S., Tilch, E., Salminen, A. V., Putz, B., et al. (2017). Identification of novel risk loci for restless legs syndrome in genome-wide association studies in individuals of European ancestry: A meta-analysis. *Lancet Neurology*, *16*(11), 898–907. https://doi.org/10.1016/S1474-4422(17)30327-7.

Sharples, S. A., Humphreys, J. M., Jensen, A. M., Dhoopar, S., Delaloye, N., Clemens, S., et al. (2015). Dopaminergic modulation of locomotor network activity in the neonatal mouse spinal cord. *Journal of Neurophysiology*, *113*(7), 2500–2510. https://doi.org/10.1152/jn.00849.2014.

Shin, R. M., Masuda, M., Miura, M., Sano, H., Shirasawa, T., Song, W. J., et al. (2003). Dopamine D4 receptor-induced postsynaptic inhibition of GABAergic currents in mouse globus pallidus neurons. *The Journal of Neuroscience*, *23*(37), 11662–11672.

Silvestre, J. S., & Prous, J. (2005). Research on adverse drug events. I. Muscarinic M-3 receptor binding affinity could predict the risk of antipsychotics to induce type 2 diabetes. *Methods and Findings in Experimental and Clinical Pharmacology, 27*(5), 289–304.

Skagerberg, G., Bjorklund, A., Lindvall, O., & Schmidt, R. H. (1982). Origin and termination of the diencephalo-spinal dopamine system in the rat. *Brain Research Bulletin, 9*(1-6), 237–244.

Stefansson, H., Rye, D. B., Hicks, A., Petursson, H., Ingason, A., Thorgeirsson, T. E., et al. (2007). A genetic risk factor for periodic limb movements in sleep. *The New England Journal of Medicine, 357*(7), 639–647. https://doi.org/10.1056/NEJMoa072743.

Swant, J., Stramiello, M., & Wagner, J. J. (2008). Postsynaptic dopamine D3 receptor modulation of evoked IPSCs via GABA(A) receptor endocytosis in rat hippocampus. *Hippocampus, 18*(5), 492–502. https://doi.org/10.1002/hipo.20408.

Tamae, A., Nakatsuka, T., Koga, K., Kato, G., Furue, H., Katafuchi, T., et al. (2005). Direct inhibition of substantia gelatinosa neurones in the spinal cord by activation of dopamine D2-like receptors. *The Journal of Physiology, 568*(Pt 1), 243–253.

Thirumalai, V., & Cline, H. T. (2008). Endogenous dopamine suppresses initiation of swimming in prefeeding zebrafish larvae. *Journal of Neurophysiology, 100*(3), 1635–1648. doi:90568.2008 [pii]. https://doi.org/10.1152/jn.90568.2008.

Trenkwalder, C., Allen, R., Hogl, B., Clemens, S., Patton, S., Schormair, B., et al. (2018). Comorbidities, treatment, and pathophysiology in restless legs syndrome. *Lancet Neurology, 17*(11), 994–1005. https://doi.org/10.1016/S1474-4422(18)30311-9.

Trenkwalder, C., Canelo, M., Lang, M., Schroeder, H., Kelling, D., Berkels, R., et al. (2017). Management of augmentation of restless legs syndrome with rotigotine: A 1-year observational study. *Sleep Medicine, 30*, 257–265. https://doi.org/10.1016/j.sleep.2015.10.006.

Trotti, L. M., Bhadriraju, S., & Rye, D. B. (2008). An update on the pathophysiology and genetics of restless legs syndrome. *Current Neurology and Neuroscience Reports, 8*(4), 281–287.

Verma, V., Hasbi, A., O'Dowd, B. F., & George, S. R. (2010). Dopamine D1–D2 receptor heteromer-mediated calcium release is desensitized by D1 receptor occupancy with or without signal activation: Dual functional regulation by G protein-coupled receptor kinase 2. *The Journal of Biological Chemistry, 285*(45), 35092–35103. https://doi.org/10.1074/jbc.M109.088625.

Walters, A. S., LeBrocq, C., Passi, V., Patel, S., Hanna, P. A., Cohen, B., et al. (2003). A preliminary look at the percentage of patients with Restless Legs Syndrome who also have Parkinson Disease, Essential Tremor or Tourette Syndrome in a single practice. *Journal of Sleep Research, 12*(4), 343–345.

Waters, N., Svensson, K., Haadsma-Svensson, S. R., Smith, M. W., & Carlsson, A. (1993). The dopamine D3-receptor: A postsynaptic receptor inhibitory on rat locomotor activity. *Journal of Neural Transmission. General Section, 94*(1), 11–19.

Williams, A. M., & Garcia-Borreguero, D. (2009). Management of restless legs syndrome augmentation. *Current Treatment Options in Neurology, 11*(5), 327–332.

Willis, T. (1685). Of the diseases of the brain and the genus nervosum. In *The London Practice of Physick*. London: Bassett and Crooke.

Winkelman, J. W., & Johnston, L. (2004). Augmentation and tolerance with long-term pramipexole treatment of restless legs syndrome (RLS). *Sleep Medicine, 5*(1), 9–14.

Winkelman, J. W., Redline, S., Baldwin, C. M., Resnick, H. E., Newman, A. B., & Gottlieb, D. J. (2009). Polysomnographic and health-related quality of life correlates of restless legs syndrome in the Sleep Heart Health Study. *Sleep, 32*(6), 772–778.

Winkelmann, J., & Ferini-Strambi, L. (2006). Genetics of restless legs syndrome. *Sleep Medicine Reviews, 10*(3), 179–183. https://doi.org/10.1016/j.smrv.2006.01.003.

Winkelmann, J., Schormair, B., Lichtner, P., Ripke, S., Xiong, L., Jalilzadeh, S., et al. (2007). Genome-wide association study of restless legs syndrome identifies common variants in three genomic regions. *Nature Genetics, 39*(8), 1000–1006.

Winkelmann, J., Schormair, B., Xiong, L., Dion, P. A., Rye, D. B., & Rouleau, G. A. (2017). Genetics of restless legs syndrome. *Sleep Medicine*, *31*, 18–22. https://doi.org/10.1016/j.sleep.2016.10.012.

Wu, J., Dougherty, J. J., & Nichols, R. A. (2006). Dopamine receptor regulation of Ca2+ levels in individual isolated nerve terminals from rat striatum: Comparison of presynaptic D1-like and D2-like receptors. *Journal of Neurochemistry*, *98*(2), 481–494. doi:JNC3901 [pii]. https://doi.org/10.1111/j.1471-4159.2006.03901.x.

Yang, H. W., Zhou, L. J., Hu, N. W., Xin, W. J., & Liu, X. G. (2005). Activation of spinal d1/d5 receptors induces late-phase LTP of C-fiber-evoked field potentials in rat spinal dorsal horn. *Journal of Neurophysiology*, *94*(2), 961–967. https://doi.org/10.1152/jn.01324.2004.

Yang, S. N. (2000). Sustained enhancement of AMPA receptor- and NMDA receptor-mediated currents induced by dopamine D1/D5 receptor activation in the hippocampus: An essential role of postsynaptic Ca2+. *Hippocampus*, *10*(1), 57–63. https://doi.org/10.1002/(SICI)1098-1063(2000)10:1<57::AID-HIPO6>3.0.CO;2-0.

Yepes, G., Guitart, X., Rea, W., Newman, A. H., Allen, R. P., Earley, C. J., et al. (2017). Targeting hypersensitive corticostriatal terminals in restless legs syndrome. *Annals of Neurology*, *82*(6), 951–960. https://doi.org/10.1002/ana.25104.

Zeng, C., Wang, D., Yang, Z., Wang, Z., Asico, L. D., Wilcox, C. S., et al. (2004). Dopamine D1 receptor augmentation of D3 receptor action in rat aortic or mesenteric vascular smooth muscles. *Hypertension*, *43*(3), 673–679.

Zhao, H., Zhu, W., Pan, T., Xie, W., Zhang, A., Ondo, W. G., et al. (2007). Spinal cord dopamine receptor expression and function in mice with 6-OHDA lesion of the A11 nucleus and dietary iron deprivation. *Journal of Neuroscience Research*, *85*(5), 1065–1076. https://doi.org/10.1002/jnr.21207.

Zhu, H., Clemens, S., Sawchuk, M., & Hochman, S. (2007a). Expression and distribution of all dopamine receptor subtypes (D1–D5) in the mouse lumbar spinal cord: A real-time polymerase chain reaction and non-autoradiographic in situ hybridization study. *Neuroscience*, *149*, 885–897.

Zhu, H., Clemens, S., Sawchuk, M., & Hochman, S. (2007b). Expression and distribution of all dopamine receptor subtypes (D(1)-D(5)) in the mouse lumbar spinal cord: A real-time polymerase chain reaction and non-autoradiographic in situ hybridization study. *Neuroscience*, *149*(4), 885–897.

Zhu, H., Clemens, S., Sawchuk, M., & Hochman, S. (2008). Unaltered D1, D2, D4, and D5 dopamine receptor mRNA expression and distribution in the spinal cord of the D3 receptor knockout mouse. *Journal of Comparative Physiology. A, Neuroethology, Sensory, Neural, and Behavioral Physiology*, *194*(11), 957–962.

Zucconi, M., Ferri, R., Allen, R., Baier, P. C., Bruni, O., Chokroverty, S., et al. (2006). The official World Association of Sleep Medicine (WASM) standards for recording and scoring periodic leg movements in sleep (PLMS) and wakefulness (PLMW) developed in collaboration with a task force from the International Restless Legs Syndrome Study Group (IRLSSG). *Sleep Medicine*, 7(2), 175–183. https://doi.org/10.1016/j.sleep.2006.01.001.

CHAPTER FIVE

The neurophysiology of hyperarousal in restless legs syndrome: Hints for a role of glutamate/GABA

Giuseppe Lanza*, Raffale Ferri
Oasi Research Institute—IRCCS, Troina, Italy
*Corresponding author: e-mail address: glanza@oasi.en.it

Contents

Abstract

Restless legs syndrome (RLS) is a common sensory-motor circadian disorder, whose basic components include urge to move the legs, unpleasant sensory experience, and periodic leg movements during sleep, all associated with an enhancement of the individual's arousal state. Brain iron deficiency (BID) is considered to be a key initial pathobiological factor, based on alterations of iron acquisition by the brain, also moderated by genetic factors. In addition to the well-known dopaminergic involvement in RLS, previous studies pointed out that BID brings also a hyperglutamatergic state that influences a dysfunctional cortico-striatal-thalamic-cortical circuit in genetically vulnerable individuals. However, the enhancement of arousal mechanisms in RLS may also be explained by functional changes of the ascending arousal systems and by deficitary GABA-mediated inhibitory control. Very recently, it was also suggested that BID induces a hypoadenosinergic state in RLS, thus possibly providing a link for a putative unified pathophysiological mechanism accounting for both hyperarousal and sensory-motor

Advances in Pharmacology, Volume 84
ISSN 1054-3589
https://doi.org/10.1016/bs.apha.2018.12.002
© 2019 Elsevier Inc.
All rights reserved.

signs. Consequently, RLS might be viewed as a multitransmitter neurochemical disorder, globally resulting in enhanced excitability and decreased inhibition. In this framework, understanding the complex interaction of different neuronal circuits in generating the symptoms of RLS is mandatory both for a better diagnostic refinement and for an innovative therapeutic support. Notably, multiple neurotransmission dysfunction, either primary or triggered by BID, may also bridge the gap between RLS and other chronic pain disorders. This chapter summarizes the current experimental and clinical findings into a heuristic model of the electrophysiology and neurochemistry underlying RLS.

Abbreviations

ACC anterior cingulate cortex
BID brain iron deficiency
CSP cortical silent period
DA dopamine
DOPA L-3,4-dihydroxyphenylalanine
GABA γ-aminobutyric acid
GLU glutamate
LTD long-term depression
M1 primary motor cortex
MRS magnetic resonance spectroscopy
NAA *N*-acetyl-aspartate
NMDA *N*-methyl-D-aspartate
PLMS periodic leg movements during sleep
rTMS repetitive transcranial magnetic stimulation
S1 primary somatosensory cortex
tDCS transcranial direct current stimulation
TMS transcranial magnetic stimulation
tsDCS transcutaneous spinal direct current stimulation

1. Introduction

Restless legs syndrome (RLS) defines a rest-induced, mainly nocturnal, sensory-prompted urge to move the legs during sleep. RLS can be conceptualized as an enhanced biological "drive" whose primary purpose is to keep the individual alert, active, and moving. Approximately 88% of individuals with RLS have an objective motor sign of repetitive periodic leg movements during sleep (PLMS) (Ferré, García-Borreguero, Allen, & Earley, 2018). Moderate-to-severe RLS also presents with an enhanced arousal state (Ferri, Rundo, et al., 2015). This "hyperarousal" likely reflects specific changes in neural mechanisms that govern both the sensory-motor system and the sleep-wake pattern (Trenkwalder & Paulus, 2010).

In RLS, changes in iron homeostasis might play a major role, at least in a number of cases, and seem also to influence the activity of the dopamine (DA) system, as well as that of glutamate (GLU), γ-aminobutyric acid (GABA), adenosine, opioids, and other neurotransmitters. Moreover, the possibility that DAergic dysfunction itself is associated with alterations of iron metabolism within the brain is also reasonable. In addition, experimental evidence in iron-depleted animals shows that disruption in brain iron homeostasis produces an impairment of DA transmission within multiple brain areas (Ferré, García-Borreguero, et al., 2018). Lastly, low ferritin serum concentration is a risk factor for the so-called augmentation, defined as a worsening of symptoms under DAergic therapy (Hyacinthe et al., 2015; Unger, Bianco, Jones, Allen, & Earley, 2014). Overall, these abnormalities may lead to a dysfunctional cortico-striatal-thalamic-cortical circuit and to a defective brain iron homeostasis. However, although the genetic contribution seems to be relevant, at least in some RLS patients, simply an involvement of the above mentioned network only fails to explain the hyperarousal state.

Currently, the pathophysiology of RLS can be seen as a continuous spectrum, with a major genetic contribution at one end and a major environmental or comorbid disease contribution at the other (Trenkwalder, Allen, Högl, Paulus, & Winkelmann, 2016). Although the link to DA is widely documented by a number of genetic studies, DAergic pathways play also a pivotal role in daily clinical practice, given that RLS symptoms typically improve under low-dose DAergic therapy and worsen under neuroleptic/anti-DAergic drugs. Nonetheless, until now, the anatomical locus where the RLS-involved DAergic dysfunction is located has not been identified. The L-3,4-dihydroxyphenylalanine(DOPA)ergic and the A11 diencephalic system dysfunction have been assumed in animal models, considering this area as the major DAergic innervation source for the spinal cord (Barraud et al., 2010; Ondo, Zhao, & Le, 2007). Nevertheless, to date, no neuropathologic alteration in humans A11 region has been demonstrated by the autopsy study (Earley, Allen, Connor, Ferrucci, & Troncoso, 2009).

It is intriguing how current evidences recommend a more widespread involvement in RLS symptomatology and pathophysiology, impacting not only sleep and its circadian pattern, but also mood/affect regulation (Lee et al., 2014), personality traits (Antelmi et al., 2014), cortical-spinal excitability (Allen, 2015), and thalamo-cortical connectivity (Ku et al., 2014). Hence, the application of neuroimaging and electrophysiological methods in RLS has recently enabled to further explore the underlying pathomechanisms, to analyze various neurochemical circuits and, possibly, to enlarge the therapeutic arsenal on a more rational basis and evidence-based findings.

2. RLS as an enhanced cortico-spinal excitability disorder

RLS patients, especially those with moderate-to-severe symptoms, usually experience a considerably lower threshold of their flexor reflexes during sleep, which are qualitatively similar to RLS-related PLMS (Bara-Jimenez, Aksu, Graham, Sato, & Hallett, 2000). This can be supposed to be the electrophysiological correlate of hyperexcitability of the spinal cord, which is likely to be involved in PLMS generation as well (Ferré, García-Borreguero, et al., 2018). However, it has been reported that patients with totally absent voluntary activity in their legs after a severe injury of the spinal cord experience leg movements with similar periodicity, duration, and qualitative pattern of PMLS (Ferri, Proserpio, et al., 2015). Therefore, these leg movements cannot be related to cortical arousal episodes, being also circadian-independent.

The spinal component of RLS hyperexcitability most probably depends on altered supraspinal-mediated mechanisms, due to either a hyperfunctioning of an excitatory mechanism or a hypofunctioning of the inhibitory control. Both situations seem to be the case, since cortical hyperexcitability and disinhibition in RLS have been well documented by several transcranial magnetic stimulation (TMS) studies (Lanza, Cantone, et al., 2015; Lanza, Lanuzza, et al., 2015; Magalhães et al., 2015). The distinctive alterations in some of TMS parameters, namely, a decrease in cortical silent period (CSP) and short-latency intracortical inhibition, favored abnormalities in sensory-motor integration within the cortico-striatal-thalamic-cortical circuit (Lanza et al., 2017). The finding of increased electroencephalography (EEG) high frequencies during the sleep onset period also supports the concept of RLS as an enhancement of the arousal drive (Ferri et al., 2014).

Finally, it is worth mentioning that Allen and coworkers found that the cerebrospinal fluid (CSF) content of hypocretin-1/orexin A, a well-known wake-enhancing neuropeptide, was considerably higher in RLS patients in comparison to healthy controls (Allen, Mignot, Ripley, Nishino, & Earley, 2002). However, other authors described normal CSF hypocretin levels (Mignot et al., 2002; Stiasny-Kolster et al., 2003), lack of correlation between CSF hypocretin and RLS severity (Stiasny-Kolster et al., 2003), and lack of evidence of significant circadian rhythms for CSF hyprocretin-1 in RLS patients (Poceta, Parsons, Engelland, & Kripke, 2009).

A recent functional magnetic resonance imaging (fMRI) study agrees with this interpretation given that, compared to controls, RLS patients showed highly significant changes in regional spontaneous activity of the striatum and thalamus, and, although less pronounced, in the frontal cortex (Zhuo et al., 2017). An even more recent study in RLS has noted a significant decrease of the cortical thickness of the primary somatosensory cortex (S1) and the corpus callosum, including the callosal fibers that link the two somatosensory cortices (Lee et al., 2018). Anatomical data indicate that somatosensory and motor cortical areas are greatly and directly inter-linked through reciprocal projections and, indirectly, through projections to similar striatal neurons (Ramanathan, Hanley, Deniau, & Bolam, 2002). In addition, motor and somatosensory cortical areas also project to the same specific thalamic areas, giving the framework for a sensory-motor integration by tightly interconnected cortical, striatal, and thalamic areas. Consequently, the PLMS and akathisia components of RLS seem to ascend as a sensory-motor network that involves both S1 and primary motor cortex (M1) through a dysfunctional cortico-striatal-thalamic-cortical circuit (Ferré, García-Borreguero, et al., 2018).

3. The complex role of iron in RLS hyperarousal

Brain iron deficiency (BID) is probably a major mechanism in the development of RLS, as demonstrated by a number of studies showing a high prevalence of RLS in situations with insufficient iron availability (Earley et al., 2014). Indeed, the predominance of RLS in patients suffering from iron-deficiency anemia goes up to 30%, which is six times higher than the prevalence of RLS in the general population (Allen, Auerbach, Bahrain, Auerbach, & Earley, 2013). However, most patients do not show total deficiency of iron, rather they have a particular deficiency of iron within the brain. This CNS iron metabolism deficiency, that basically consists of a dysregulated iron transportation through the blood-brain barrier (Ferré, García-Borreguero, et al., 2018), was first demonstrated by elevated transferrin levels and reduced ferritin in the CSF of RLS patients (Earley et al., 2000). This finding was further supported by several imaging studies with all, except two, showing reduced iron in particular brain regions and especially in the substantia nigra (Earley et al., 2014).

BID in rodents can be induced by a severe iron-deficient diet during the postweaning period, thus representing a reliable model of RLS (Earley et al., 2014). It has been observed that diet-induced BID in rats reduces sleep and increase PLMS and arousal activity (Lai et al., 2017). Moreover, BID-induced rodents reproduce the RLS circadian course, along with an increased wakefulness at the end of the period that one is awake (Allen et al., 2017; Dean, Allen, O'Donnell, & Earley, 2006). However, more importantly and differently from the genetic mouse models of RLS, BID provided a valuable model to understand the neurochemical alterations in RLS, including changes not only in DAergic, but also in the glutamatergic, adenosinergic, and, to a lesser extent, GABAergic systems (for reviews, see Earley et al., 2014; Ferré, Quiroz, et al., 2018).

4. Not only dopamine: The glutamate involvement in RLS

The clinically based evidence for an altered glutamatergic neurotransmission in RLS comes from many independent sources. For instance, ketamine, a noncompetitive inhibitor of *N*-methyl-D-aspartate (NMDA) receptor, has been shown in a limited case study to improve RLS (Kapur & Friedman, 2002). The μ-opioid receptor agonist methadone, another noncompetitive NMDA antagonist, is highly effective for RLS at low, nonanalgesic doses (Silver, Allen, Senerth, & Earley, 2011). A previous study using magnetic resonance spectroscopy (MRS) noted a rise in basal levels of GLU in the thalamus of RLS patients (Allen, Barker, Horská, & Earley, 2013). Lastly, medications that are able to treat RLS by binding the α2δ auxiliary subunit of the voltage-gated Ca^{2+} channel, such as gabapentin, are likely to produce benefits by acting on the glutamatergic system (García-Borreguero et al., 2014).

The α2δ subunit is specially localized in glutamatergic terminals, through which α2δ ligands exert a GLU-mediated presynaptic inhibition (Dooley, Taylor, Donevan, & Feltner, 2007). Additionally, medications that bind the α2δ protein are also more effective in improving sleep compared to DA receptor agonists (García-Borreguero et al., 2014). As a matter of fact, clinical trials have shown that, although DA receptor agonists markedly improve PLMS, the general efficiency of sleep does not change significantly (Inoue et al., 2010; Oertel et al., 2010). This finding can be interpreted with the activity of two interacting, thought distinct, mechanisms underlying RLS: a DAergic component, mostly involved in PLMS and akathisia, and a glutamatergic component, which is part of the hyperarousal state (Ferré, García-Borreguero, et al., 2018).

In agreement with the concept of iron as a pathomechanism of RLS, BID in rodents results to alterations in the glutamatergic system (McGahan et al., 2005; Shukla, Agarwal, & Shukla, 1989). The experimental proof for a BID-dependent change in glutamatergic transmission was also found in a recent optogenetic-microdialysis research on rodents with BID (Yepes et al., 2017). This methodology allowed the measurement of the striatal extracellular concentration of GLU on local light-induced stimulation of cortico-striatal glutamatergic terminals, suggesting that BID produces hypersensitivity of the cortico-striatal glutamatergic terminals (Yepes et al., 2017).

On the other hand, the DA receptor agonists pramipexole and ropinirole, as well as the α2δ ligand gabapentin, completely block the optogenetic-induced GLU release both in BID rats and controls (Yepes et al., 2017). This implies that DA receptors and voltage-gated Ca^{2+} channels, localized in the striatal glutamatergic terminals, represent real targets for both DA receptor agonists and α2δ ligands in RLS (Yepes et al., 2017). The differential effect of several DA receptor antagonists in counteracting the ability of pramipexole to inhibit cortico-striatal GLU release pointed to the involvement of the D2 and D4 receptor subtypes (Yepes et al., 2017). Bearing in mind that DA receptor agonists and α2δ ligands produce approximately the same clinical outcome, this finding seems to support the hypothesis that the BID-induced hypersensitivity of the cortico-striatal terminals represents a major pathogenetic mechanism underlying RLS (Ferré, García-Borreguero, et al., 2018).

The question here is whether the hypersensitivity of the cortico-striatal glutamatergic terminals is a primary determinant of the dysfunctional cortico-striatal-thalamic-cortical circuits in RLS or not. In this context, it is reasonable to speculate that the hypersensitivity induced by BID may occur not only at the level of cortico-striatal terminals of pyramidal tract neurons but also at other glutamatergic terminals in the spinal cord, thalamus, and mesencephalon, which eventually results in an impaired dopaminergic state, a thalamic increase of GLU levels, and a cortico-spinal hyperexcitability (Ferré, García-Borreguero, et al., 2018). Additionally, the BID-induced altered dopaminergic state might also be associated with the ability of the striatal GLU to control the local release of DA. Consequently, optogenetically induced GLU release from cortico-striatal terminals may locally induce striatal DA release (Quiroz et al., 2016).

Finally, the tonic release of DA in the spinal cord during naturally occurring wakefulness and nonrapid eye movement (NREM) sleep in intact animals needs consideration (Taepavarapruk et al., 2008). From this finding, one may conclude that the A11-DA area neurons exert a major role in protecting against RLS. As known, the RLS sensory dysesthesias, partially managed by DAergic drugs, are thought to be prompted by the disinhibition of the spinal sensory tract neurons due to impaired supraspinal DA activity (namely, the A11 cell group) (Clemens, Rye, & Hochman, 2006). Indeed, recent findings have indicated that, when the A11-DA cell groups are ablated by the neurotoxin 6-hydroxydopamine, sensory thresholds in awake rats are markedly and permanently reduced (Wang, Sutherland, McErlane, & Soja, 2005). Taken together, these evidences suggest that, under normal conditions, A11-DA neurons provide a tonic DAergic inhibitory input to the spinal sensory neurons during wakefulness and NREM sleep, which, during REM sleep, is not only diminished but also compensated by an increased inhibition by GABA and glycine (Taepavarapruk et al., 2008). If the A11-DA diencephalon-spinal neurons become dysfunctional, as in RLS, such an imbalance in the release of spinal DA during wakefulness just prior to the onset of sleep may contribute to the sensory dysesthesias experienced in RLS and, likely, even in other forms of chronic pain (Soja, 2007).

5. GABA and RLS

As mentioned above, TMS has revealed changes in cortical excitability, namely, dysfunctional GABA-mediated inhibitory control and sensory-motor integration, which have been proposed to be part of RLS pathophysiology (Lanza et al., 2017). Overall, these results identify a pattern that seems to be disease-specific rather than a general consequence of the sleep architecture changes (Lanza, Cantone, et al., 2015; Lanza, Lanuzza, et al., 2015). Neurophysiologically, this finding was considered as the correlate of GABA involvement in RLS (Lanza, Lanuzza, et al., 2018), being also in accordance with the occurrence of recurrent CSPs in RLS (increased number of separate compounds of CSP, which could be interpreted as an additional sign of dysfunctional inhibitory system) (Ahlgrén-Rimpiläinen, Lauerma, Kähkönen, Markkula, & Rimpiläinen, 2012). Nonetheless, the arousal system has a more complex pathophysiology, also involving subcortical structures that cannot be directly probed by TMS of M1 or other cortically located targets. Thus, there is a need for further data from different diagnostic approaches.

By using proton MRS at 4 T, it was found that thalamic GLU in RLS was 50% higher than in controls (Allen, Auerbach, et al., 2013; Allen, Barker, et al., 2013) and the neuronal marker *N*-acetyl aspartate (NAA) was reduced in the thalamus (Rizzo et al., 2012). However, very few studies tested the levels of GABA, the major CNS inhibitory neurotransmitter, in patients with RLS. A previous investigation (Winkelman, Schoerning, Platt, & Jensen, 2014) hypothesized that GABA levels would be lower in the thalamus and anterior cingulated cortex (ACC) of RLS subjects because these areas participate in the ascending pain modulatory systems (Shackman et al., 2011). Similarly, a lower levels of GABA in the cerebellum would be expected, since previous fMRI data suggest that this structure is normally active during RLS-related leg movements and dysesthesias (Margariti et al., 2012). Unexpectedly, however, the authors were unable to note differences between patients and controls, although they demonstrated an association between the levels of GABA and both the actigraphy-derived PLM indices and RLS severity, with a positive correlation in the thalamus and a negative correlation in the cerebellum. Moreover, NAA levels were increased in ACC of patients in comparison to controls (Winkelman et al., 2014).

There is a number of possible explanations for the lack of variations of GABA levels in RLS in this study. First, the sample size was small. Second, the wash-out period from RLS medications was probably too short. Finally, it is possible that differences between groups may have been apparent if acquisition had occurred later in the day, when RLS patients were more symptomatic; the strong correlation of symptom severity during the nights immediately prior to MRS scans with cerebellar and thalamic GABA levels supports this possibility (Winkelman et al., 2014).

The association of GABA levels with actigraphy-related RLS severity and PLMS that were in conflicting directions in the cerebellum and thalamus deserves comment. Connections between the intralaminar nuclei of the thalamus and the cerebellum are well established and are part of the neural traffic that leads to the striatum (Hoshi, Tremblay, Feger, Carras, & Strick, 2005). The striatum has been implicated in RLS pathophysiology (both awake and asleep) by using positron emission tomography (PET), single-photon emission computed tomography, and fMRI (Cervenka et al., 2006; Margariti et al., 2012; Staedt et al., 1993). From this perspective, overactivity of the cerebellum (which is associated with reduced GABA activity) might contribute to RLS symptoms through its influence on the striatum via the thalamic nuclei. Notably, a recent PET study on Tourette syndrome (which shares compulsive movements and premonitory sensory experiences similar to those complained by RLS patients) (Winkelman, Gagnon, & Clair, 2013) also found GABA binding abnormalities in opposite directions in the cerebellum and thalamus (Lerner et al., 2012). Likewise, the authors hypothesized that tics may be generated by an abnormal cerebellar activity transmitted through the thalamus to the striatum.

6. Further insights from neuromodulatory interventions

Repetitive TMS (rTMS) and transcranial direct current stimulation (tDCS) are emerging tools able to transiently modulate CNS excitability in different neuropsychiatric diseases, including sleep disorders. Furthermore, the capability to prompt neuronal plasticity in the motor cortex and connected areas underlies the interest for therapeutic and rehabilitative purposes (Rossini et al., 2015). The rTMS, where magnetic stimuli are delivered in trains on the same cortical region, is able to induce cortical plasticity via complex phenomena, mainly dependent on mechanisms of long-term depression (LTD) and long-term potentiation (Di Lazzaro et al., 2002; Hallett, 2000). Additionally, the modulation of specific neural circuits is likely to promote changes in regional cerebral blood flow, synaptic plasticity, and neurotransmitter release (Lefaucheur et al., 2014). Finally, remote neurochemical effects in deep areas following cortical stimulation are possible; for instance, rTMS of M1 induces release of striatal DA, thus emphasizing the role of subcortical DA and the potential experimental applications in a number of sleep diseases and movement disorders (Strafella, Paus, Fraraccio, & Dagher, 2003).

The modulation of the sensory-motor cortex induced by low-frequency (inhibitory) rTMS has been recently tested in RLS, resulting in amelioration of sensory complaints (Lanza, Cantone, et al., 2018). However, at a pure electrophysiological level, RLS subjects exhibited only partially inhibitory rTMS-induced cortical plasticity over S1, and did not respond to M1 stimulation. The authors concluded that both the shortening of CSP at baseline and the lack of rTMS-induced phenomena of LTD might be considered as "proof of evidence" for impaired GABA mechanisms of cortical excitability (Lanza, Cantone, et al., 2018) and synaptic plasticity in RLS (Lanza, Lanuzza, et al., 2018). Regarding measures of excitation, resting motor threshold (rMT) is a global TMS index reflecting the excitation state of the cortico-spinal cells and intracortical interneurons, mainly mediated by GLU transmission (Paulus et al., 2008; Ziemann et al., 2015). Although baseline rMT was similar between patients and controls, it did not increase in patients after the rTMS-induced inhibition of M1. Similarly, the latency of the motor responses, which reflects the balance between excitatory/inhibitory intracortical circuits and the intracortical projections into the cortico-spinal neurons (Rossini et al., 2015), changed consistently with the different stimulation modalities in controls but not in patients. Taken together, these data support the possibility that also GLU circuitry is involved in RLS (Lanza, Cantone, et al., 2018).

In tDCS, two sponge electrodes are fixed to the subject's head, and a constant electrical current generated by the stimulator is usually applied over a few minutes. DCS modulates spontaneous cell firing and related motor evoked potentials, and its plastic after-effects are comparable to those of rTMS (Nitsche & Paulus, 2000). According to these principles, a randomized, double blind, sham-controlled trial with the use of cathodal (−), anodal (+), and sham (simulated) stimulation on the primary sensory-motor areas was performed in drug-naïve RLS patients (Koo et al., 2015). Given that neither of these two montages was effective, the authors hypothesized that hyperexcitability of S1 might be an epiphenomenon rather than a primary cause of RLS (Koo et al., 2015). However, the extracephalic electrode used in this study may have possibly needed higher intensities than the cephalic return electrodes (Moliadze, Antal, & Paulus, 2010). Moreover, given that a pure tangential current flow might be ineffective, as long as the authors did not prove a modulation of excitability by TMS, the negative outcome cannot be generalized (Krieg, Salinas, Narayana, Fox, & Mogul, 2013).

Finally, transcutaneous spinal DCS (tsDCS) was recently applied in a placebo-controlled, double-blinded investigation in idiopathic RLS (Heide et al., 2014). Each participant received one session of cathodal, anodal, and sham stimulation of the thoracic spinal cord for 15 min at 2.5 mA, in a randomized order and in the evening or at nighttime. The administration of anodal tsDCS in patients resulted in a substantial alleviation of symptoms and a decrease of spinal excitability, as indicated by the Hoffmann reflex parameters. Application of cathodal stimulation also led to a significant clinical improvement, whereas sham tsDCS did not produce clinical or neurophysiological effects (Heide et al., 2014).

7. Summary remarks and future directions

Overall, RLS is likely to arise at different levels of a complex CNS networks and transmission pathways, encompassing somatosensory perception, autonomic processes, and motion, eventually resulting in a modified, possibly temporary and circadian, excitability of a multifaceted cortical-subcortical-spinal drive (Fig. 1).

Quite a number of TMS studies have noted alterations of both cortical-subcortical functioning and spinal circuits, bringing about increased excitation and decreased inhibition. It is notable that a reduced central inhibition is likely to influence the excitation state of segmental spinal pathways more than an increased primary excitability. Several TMS evidences, indeed, highlight a supra-spinal disinhibition, mainly GABA-mediated, in RLS (Lanza et al., 2017; Lanza, Cantone, et al., 2018; Lanza, Lanuzza, et al., 2018; Magalhães et al., 2015), and, at the same time, make a PLMS cortical

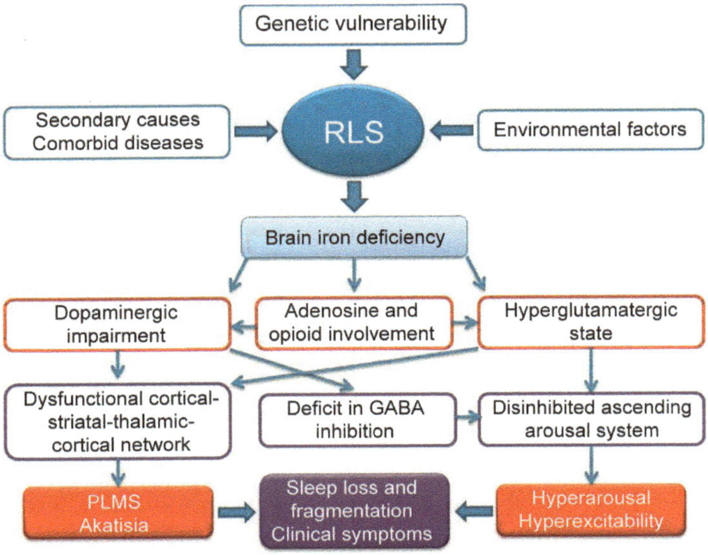

Fig. 1 Integrative scheme summarizing the electrophysiological mechanisms and related neurochemical basis involved in the generation of periodic leg movements during sleep (PLMS), akathisia, and hyperarousal/hyperexcitability state of restless legs syndrome (RLS).

origin rather unlikely (Plazzi, Vetrugno, Meletti, & Provini, 2002; Provini et al., 2001; Trenkwalder et al., 1993). In addition, a connection between RLS and GABA has been established (Winkelman et al., 2014), adding support to the "disinhibition hypothesis" in RLS. Compromised inhibition also agrees with the hyperarousal state also at the EEG level (Ferri et al., 2014), which is in line with the increased arousal-related transient events during sleep (Ferri et al., 2010) that can be reduced by clonazepam but not by pramipexole, indicating their independence from PLMS (Manconi et al., 2012).

The increase in EEG high frequency oscillations may be related to the observation of enhanced connectivity at the resting-state fMRI in RLS. Very recent mapping studies have indicated that abnormally increased synchronization of regional blood oxygenation level-dependent (BOLD) in distinct brain areas may be a key feature of the intrinsic architecture of RLS (Gorges et al., 2016), and probably due to inhibitory influence loss. This was witnessed in the ventral and dorsal columns, thalamus, basal ganglia, and cingulate networks, while no variation has been demonstrated for the brainstem and sensory-motor system. Therefore, the pathophysiology underlying RLS should be viewed beyond the traditional view of brainstem and sensory-motor system only, given that it encompasses much broader CNS areas (Gorges et al., 2016).

Structural MRI findings of white matter changes in RLS support the involvement of different cerebral regions (Earley, Barker, Horská, & Allen, 2006). Similarly, functional neuroimaging studies indicate a decreased iron concentration in multiple brain areas, including the substantia nigra (Allen, Barker, Wehrl, Song, & Earley, 2001; Unrath, Müller, Ludolph, Riecker, & Kassubek, 2008), the thalamus (Schmidauer et al., 2005), and the striatum, particularly the putamen (Godau, Klose, Di Santo, Schweitzer, & Berg, 2008; Rizzo et al., 2013). Therefore, several anatomic loci have been suggested and, in particular, much has been made of a "spinal theory" of RLS that focuses on the A11 descending DOPAergic system, although scant neuropathological data have been provided in support. Another fMRI study noted that both augmentation and reduction in the connectivity between some cortical areas and the thalamus were observed in RLS patients even during the asymptomatic period (Ku et al., 2014). This finding indicates that connectivity changes possibly reflect the pathways involved in producing RLS symptoms and suggests that these patients may have deficits in controlling and managing sensory information (Ku et al., 2014).

Very recently, an adenosine involvement, possibly induced by BID, appears to be the next pathogenetic step. Interestingly, hyperarousal itself might be determined by the hypoadenosinergic state, which may disinhibit the ascending arousal systems, including the glutamatergic component of the ascending reticular activating system (Ferré, García-Borreguero, et al., 2018). Even abnormal peripheral nerve function can affect both spinal and supraspinal activity, supporting the hyperexcitability hypothesis. Nevertheless, findings from a single technique should always be considered in the context of the whole networks proposed for RLS (Lanza et al., 2016). Lastly, further understandings come from recent investigations using noninvasive stimulation techniques: DCS has proved to be a painless way of reducing spinal cord excitability (Heide et al., 2014); rTMS may restore the normal balance between descending excitatory and inhibitory pathways, hence preventing abnormal central somatosensory processing (Lin et al., 2015). Given the subjective clinical improvement produced (Altunrende, Yildiz, Cevik, & Yildiz, 2014; Lanza, Cantone, et al., 2018; Lin et al., 2015), these approaches might represent a new nonpharmacological option for RLS.

In this scenario, the future and continued exploration of different neurotransmission systems will shed light on the neurochemical basis underlying

RLS. At the same time, evaluating the effect of agents acting on different pathways (DA, GLU, GABA, adenosine, opioids) may disclose biomarkers of drug responsiveness. The association between clinical neurophysiology and functional neuroimaging also requires to be examined in more details. For instance, the use of fMRI is useful to probe connectivity within the human brain in both normal and pathological conditions. Real-time integration of TMS with high-density EEG can offer valuable information on reactivity of loco-regional cortical networks and their dynamics. Indeed, without concurrent EEG recording (that has an excellent temporal resolution), TMS is largely limited to M1; though, the possibility to extend the analysis to nonmotor cortical regions may offer additional pathophysiological insights.

8. Conclusion

At this moment, we are in particular need for alternative treatments for RLS. The initially efficacious DAergic agonists, after a continued use, produce side effects that often lead to discontinuation of therapy in a nonnegligible proportion of cases. On the other hand, the mechanism of action responsible for the therapeutic effects of many other drugs for RLS still remains rather unclear. Based on what is reported in this chapter, the mechanisms of action of these drugs may be related, at least in part, to their capability to directly or indirectly temper the hyperexcitability/hyperarousal state of RLS (Clemens et al., 2006; Kumru et al., 2015). Further efforts should be devoted to the elucidation of the initial pathogenetic mechanisms that eventually lead to changes of different neurotransmitter systems. This will also allow the development of new targeted drugs for RLS and other sleep disorders.

Acknowledgments

None.

Conflict of interest

The authors have no conflicts of interest to declare.

References

Ahlgrén-Rimpiläinen, A., Lauerma, H., Kähkönen, S., Markkula, J., & Rimpiläinen, I. (2012). Recurrent CSPs after transcranial magnetic stimulation of motor cortex in restless legs syndrome. *Neurology Research International*, *2012*, 628949.

Allen, R. P. (2015). Restless leg syndrome/Willis-Ekbom disease pathophysiology. *Sleep Medicine Clinics*, *10*, 207–214.

Allen, R. P., Auerbach, S., Bahrain, H., Auerbach, M., & Earley, C. J. (2013). The prevalence and impact of restless legs syndrome on patients with iron deficiency anemia. *American Journal of Hematology*, *88*, 261–264.

Allen, R. P., Barker, P. B., Horská, A., & Earley, C. J. (2013). Thalamic glutamate/glutamine in restless legs syndrome: Increased and related to disturbed sleep. *Neurology*, *80*, 2028–2034.

Allen, R. P., Barker, P. B., Wehrl, F. W., Song, H. K., & Earley, C. J. (2001). MRI measurement of brain iron in patients with restless legs syndrome. *Neurology*, *56*, 263–265.

Allen, R. P., Donelson, N. C., Jones, B. C., Li, Y., Manconi, M., Rye, D. B., et al. (2017). Animal models of RLS phenotypes. *Sleep Medicine*, *31*, 23–28.

Allen, R. P., Mignot, E., Ripley, B., Nishino, S., & Earley, C. J. (2002). Increased CSF hypocretin-1 (orexin-A) in restless legs syndrome. *Neurology*, *59*, 639–641.

Altunrende, B., Yildiz, S., Cevik, A., & Yildiz, N. (2014). Repetitive transcranial magnetic stimulation in restless legs syndrome: Preliminary results. *Neurological Sciences*, *35*, 1083–1088.

Antelmi, E., Vinai, P., Pizza, F., Marcatelli, M., Speciale, M., & Provini, F. (2014). Nocturnal eating is part of the clinical spectrum of restless legs syndrome and an underestimated risk factor for increased body mass index. *Sleep Medicine*, *15*, 168–172.

Bara-Jimenez, W., Aksu, M., Graham, B., Sato, S., & Hallett, M. (2000). Periodic limb movements in sleep: State-dependent excitability of the spinal flexor reflex. *Neurology*, *54*, 1609–1616.

Barraud, Q., Obeid, I., Aubert, I., Barrière, G., Contamin, H., McGuire, S., et al. (2010). Neuroanatomical study of the A11 diencephalospinal pathway in the non-human primate. *PLoS One*, *5*, e13306.

Cervenka, S., Palhagen, S. E., Comley, R. A., Panagiotidis, G., Cselenyi, Z., Matthews, J. C., et al. (2006). Support for dopaminergic hypoactivity in restless legs syndrome: A PET study on D2-receptor binding. *Brain*, *129*, 2017–2028.

Clemens, S., Rye, D., & Hochman, S. (2006). Restless legs syndrome: Revisiting the dopamine hypothesis from the spinal cord perspective. *Neurology*, *67*, 125–130.

Dean, T., Jr., Allen, R. P., O'Donnell, C. P., & Earley, C. J. (2006). The effects of dietary iron deprivation on murine circadian sleep architecture. *Sleep Medicine*, *7*, 634–640.

Di Lazzaro, V., Oliviero, A., Berardelli, A., Mazzone, P., Insola, A., Pilato, F., et al. (2002). Direct demonstration of the effects of repetitive transcranial magnetic stimulation on the excitability of the human motor cortex. *Experimental Brain Research*, *144*, 549–553.

Dooley, D. J., Taylor, C. P., Donevan, S., & Feltner, D. (2007). Ca^{2+} channel $\alpha 2\delta$ ligands: Novel modulators of neurotransmission. *Trends in Pharmacological Sciences*, *28*, 75–82.

Earley, C. J., Allen, R. P., Connor, J. R., Ferrucci, L., & Troncoso, J. (2009). The dopaminergic neurons of the A11 system in RLS autopsy brains appear normal. *Sleep Medicine*, *10*, 1155–1157.

Earley, C. J., Barker, B. P., Horská, A., & Allen, R. P. (2006). MRI-determined regional brain iron concentrations in early and late-onset restless legs syndrome. *Sleep Medicine*, *7*, 458–461.

Earley, C. J., Connor, J. R., Beard, J. L., Malecki, E. A., Epstein, D. K., & Allen, R. P. (2000). Abnormalities in CSF concentrations of ferritin and transferrin in restless legs syndrome. *Neurology*, *54*, 1698–1700.

Earley, C. J., Connor, J. R., García-Borreguero, D., Jenner, P., Winkelman, J., Zee, P. C., et al. (2014). Altered brain iron homeostasis and dopaminergic function in restless legs syndrome (Willis-Ekbom disease). *Sleep Medicine*, *15*, 1288–1301.

Ferré, S., García-Borreguero, D., Allen, R. P., & Earley, C. J. (2018). New insights into the neurobiology of restless legs syndrome. *The Neuroscientist*. https://doi.org/10.1177/1073858418791763, https://www.ncbi.nlm.nih.gov/pubmed/30047288 [Epub ahead of print].

Ferré, S., Quiroz, C., Guitart, X., Rea, W., Seyedian, A., Moreno, E., et al. (2018). Pivotal role of adenosine neurotransmission in restless legs syndrome. *Frontiers in Neuroscience*, *11*, 722.
Ferri, R., Cosentino, F. I., Manconi, M., Rundo, F., Bruni, O., & Zucconi, M. (2014). Increased electroencephalographic high frequencies during the sleep onset period in patients with restless legs syndrome. *Sleep*, *37*, 1375–1381.
Ferri, R., Manconi, M., Aricò, D., Sagrada, C., Zucconi, M., Bruni, O., et al. (2010). Acute dopamine-agonist treatment in restless legs syndrome. Effects on sleep architecture and NREM sleep instability. *Sleep*, *3*, 793–800.
Ferri, R., Proserpio, P., Rundo, F., Lanza, A., Sambusida, K., Redaelli, T., et al. (2015). Neurophysiological correlates of sleep leg movements in acute spinal cord injury. *Clinical Neurophysiology*, *126*, 333–338.
Ferri, R., Rundo, F., Zucconi, M., Manconi, M., Bruni, O., Ferini-Strambi, L., et al. (2015). An evidence-based analysis of the association between periodic leg movements during sleep and arousals in restless legs syndrome. *Sleep*, *38*, 919–924.
García-Borreguero, D., Patrick, J., DuBrava, S., Becker, P. M., Lankford, A., Chen, C., et al. (2014). Pregabalin versus pramipexole: Effects on sleep disturbance in restless legs syndrome. *Sleep*, *37*, 635–643.
Godau, J., Klose, U., Di Santo, A., Schweitzer, K., & Berg, D. (2008). Multiregional brain iron deficiency in restless legs syndrome. *Movement Disorders*, *23*, 1184–1187.
Gorges, M., Rosskopf, J., Müller, H. P., Lindemann, K., Hornyak, M., & Kassubek, J. (2016). Patterns of increased intrinsic functional connectivity in patients with restless legs syndrome are associated with attentional control of sensory inputs. *Neuroscience Letters*, *617*, 264–269.
Hallett, M. (2000). Transcranial magnetic stimulation and the human brain. *Nature*, *406*, 147–150.
Heide, A. C., Winkler, T., Helms, H. J., Nitsche, M. A., Trenkwalder, C., Paulus, W., et al. (2014). Effects of transcutaneous spinal direct current stimulation in idiopathic restless legs patients. *Brain Stimulation*, *7*, 636–642.
Hoshi, E., Tremblay, L., Feger, J., Carras, P. L., & Strick, P. L. (2005). The cerebellum communicates with the basal ganglia. *Nature Neuroscience*, *8*, 1491–1493.
Hyacinthe, C., De Deurwaerdere, P., Thiollier, T., Li, Q., Bezard, E., & Ghorayeb, I. (2015). Blood withdrawal affects iron store dynamics in primates with consequences on monoaminergic system function. *Neuroscience*, *290*, 621–635.
Inoue, Y., Hirata, K., Kuroda, K., Fujita, M., Shimizu, T., Emura, N., et al. (2010). Efficacy and safety of pramipexole in Japanese patients with primary restless legs syndrome: A polysomnographic randomized, double-blind, placebo controlled study. *Sleep Medicine*, *11*, 11–16.
Kapur, N., & Friedman, R. (2002). Oral ketamine: A promising treatment for restless legs syndrome. *Anesthesia & Analgesia*, *94*, 1558–1559.
Koo, Y. S., Kim, S. M., Lee, C., Lee, B. U., Moon, Y. J., Cho, Y. W., et al. (2015). Transcranial direct current stimulation on primary sensorimotor area has no effect in patients with drug-naïve restless legs syndrome: A proof-of-concept clinical trial. *Sleep Medicine*, *16*, 280–287.
Krieg, T. D., Salinas, F. S., Narayana, S., Fox, P. T., & Mogul, D. J. (2013). PET-based confirmation of orientation sensitivity of TMS-induced cortical activation in humans. *Brain Stimulation*, *6*, 898–904.
Ku, J., Cho, Y. W., Lee, Y. S., Moon, H. J., Chang, H., Earley, C. J., et al. (2014). Functional connectivity alternation of the thalamus in restless legs syndrome patients during the asymptomatic period: A resting state connectivity study using functional magnetic resonance imaging. *Sleep Medicine*, *15*, 289–294.
Kumru, H., Vidal, J., Benito, J., Barrio, M., Portell, E., Valles, M., et al. (2015). Restless leg syndrome in patients with spinal cord injury. *Parkinsonism & Related Disorders*, *21*, 1461–1464.

Lai, Y. Y., Cheng, Y. H., Hsieh, K. C., Nguyen, D., Chew, K. T., Ramanathan, L., et al. (2017). Motor hyperactivity of the iron-deficient rat—An animal model of restless legs syndrome. *Movement Disorders*, *32*, 1687–1693.

Lanza, G., Bachmann, C. G., Ghorayeb, I., Wang, Y., Ferri, R., & Paulus, W. (2017). Central and peripheral nervous system excitability in restless legs syndrome. *Sleep Medicine*, *31*, 49–60.

Lanza, G., Cantone, M., Aricò, D., Lanuzza, B., Cosentino, F. I. I., Paci, D., et al. (2018). Clinical and electrophysiological impact of repetitive low-frequency transcranial magnetic stimulation on the sensory-motor network in patients with restless legs syndrome. *Therapeutic Advances in Neurological Disorders*, *11*, 1–12. https://doi.org/10.1177/1756286418759973.

Lanza, G., Cantone, M., Lanuzza, B., Pennisi, M., Bella, R., Pennisi, G., et al. (2015). Distinctive patterns of cortical excitability to transcranial magnetic stimulation in obstructive sleep apnea syndrome, restless legs syndrome, insomnia, and sleep deprivation. *Sleep Medicine Reviews*, *19*, 39–50.

Lanza, G., Lanuzza, B., Aricò, D., Cantone, M., Cosentino, F. I. I., Bella, R., et al. (2018). Impaired short-term plasticity in restless legs syndrome: A pilot rTMS study. *Sleep Medicine*, *46*, 1–4.

Lanza, G., Lanuzza, B., Aricò, D., Cantone, M., Cosentino, F. I., Pennisi, M., et al. (2015). Direct comparison of cortical excitability to transcranial magnetic stimulation in obstructive sleep apnea syndrome and restless legs syndrome. *Sleep Medicine*, *16*, 138–142.

Lanza, G., Lanuzza, B., Aricò, D., Cantone, M., Cosentino, F. I., Pennisi, M., et al. (2016). Response to the letter to the editor "cortical excitability in restless legs syndrome". *Sleep Medicine*, *21*, 175.

Lee, B. Y., Kim, J., Connor, J. R., Podskalny, G. D., Ryu, Y., & Yang, Q. X. (2018). Involvement of the central somatosensory system in restless legs syndrome: A neuroimaging study. *Neurology*, *90*, e1834–e1841.

Lee, H. B., Ramsey, C. M., Spira, A. P., Vachon, J., Allen, R., & Munro, C. A. (2014). Comparison of cognitive functioning among individuals with treated restless legs syndrome (RLS), untreated RLS, and no RLS. *The Journal of Neuropsychiatry and Clinical Neurosciences*, *26*, 87–91.

Lefaucheur, J. P., André-Obadia, N., Antal, A., Ayache, S. S., Baeken, C., Benninger, D. H., et al. (2014). Evidence-based guidelines on the therapeutic use of repetitive transcranial magnetic stimulation (rTMS). *Clinical Neurophysiology*, *125*, 2150–2206.

Lerner, A., Bagic, A., Simmons, J. M., Mari, Z., Bonne, O., Xu, B., et al. (2012). Widespread abnormality of the gamma-aminobutyric acid-ergic system in Tourette syndrome. *Brain*, *135*, 1926–1936.

Lin, Y. C., Feng, Y., Zhan, S. Q., Li, N., Ding, Y., Hou, Y., et al. (2015). Repetitive transcranial magnetic stimulation for the treatment of restless legs syndrome. *Chinese Medical Journal*, *128*, 1728–1731.

Magalhães, S. C., Kaelin-Lang, A., Sterr, A., do Prado, G. F., Eckeli, A. L., & Conforto, A. B. (2015). Transcranial magnetic stimulation for evaluation of motor cortical excitability in restless legs syndrome/Willis-Ekbom disease. *Sleep Medicine*, *16*, 1265–1273.

Manconi, M., Ferri, R., Zucconi, M., Bassetti, C. L., Fulda, S., Aricò, D., et al. (2012). Dissociation of periodic leg movements from arousals in restless legs syndrome. *Annals of Neurology*, *71*, 834–844.

Margariti, P. N., Astrakas, L. G., Tsouli, S. G., Hadjigeorgiou, G. M., Konitsiotis, S., & Argyropoulou, M. I. (2012). Investigation of unmedicated early onset restless legs syndrome by voxel-based morphometry, T2 relaxometry, and functional MR imaging during the night-time hours. *American Journal of Neuroradiology*, *33*, 667–672.

McGahan, M. C., Harned, J., Mukunnemkeril, M., Goralska, M., Fleisher, L., & Ferrell, J. B. (2005). Iron alters glutamate secretion by regulating cytosolic aconitase activity. *American Journal of Physiology. Cell Physiology*, *288*, C1117–C1124.

Mignot, E., Lammers, G. J., Ripley, B., Okun, M., Nevsimalova, S., Overeem, S., et al. (2002). The role of cerebrospinal fluid hypocretin measurement in the diagnosis of narcolepsy and other hypersomnias. *Archives of Neurology*, *59*, 1553–1562.

Moliadze, V., Antal, A., & Paulus, W. (2010). Electrode-distance dependent after-effects of transcranial direct and random noise stimulation with extracephalic reference electrodes. *Clinical Neurophysiology*, *121*, 2165–2171.

Nitsche, M. A., & Paulus, W. (2000). Excitability changes induced in the human motor cortex by weak transcranial direct current stimulation. *The Journal of Physiology*, *527*, 633–639.

Oertel, W. H., Benes, H., Garcia-Borreguero, D., Hogl, B., Poewe, W., Montagna, P., et al. (2010). Rotigotine transdermal patch in moderate to severe idiopathic restless legs syndrome: A randomized, placebo-controlled polysomnographic study. *Sleep Medicine*, *11*, 848–856.

Ondo, W. G., Zhao, H. R., & Le, W. D. (2007). Animal models of restless legs syndrome. *Sleep Medicine*, *8*, 344–348.

Paulus, W., Classen, J., Cohen, L. G., Large, C. H., Di Lazzaro, V., Nitsche, M., et al. (2008). State of the art: Pharmacologic effects on cortical excitability measures tested by transcranial magnetic stimulation. *Brain Stimulation*, *1*, 151–163.

Plazzi, G., Vetrugno, R., Meletti, S., & Provini, F. (2002). Motor pattern of periodic limb movements in sleep in idiopathic RLS patients. *Sleep Medicine*, *3*, S31–S34.

Poceta, J. S., Parsons, L., Engelland, S., & Kripke, D. F. (2009). Circadian rhythm of CSF monoamines and hypocretin-1 in restless legs syndrome and Parkinson's disease. *Sleep Medicine*, *10*, 129–133.

Provini, F., Vetrugno, R., Meletti, S., Plazzi, G., Solieri, L., Lugaresi, E., et al. (2001). Motor pattern of periodic limb movements during sleep. *Neurology*, *57*, 300–304.

Quiroz, C., Orrú, M., Rea, W., Ciudad-Roberts, A., Yepes, G., Britt, J. P., et al. (2016). Local control of extracellular dopamine levels in the medial nucleus accumbens by a glutamatergic projection from the infralimbic cortex. *The Journal of Neuroscience*, *36*, 851–859.

Ramanathan, S., Hanley, J. J., Deniau, J. M., & Bolam, J. P. (2002). Synaptic convergence of motor and somatosensory cortical afferents onto GABAergic interneurons in the rat striatum. *The Journal of Neuroscience*, *22*, 8158–8169.

Rizzo, G., Manners, D., Testa, C., Tonon, C., Vetrugno, R., Marconi, S., et al. (2013). Low brain iron content in idiopathic restless legs syndrome patients detected by phase imaging. *Movement Disorders*, *28*, 1886–1890.

Rizzo, G., Tonon, C., Testa, C., Manners, D., Vetrugno, R., Pizza, F., et al. (2012). Abnormal medial thalamic metabolism in patients with idiopathic restless legs syndrome. *Brain*, *135*, 3712–3720.

Rossini, P. M., Burke, D., Chen, R., Cohen, L. G., Daskalakis, Z., Di Iorio, R., et al. (2015). Non-invasive electrical and magnetic stimulation of the brain, spinal cord, roots and peripheral nerves: Basic principles and procedures for routine clinical and research application. An updated report from an I.F.C.N. committee. *Clinical Neurophysiology*, *126*, 1071–1107.

Schmidauer, C., Sojer, M., Seppi, K., Stockner, H., Högl, B., Biedermann, B., et al. (2005). Transcranial ultrasound shows nigral hypoechogenicity in restless legs syndrome. *Annals of Neurology*, *5*, 630–634.

Shackman, A. J., Salomons, T. V., Slagter, H. A., Fox, A. S., Winter, J. J., & Davidson, R. J. (2011). The integration of negative affect, pain and cognitive control in the cingulate cortex. *Nature Reviews. Neuroscience*, *12*, 154–167.

Shukla, A., Agarwal, K. N., & Shukla, G. S. (1989). Latent iron deficiency alters gamma-aminobutyric acid and glutamate metabolism in rat brain. *Experientia*, *45*, 343–345.

Silver, N., Allen, R. P., Senerth, J., & Earley, C. J. (2011). A 10-year, longitudinal assessment of dopamine agonists and methadone in the treatment of restless legs syndrome. *Sleep Medicine*, *12*, 440–444.

Soja, P. (2007). Modulation of prethalamic sensory inflow during sleep versus wakefulness. In G. Lavigne, B. Sessle, M. Choiniere, & P. Soja (Eds.), *Sleep and pain* (pp. 45–76). Seattle, WA: IASP Press.

Staedt, J., Stoppe, G., Kogler, A., Munz, D., Riemann, H., Emrich, D., et al. (1993). Dopamine D2 receptor alteration in patients with periodic movements in sleep (nocturnal myoclonus). *Journal of Neural Transmission, 93*, 71–74.

Stiasny-Kolster, K., Mignot, E., Ling, L., Möller, J. C., Cassel, W., & Oertel, W. H. (2003). CSF hypocretin-1 levels in restless legs syndrome. *Neurology, 61*, 1426–1429.

Strafella, A. P., Paus, T., Fraraccio, M., & Dagher, A. (2003). Striatal dopamine release induced by repetitive transcranial magnetic stimulation of the human motor cortex. *Brain, 126*, 2609–2615.

Taepavarapruk, N., Taepavarapruk, P., John, J., Lai, Y. Y., Siegel, J. M., Phillips, A. G., et al. (2008). State-dependent changes in glutamate, glycine, GABA, and dopamine levels in cat lumbar spinal cord. *Journal of Neurophysiology, 100*, 598–608.

Trenkwalder, C., Allen, R., Högl, B., Paulus, W., & Winkelmann, J. (2016). Restless legs syndrome associated with major diseases: A systematic review and new concept. *Neurology, 86*, 1336–1343.

Trenkwalder, C., Bucher, S. F., Oertel, W. H., Proeckl, D., Plendl, H., & Paulus, W. (1993). Bereitschaftspotential in idiopathic and symptomatic restless legs syndrome. *Electroencephalography and Clinical Neurophysiology, 89*, 95–103.

Trenkwalder, C., & Paulus, W. (2010). Restless legs syndrome: Pathophysiology, clinical presentation and management. *Nature Reviews. Neurology, 6*, 337–346.

Unger, E. L., Bianco, L. E., Jones, B. C., Allen, R. P., & Earley, C. J. (2014). Low brain iron effects and reversibility on striatal dopamine dynamics. *Experimental Neurology, 261*, 462–468.

Unrath, A., Müller, H. P., Ludolph, A. C., Riecker, A., & Kassubek, J. (2008). Cerebral white matter alterations in idiopathic restless legs syndrome, as measured by diffusion tensor imaging. *Movement Disorders, 23*, 1250–1255.

Wang, D., Sutherland, D., McErlane, S., & Soja, P. (2005). Long-lasting reduction in rat sensory thresholds following ablation of diencephalic A11 dopamine (DA) nuclei. *Society for Neuroscience, 623*, 21.

Winkelman, J. W., Gagnon, A., & Clair, A. G. (2013). Sensory symptoms in restless legs syndrome: The enigma of pain. *Sleep Medicine, 14*, 934–942.

Winkelman, J. W., Schoerning, L., Platt, S., & Jensen, J. E. (2014). Restless legs syndrome and central nervous system gamma-aminobutyric acid: Preliminary associations with periodic limb movements in sleep and restless leg syndrome symptom severity. *Sleep Medicine, 15*, 1225–1230.

Yepes, G., Guitart, X., Rea, W., Newman, A. H., Allen, R. P., Earley, C. J., et al. (2017). Targeting hypersensitive corticostriatal terminals in restless legs syndrome. *Annals of Neurology, 82*, 951–960.

Zhuo, Y., Wu, Y., Xu, Y., Lu, L., Li, T., Wang, X., et al. (2017). Combined resting state functional magnetic resonance imaging and diffusion tensor imaging study in patients with idiopathic restless legs syndrome. *Sleep Medicine, 38*, 96–103.

Ziemann, U., Reis, J., Schwenkreis, P., Rosanova, M., Strafella, A., Badawy, R., et al. (2015). TMS and drugs revisited 2014. *Clinical Neurophysiology, 126*, 1847–1868.

Further reading

Bosco, G., & Poppele, R. E. (2001). Proprioception from a spinocerebellar perspective. *Physiological Reviews, 81*, 539–568.

SECTION II

Disease models/ genetics

CHAPTER SIX

Iron uptake at the blood-brain barrier is influenced by sex and genotype

Quinn W. Wade, Brian Chiou, James R. Connor*
Department of Neurosurgery, Penn State College of Medicine, Hershey, PA, United States
*Corresponding author: e-mail address: jconnor@pennstatehealth.psu.edu

Contents

Abstract

Iron transport to the brain is a critically important and highly regulated process necessary for proper brain function. This review aims to summarize iron uptake mechanisms in the brain and the importance of sex and genotype on this uptake. In restless legs syndrome (RLS), brain iron uptake has been hypothesized to be dysregulated, leading to the clinically observed brain iron deficiency, so this review specifically comments on this disorder. The review covers transferrin-bound transport and the more recently discovered role of ferritin in brain iron delivery. Studies on the impact of sex, MEIS1 (associated with RLS), and H63D gene variants have revealed critical regulatory mechanisms and driving factors that significantly impact iron transport that may considerably affect the clinical treatment of RLS. RLS has provided insights into the gaps in knowledge underlying brain iron uptake mechanisms and their regulation, which in turn have provided insights into the pathophysiology of RLS.

Advances in Pharmacology, Volume 84
ISSN 1054-3589
https://doi.org/10.1016/bs.apha.2019.02.005
© 2019 Elsevier Inc.
All rights reserved.

Abbreviations

AD Alzheimer's disease
BBB blood-brain barrier
BREC bovine retinal endothelial cells
BTBD9 BTB/POZ domain-containing protein 9
CNS central nervous system
CSF cerebral spinal fluid
CXCR4 C-X-C chemokine receptor type 4
DMT1 divalent metal transporter 1
FDRI field-dependent relaxation rate increase
HD Huntington's disease
HFE hemachromatosis protein
Hft H-ferritin
IV intravenous
MEIS1 myeloid ectopic integration site 1 homolog
PD Parkinson's disease
QSM quantitative susceptibility mapping
RLS restless legs syndrome
Scara5 scavenger receptor class A member 5
SWI susceptibility-weighted imaging
Tf transferrin
TfR1 transferrin receptor 1
Tim T-cell immunoglobulin and mucin domain receptor

1. Introduction

Iron is a critical micronutrient that is essential for a wide variety of cellular mechanisms such as DNA synthesis, mitochondrial function, and oxygen transport (Beard, Dawson, & Piñero, 1996). Interestingly, the brain has unique requirements for iron and retains its own differential iron milieu that is vital for its function separate from that of systemic iron. Iron is especially abundant and important in the brain because it is required for myelin production and is a cofactor involved in neurotransmitter synthesis, such as for tyrosine hydroxylase, the rate-limiting enzyme for dopamine biosynthesis (Rajan, Colburn, & Davis, 1976; Youdim, Ben-Shachar, Ashkenazi, & Yehuda, 1983). Moreover, the brain consumes more oxygen for energy production than any other organ and consequently has a higher iron requirement for utilization of the oxygen (Connor & Menzies, 1996; Ikeda & Long, 1990). As a result, it is extremely detrimental when iron homeostasis in the brain is disrupted. Dysregulated brain iron homeostasis has been implicated in conditions such as Alzheimer's disease (AD) (Connor, Snyder, Beard, Fine, & Mufson, 1992; Tanzi & Hyman, 1991), Huntington's disease (HD) (Bartzokis, Cummings, Perlman, Hance, & Mintz, 1999; Hilditch-Maguire et al., 2000), Parkinson's disease (PD) (Dexter et al., 1989; Earle, 1968; Sofic et al., 1988), and restless legs syndrome (RLS) (Allen, Barker, Wehrl, Song, & Earley, 2001). Therefore, regulating iron uptake into the brain is a crucial part of maintaining proper neural function.

In addition to the importance of iron in the brain, the presence of the blood-brain barrier (BBB) poses further complications to its uptake because most cells in the brain do not have direct access to circulating iron (Bradbury, 1997; Brightman & Reese, 1969). Tight junctions present between endothelial cells that line the vasculature of the brain preclude significant paracellular transport of iron; therefore, iron delivery must occur through transport-mediated mechanisms across the BBB (Bradbury, 1997). Evidence shows that there are significant regional differences in the distribution of iron within the brain (Connor & Menzies, 1995). Specifically, the substantia nigra, red nucleus, and striatum are more enriched with iron than other brain regions (Hallgren & Sourander, 1958; Hill & Switzer, 1984). This observation indicates that there is regional regulation of iron delivery to the brain. Thus, the uptake mechanisms for iron into the brain are not only tightly regulated but also complicated further to ensure heterogeneous delivery to areas with higher iron requirements.

Restless legs syndrome (RLS), also known as Willis–Ekbom disease, is a condition associated with an irresistible urge to move one's legs, which is greatly exacerbated during periods of rest (Trenkwalder et al., 1999) and is hypothesized to be correlated with iron deficiency (Norlander, 1953). Several studies have shown that iron levels are decreased in RLS brains specifically, especially the substantia nigra (Allen et al., 2001). Evidence shows that transferrin is increased in the cerebrospinal fluid (CSF) from RLS individuals while ferritin levels are decreased (Clardy, Earley, Allen, Beard, & Connor, 2006; Mizuno, Mihara, Miyaoka, Inagaki, & Horiguchi, 2005). Moreover, prohepcidin, a prohormone that regulates iron efflux, is decreased in the CSF from RLS individuals (Clardy et al., 2006). Furthermore, iron regulatory protein expression was also found to be decreased in the microvasculature of RLS brains, further demonstrating the importance of iron regulation at the level of the BBB (Connor, Ponnuru, Lee, et al., 2011) but also indicating that decreased brain iron in RLS could be initiated at the level of the BBB. Additionally, decreased iron uptake into the brain aligns with the observation that myelin expression is decreased in the brains of individuals with RLS, as myelination is known to be highly dependent on iron (Connor, Ponnuru, Wang, et al., 2011). Therefore, it can be postulated that brain iron uptake is altered in RLS patients.

Delineating the methods of iron uptake in the brain in differing health states across biological classifications can aid in elucidating the process of iron homeostasis and even help identify those at risk of developing certain conditions, such as RLS. As a result of myriad studies, it has been revealed that certain genotypes can affect how the brain handles iron and to a lesser extent, there are significant differences in iron between males and females, which are explored in this review.

2. Characterization of iron uptake mechanisms

Dysregulated iron uptake may result in a number of diseases, including RLS; the concept of iron uptake is a crucial point of interest in understanding normal iron homeostasis. However, the mechanisms of iron uptake differ depending on cell type, and iron uptake into the brain is further complicated by the presence of the blood-brain barrier that serves to regulate this uptake (Simpson et al., 2015). In this section, we will outline the major forms of iron uptake across the BBB: transferrin (Tf)-bound iron and ferritin-bound iron (Fig. 1).

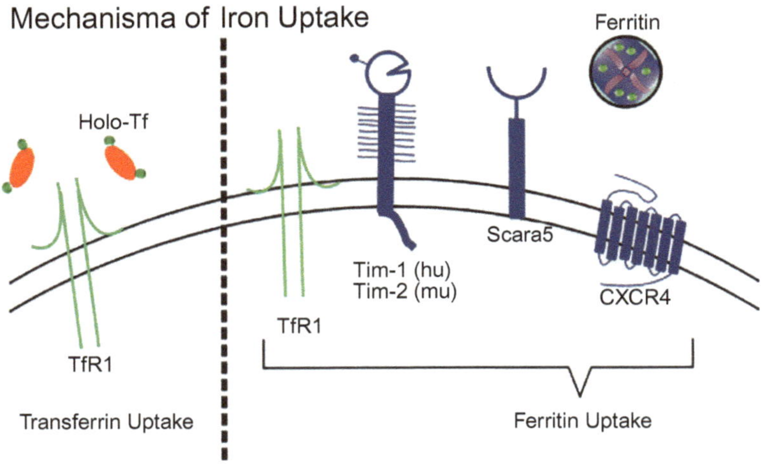

Fig. 1 Mechanisms of iron uptake. While transferrin (Tf) is taken up by transferrin receptor 1 (TfR1), ferritin can be taken up by TfR1, T-cell immunoglobulin and mucin domain receptor 1/2 (Tim-1/2), scavenger receptor class A member 5 (Scara5), and CXCR4.

2.1 Uptake of free iron

Free iron plays an important role both during dietary absorption as well as during iron release from cells. Typically, iron exists in either the ferrous (Fe^{2+}) or ferric (Fe^{3+}) form; extracellular iron typically exists in the ferric state while intracellular iron typically exists in the ferrous state. For the uptake of free iron, there are three major transport proteins: ZIP8, ZIP14, and divalent metal transporter 1 (DMT1) (Garrick, Dolan, Romano, & Garrick, 1999; Liuzzi, Aydemir, Nam, Knutson, & Cousins, 2006; Wang et al., 2012). Though these three proteins are all transmembrane proteins and require symport of H^+ ions to function, the tissue distribution and cellular expression differ throughout the body (Knutson, 2018). ZIP protein expression in the BBB endothelial cells has not been reported to our knowledge, and no studies exist that demonstrate direct uptake of free iron at the BBB *via* DMT1 or any other mechanism.

2.2 Uptake of transferrin-bound iron

A significant mechanism for protein-mediated uptake of iron is through Tf. The level of Tf saturation in the blood coupled with the binding capacity of the Tf receptor suggests that Tf occupies almost 100% of transferrin receptor 1 (TfR1) at a normal physiological level, likening Tf-mediated iron delivery as a slow but steady drip of iron to almost every cell type. A non-classical pathway demonstrates the reduction of the iron contained by transferrin directly at the cell surface, potentially by the Steap family of metalloreductases, where it is thereafter taken up into the cell either as bound iron or free iron (McCarthy & Kosman, 2012, 2015b). In the more well-defined pathway, holo-Tf binds to TfR1 and is endocytosed *via* a clathrin-dependent mechanism (Roberts, Fine, & Sandra, 1993). Due to the endosomal pH, the iron on Tf is released to be reduced by a ferroreductase such as STEAP3. Following endocytosis, the Tf/TfR1 complex is found in the endosome and may transport to a number of different subcellular structures. The endosome containing the Tf/TfR1 complex has been shown to make contact with mitochondria in a process termed "kiss-and-run," delivering iron directly to the mitochondria through a yet-unknown transporter (Das, Nag, Mason, & Barroso, 2016). Alternatively, the free iron found in the endosome can be transported to the cytosol *via* DMT1, ZIP8, or ZIP14 (Garrick et al., 1999; Liuzzi et al., 2006; Wang et al., 2012). These processes make the free iron readily available to the cell, either as Fe^{2+} to be used in metabolic reactions or as ferric iron stored in intracellular ferritin.

With regard to endothelial cells of the brain, our recent studies have changed the paradigm for the way the brain acquires iron. Historically, the transcytosis hypothesis put forth the idea that the Tf/TfR1 complex transcytoses across the endothelial cells of the BBB and deposits holo-Tf into the brain parenchyma thereafter (Fishman, Rubin, Handrahan, Connor, & Fine, 1987; Xu & Ling, 1994). In fact, many therapies have attempted to take advantage of this pathway to use in the treatment of brain disorders by either conjugating a molecule to transferrin or by using a bi-specific antibody targeting TfR1 and a second therapeutic target in the brain (Yu et al., 2014; Zuchero et al., 2016). While these molecules have had a measure of success in BBB penetration in mice and monkey models (Yu et al., 2014), these molecules have typically failed to produce significant results in clinical trials. In the assumption of the transcytosis hypothesis, many scientists are discounting the important contributions of Tf and the iron it carries to the endothelial cell itself. Specifically, they are overlooking the fact that a large part of the endocytosed Tf-iron is used by the endothelial cell for its own metabolic requirements and the apo-Tf is recycled back out to circulation.

The mechanism for release of iron from Tf and into the endothelial cell is transport through DMT1. There was initial lack of agreement regarding expression of DMT1 in the endothelial cells of the BBB although there was agreement that the endothelial cells had to have some mechanism to acquire iron (Burdo et al., 2001; Gunshin et al., 1997; Moos, Skjoerringe, Gosk, & Morgan, 2006; Siddappa et al., 2002; Skjørringe, Burkhart, Johnsen, & Moos, 2015). Some research suggests that DMT1 isoforms minimally contribute to iron uptake or regulation within the endothelial cells (Moos & Morgan, 2003; Moos, Nielsen, Skjørringe, & Morgan, 2007). This research postulates that DMT1 is either found in such low abundance (Enerson & Drewes, 2006) or is segregated only to neurons that it does not impact iron uptake into the brain (Moos et al., 2007). Conversely, others have shown the importance of endosomal DMT1 in Tf-mediated transport across the BBB (Chiou, Neal, et al., 2018a; Duck, Simpson, & Connor, 2017; Simpson et al., 2015). Specifically, iron uptake into the brain is diminished in the Belgrade rat model that has a deficit in DMT1 (Burdo et al., 2001; Moos & Morgan, 2003; Simpson et al., 2015), and recent studies have demonstrated reduced iron transport in a cell culture model of the human BBB when DMT1 is inhibited (Chiou, Neal, et al., 2018b). If transcytosis was the only option available to Tf after endocytosis, there should be no contribution of DMT1 to endothelial iron status. However, DMT1 significantly alters the kinetics of Tf-mediated uptake by changing the rate at which Tf is taken up by the endothelial cells. This provides strong evidence for a crucial intracellular pathway that is not explained by and contrary to transcytosis. Compounding this, regulation of iron uptake by brain-side signals or other intracellular proteins changes the amount of iron loading by the endothelial cells (Chiou, Neal, et al., 2018a).

2.3 Uptake of Ferritin

Another method of iron delivery is through ferritin. Fisher and colleagues have demonstrated uptake of ferritin into the brain *in vivo* (Fisher et al., 2007), while many other studies have shown the transport of ferritin across the BBB *in vitro* (Chiou, Neal, et al., 2018a, 2018b; Fiandra et al., 2016). Typically, ferritin can be found circulating in the serum (Cohen et al., 2010) or in the CSF (Patton et al., 2017), but the biological role of this circulating ferritin has been hypothesized as a product of cell damage (Kell & Pretorius, 2014), a marker for inflammation, or as an alternative iron delivery mechanism (Chiou & Connor, 2018). In RLS, where a decrease in iron uptake has been hypothesized, it has been shown that the endothelial cells of the brain have decreased levels of H-ferritin (Hft) (Connor, Ponnuru, Lee, et al., 2011), suggesting further limited acquisition of iron by the BBB. Decreased H-ferritin and iron were also found in the substantia nigra pars compacta in RLS brains (Snyder & Connor, 2009).

When making the distinction between serum/CSF ferritin, it is important to consider the ratio of the H- and L-ferritin subunits that comprise the 24-mer mature ferritin protein. This ratio generally is dependent upon the cell type that secreted the ferritin into circulation. While the H subunit contains ferroxidase activity, the L subunit is responsible for iron turnover at the ferroxidase site and in the nucleation of iron within the ferritin core. A major difference between serum and secreted ferritin is that serum ferritin is largely comprised of the L subunit with 1 or 2 H subunits while secreted ferritin prefers a higher proportion of H:L ratio, typically around a 10:14 ratio (Arosio, Ingrassia, & Cavadini, 2009). This has major implications for the dynamic properties of the fully assembled molecule—a proper balance between the H and L subunit is necessary to facilitate maximum entry of iron into the core. It has also been shown that Hft is taken up by all organs at a higher rate than L-ferritin (Fisher et al., 2007). This suggests that in times of high iron demand, a 24-mer comprised of more H subunits will contribute more iron to the system after uptake.

Ferritin uptake into the brain is a significant area of research. Unlike Tf, which primarily uses TfR1 to facilitate uptake, ferritin has been shown to utilize a number of different receptors. Further complicating matters are the diversity in receptors: L-ferritin has been shown to bind to Scara5 (Li et al., 2009), a macrophage scavenger receptor, while H-ferritin has been shown to bind to TfR1 (Li et al., 2010), Tim-1 in humans (Chiou, Neal, et al., 2018a), Tim-2 in mice (Chen et al., 2005; Han et al., 2011; Todorich, Zhang, Slagle-Webb, Seaman, & Connor, 2008), and CXCR4 (Li, Luo, Mines, Zhang, & Fan, 2006). Whether multiple receptors work in tandem to facilitate uptake is currently unclear, but it is recognized that for ferritin to use all of these receptors, multiple regulatory mechanisms must exist.

As with Tf, in order for ferritin to be taken up, it must also be secreted. Important sources of secreted ferritin are cells such as macrophages and microglia, the resident macrophages of the brain, as well as hepatocytes (Connor, Zhang, Nixon, Webb, & Perno, 2015; Tran, Eubanks, Schaffer, Zhou, & Linder, 1997; Truman-Rosentsvit et al., 2018). In particular, it has been shown that acute infection as well as iron loading causes increased secretion of Hft (Meyron-Holtz, Moshe-Belizowski, & Cohen, 2011). A novel function of endothelial cells to release Hft into the abluminal side of the BBB after iron loading has also been found (Chiou, Neal, et al., 2018b). Furthermore, this Hft release is sensitive to cues such as apo-Tf and holo-Tf. Taken together, the upregulation of Hft secretion is likely to be an important indication of a bodily response to some form of challenge, either to mobilize more iron for the body to metabolize or to limit the amount of iron that is available to potential pathogens.

The mechanism of ferritin secretion has received little attention. Historically, ferritin was thought to be exclusively intracellular—any extracellular ferritin found was a byproduct of damaged cells releasing its content to circulation. Corroborating this is the lack of glycosylation of ferritin as well as the fact that ferritin does not enter the ER even when translated by the rough ER (Cohen et al., 2010). However, recent literature has demonstrated that ferritin is secreted through two non-classical mechanisms: secretory autophagy and through exosomes (Truman-Rosentsvit et al., 2018). In secretory autophagy, an autophagosome is formed as in normal autophagy. However, instead of trafficking to the lysosome, this secretory autophagosome is transported to the cell surface and releases its contents (Ponpuak et al., 2015). This route of secretion would explain why ferritin can be assayed for directly from the circulation and serum. The presence of ferritin in exosomes has been shown in a number of recent publications (Mrowczynski et al., 2017; Truman-Rosentsvit et al., 2018).

Ferritin-containing exosomes may be a more targeted way for the body to deliver iron. Importantly, it is still unclear which secretion pathway is the major contributor to extracellular ferritin.

3. Contributions of sex to brain iron uptake

There is evidence that the brain is a sexually dimorphic organ with reports of higher levels of myelination in female brains and dopamine synthesis compared to males (Bazzett & Becker, 1994; McDermott, Liu, & Dluzen, 1994; Munro et al., 2006) and these processes are highly dependent on iron. Additionally, it is well accepted that females generally have lower levels of peripheral iron compared to males (Fleming et al., 2001; Whitfield, Treloar, Zhu, Powell, & Martin, 2003). However, it is currently unclear whether there are actual differences in brain iron levels and altered handling between males and females. The BBB isolates and protects the brain from systemic fluctuations, thus alterations in the iron levels of peripheral organs do not significantly affect brain iron levels. Despite this tight regulation and distinct compartmentalization separate from that of the periphery, there is evidence that the brain is responsive to systemic circulating iron (Bartzokis et al., 2007; Beard & Connor, 2003; Piñero, Jones, & Beard, 2000). Hallgren and Sourander first acknowledged this possibility that iron within the brain is responsive to iron in the periphery in their histological analysis of brain iron levels *post mortem* (Hallgren & Sourander, 1958). Thus, the differences in peripheral iron levels among males and females could translate to alterations in brain iron levels.

One neuroimaging study found that females had statistically significantly lower levels of iron in the caudate compared to males when using a susceptibility-weighted phase image (SWI) process (Hagemeier et al., 2013). Hagemeier et al. used approximately 120 females and 90 males that were perhaps more adequately powered than the other studies (Hagemeier et al., 2013). Furthermore, Persson et al. estimated iron levels in approximately 200 healthy individuals with quantitative susceptibility mapping (QSM) and found that females had significantly lower susceptibility values and thus iron levels in the substantia nigra compared to males regardless of age (Persson et al., 2015). They also found a similar trend in the red nucleus, although this did not reach statistical significance (Persson et al., 2015).

Another study found that females had lower levels of ferritin in the brain compared to males (Bartzokis et al., 2007). Bartzokis et al. utilized a field-dependent relaxation rate increase (FDRI) method to determine brain ferritin levels in approximately 70 healthy females and 90 healthy males (Bartzokis et al., 2007). The thalamus, frontal white matter, and corpus callosum were all investigated, and females consistently had lower levels of ferritin in these regions (Bartzokis et al., 2007). However, it is important to note that the data were not statistically significant due to the high variability among all subjects (Bartzokis et al., 2007). Another neuroimaging study using SWI that had approximately 40 females and 40 males found no significant differences in brain iron levels (Xu, Wang, & Zhang, 2008).

In summary, previous investigations into sex differences regarding iron levels in the brain have found mixed but strongly suggestive results indicative of a sex disparity. Further research into iron and associated transport proteins is required to clarify and delineate sex differences and impact on brain iron levels and handling. In addition, the imaging analyses utilized and sample populations' biological characteristics varied among the studies, so each much be regarded separately as results from one study cannot be extrapolated and compared directly to another. There are numerous other aspects that need to be considered such as age- and sex-specific factors like childbirth and hormones that could influence the results that are obtained. For example, Tishler et al. found that frontal white matter iron levels were higher in females with pre-menopausal hysterectomies compared to age-matched female controls (Tishler, Raven, Lu, Altshuler, & Bartzokis, 2012). Additionally, no significant regional change in the level of brain iron does not discount altered distribution among different cell types, which should be further investigated.

In rodents, radioisotope experiments found that female mice had significantly higher amounts of cortical Fe^{59} accumulation compared to males (Duck, Neely, Simpson, & Connor, 2018). One study demonstrated that BALB/c and DBA/2J male mice had statistically ($P < 0.0001$) higher mean levels of iron in the brain compared to age-matched females (Hahn et al., 2009). However, there was no sex difference in brain iron levels in C57BL/6 mice (Hahn et al., 2009). This suggests strain or genotype is another level of complexity that must be considered when investigating sex differences for brain iron uptake. Another study using Sprague–Dawley rats found no statistically significant difference in brain iron concentration between males and females (Uchino, Tsuzuki, & Inoue, 1990). However, no difference in total brain iron does not exclude regional differences in iron on the basis of sex. Evidently, there are numerous confounding factors that must be acknowledged in both human subjects and rodents when examining sex differences. Overall, there remains a gap in knowledge concerning the influence of sex on brain iron levels and uptake, but studies have shown compelling data that indicate there is a difference. Further research assessing the levels of iron-associated transporters in the BBB in males and females would help reveal mechanistically why iron uptake into the brain would differ based on sex.

It is established that RLS is twice as common in females compared to males (Berger & Kurth, 2007). In addition, the prevalence of RLS among females increases with the number of pregnancies and child births (Berger, Luedemann, Trenkwalder, John, & Kessler, 2004). There appears to be a high association between pregnancy and RLS because studies have shown that pregnant females are at increased risk for developing RLS and those currently affected by RLS find symptoms worsened during pregnancy (Lee, Zaffke, & Baratte-Beebe, 2001). Moreover, it is well known that pregnant females are at risk for iron deficiency so there is correlative evidence between the difference in iron levels between males and females and also the prevalence of disorders that are suggested to have aberrant iron homeostasis (Allen, 2004). Therefore, it is important to investigate sex differences on iron uptake into the brain as this disparity can be implicated in conditions of dysregulated iron management, such as RLS.

4. Contributions of the MEIS1 genotype

Although insufficient iron is believed to play a role in the physiology of RLS, not all who are iron-deficient have RLS and many individuals with RLS have normal levels of iron and associated proteins in the periphery (Ekbom, 1960; Norlander, 1953). What may be more important is the status of iron within the brain as evidence shows that there are low levels of iron and altered associated proteins in the brains of RLS individuals (Allen et al., 2001; Earley et al., 2000). Therefore, it is hypothesized that the ability of the brain to take up iron from the periphery or maintain its iron is impaired (Bartzokis et al., 2007; Beard et al., 1996; Piñero et al., 2000). In particular, MEIS1 (myeloid ectopic integration site 1 homolog), a homeobox gene that encodes a transcription factor involved in hematopoiesis and nervous system development (Barber et al., 2013; Hisa et al., 2004; Spieler et al., 2014) has been found to be highly associated with developing RLS by genome-wide association studies (GWAS) (Winkelmann et al., 2007). MEIS1 along with other RLS-associated genes such as BTBD9, are expressed within ganglionic eminences during telencephalon development (Spieler et al., 2014). Also, Owa and colleagues found that Meis1 in the mouse is involved in granule cell development in the cerebellum (Owa et al., 2018). Xiong et al. genotyped and analyzed approximately 30 autopsy brain samples from RLS cases and discovered a single nucleotide polymorphism (C13B_2) that is associated with an increased risk of RLS (Xiong et al., 2009). This intronic variant in the MEIS1 gene was associated with reduced expression and reduced protein levels of MEIS1 (Xiong et al., 2009). Conversely, another study showed that MEIS1 protein levels are increased in the microvasculature extracted from RLS brains compared to control (Connor, Patton, Oexle, & Allen, 2017).

The link between brain iron and MEIS1 expression was more directly interrogated in cell culture models. Researchers found that inducing iron-deficient conditions utilizing HeLa and neuroblastoma cell lines resulted in a decrease in MEIS1 mRNA expression, whereas inducing iron overload had no effect on MEIS1 mRNA expression (Catoire et al., 2011). In contrast, researchers using BREC cultures in an *in vitro* model of the BBB found that iron deficiency in the culture resulted in an increase in MEIS1 expression whereas iron overload in the culture resulted in a decrease in MEIS1 expression (Connor et al., 2017), similar to what was reported in the microvasculature of the RLS tissue. It is important to acknowledge that the exact role of MEIS1 in the adult is unclear, and little is known about MEIS1 function in non-embryonic neuronal tissue (Xiong et al., 2009). Nonetheless, the evidence that MEIS1 is present in the microvasculature of the brain and in a BBB model and is responsive to iron deficiency is support that additional studies regarding mRNA expression, protein levels, along with regulation at the level of the BBB should investigate.

5. Contributions of the H67D/H63D HFE genotype

The human hemochromatosis protein encoded by the HFE gene is an iron management protein that functions to regulate transferrin binding to its cognate receptor, TfR1, and thus consequent iron uptake into the cell. The HFE protein can be found on the choroid plexus, brain microvasculature, and ependymal cells (Connor et al., 2001). The H63D and C282Y human gene variants of the HFE gene are the two most common polymorphisms in the HFE gene but only the C282Y variant is typically associated with hereditary hemochromatosis (HH) (Nandar, Neely, Unger, & Connor, 2013).

The H63D and C282Y genotypes also affect iron accumulation in the brain (Nandar et al., 2013). Because the C282Y variant is found in only 1.9% of the population and the H63D variant is much more prevalent at 8.1%, and because the H63D HFE variant is more commonly identified as a neurodegenerative disease modifier, this section of the review will focus on the H63D variant (Merryweather-Clarke, Pointon, Jouanolle, Rochette, & Robson, 2000; Merryweather-Clarke, Pointon, Shearman, & Robson, 1997; Nandar & Connor, 2011).

Neuroimaging studies have shown that individuals with the H63D HFE gene mutations have increased brain iron levels (Meadowcroft et al., 2016). *In vivo* studies using the H67D variant—the mouse homolog to H63D—have shown that there is significantly more iron present in the brains of H67D knock-in mice compared to wild-type controls as measured by atomic absorption (Duck et al., 2018). Although the mutant mice were found to have higher levels of total brain iron, radioactive Fe^{59} tracing revealed that the rate of uptake into the brain was not different between the H67D and wild-type young adult mice (Duck et al., 2018). Thus, despite the significant difference in brain iron levels, there was no significant difference in uptake over a 5-day period, which suggests that a set point has been reached and maintained (Duck et al., 2018). This further indicates that iron is not being continuously taken up in an uncontrolled fashion with the HFE mutation and that this may be attributable to the fact that the blood-brain barrier has already been established, so iron uptake is subjected to regulation. Therefore, even a genetic mutation that favors elevated iron uptake is subject to regulation.

Research is lacking into whether the H63D genotype is implicated in RLS. Since RLS is characterized by iron deficiency while H63D leads to iron overload, it is logical that this gene variant has not appeared in RLS studies, but perhaps it could offer protection against RLS. Oexle et al. examined the association of the C282Y HFE variant and RLS using several hundred human samples for genomic analysis (Oexle et al., 2013). They did not find any association between those with the C282Y variant and RLS (Oexle et al., 2013); however, it would be more informative to interrogate the much more prevalent H63D HFE variant, which is much more common than the C282Y variant. Thus, although it seems counterintuitive that a genotype that results in excess brain iron would be involved in RLS, a condition linked to iron deficiency, it is worth examining whether the H63D variant is protective against RLS or possibly even detrimental. Essentially, compensatory mechanisms and iron export may play a role that should be further investigated with regards to genotypic effects on RLS.

6. Clinical implications in RLS

Because the pathophysiology of RLS is associated with iron deficiency as evidenced by autopsy (Connor et al., 2003), MRI (Allen et al., 2001), and CSF (Earley et al., 2000; Mizuno et al., 2005) studies, iron supplementation has been used as a first line of treatment. Several clinical studies have shown that prescribing iron supplements or intravenous administration improves RLS symptoms in a number of individuals (Norlander, 1953; O'keeffe, Gavin, & Lavan, 1994). Oral supplementation has been effective in some cases, but it can take weeks for iron status to be restored, as oral supplements largely rely on the absorption of free iron as detailed above. Intravenous iron infusion is another method of delivery that can replenish iron levels more rapidly than oral supplementation. Specifically, Norlander used intravenous iron to treat individuals with RLS and recorded symptom remission that lasted months for the majority of patients (Norlander, 1953). Delivering iron to the periphery provides more access and potentially offers a greater availability of iron for the brain to take up. We have previously shown that the brain can signal at the level of the BBB in order to increase iron transport, thereby providing a mechanism by which the brain can directly regulate iron uptake based on brain iron status (Chiou, Neal, et al., 2018b). However, iron supplementation is not effective for all individuals, and many with RLS have normal levels of peripheral iron; therefore, it is not just insufficient iron levels that solely leads to RLS. In particular, a meta-analysis of four distinct studies that investigated the effects of iron therapy on RLS symptoms found that there was an average improvement in IRLS (International Restless Legs Syndrome) scores after treatment, but this did not reach clinical significance (Trotti, Bhadriraju, & Becker, 2009). There have been considerable concerns that intravenous iron supplementation may result in brain iron overload, but a study by our group using a human cell culture model of the BBB found that the IV iron formulations do not directly cross the BBB (Chiou, Neal, et al., 2018b). Our data suggest that the IV iron formulations must first be processed by macrophages and made into a bioavailable form of iron such as ferritin or free iron that can bind to Tf (Chiou, Neal, et al., 2018b). Therefore, the IV iron formulations become subjected to the same regulatory uptake parameters that already exist in the brain. Thus, it can be hypothesized that the supplemental iron supplied systemically may act through other uptake mechanisms and signals in the brain that could be dysfunctional to varying degrees in RLS. This would account for the heterogeneous effectiveness of iron supplementation in individuals who may or may not have normal peripheral iron levels.

Current research has demonstrated the brain microvascular endothelial cells (BMVECs) that line the BBB are also responsive to paracrine signals from astrocytes regarding brain iron status (McCarthy & Kosman, 2014, 2015a; Simpson et al., 2015). Thus, uptake is dually regulated on both sides of the BBB, and this communication between glial and the BBB must also be considered mechanistically when developing potential therapeutics.

Interestingly, the transport of iron into the brain can also have profound clinical implications, as these mechanisms can be harnessed to deliver therapeutics directly into the brain parenchyma. Fundamentally, the blood-brain barrier's stringent protection of the brain has posed consistent obstacles to targeted brain therapies. Specifically, H-ferritin can be employed to circumvent these obstacles as a carrier of specific therapeutics (Kim et al., 2011; Mazzucchelli et al., 2016, 2017). For example, apo-H-ferritin can be unfolded, added to the desired therapy, and then re-associated so as to cage the molecule as it is transported into the brain (Kim et al., 2011). The ferritin uptake mechanism that the body naturally utilizes for brain iron import can serve as a conduit for delivery of chemotherapies for glioblastomas and other neural cancers (Mazzucchelli et al., 2016, 2017). In the case of RLS, iron delivery to the brain could be enhanced as a potential therapeutic being as iron supplements are only efficacious in certain individuals. Therefore, understanding the mechanisms of iron uptake into the brain and biological characteristics that can affect these processes is critical for investigating and treating a variety of conditions where iron dysregulation is implicated, such as RLS.

7. Conclusion

The observation of brain iron deficiency in the pathogenesis of RLS has led to numerous promising research directions. Studies of impaired brain iron uptake coupled with an understanding of the pathophysiology of RLS have converged to shift the paradigm on brain iron uptake mechanisms and introduced the novel but not surprising concept that the mechanisms of uptake are regulated. Despite this, many patients remain unaffected by iron supplementation and the ability of pharmaceutical iron formulations to raise brain iron levels remains controversial. A more complete understanding of the various factors that play into RLS pathogenesis is required for proper and effective treatment. In particular, the importance of sex and genotype cannot be discounted, as these two factors play extremely significant roles in overall brain iron transport.

Conflict of interest

J.R.C. is the founder and chairman of the board of Sidero Biosciences LLC, a company with a product aimed towards using oral consumption of ferritin as a therapy for iron deficiency.

References

Allen, R. (2004). Dopamine and iron in the pathophysiology of restless legs syndrome (RLS). *Sleep Medicine*, *5*, 385–391. https://doi.org/10.1016/j.sleep.2004.01.012.

Allen, R. P., Barker, P. B., Wehrl, F., Song, H. K., & Earley, C. J. (2001). MRI measurement of brain iron in patients with restless legs syndrome. *Neurology*, *56*, 263–265. https://doi.org/10.1212/WNL.56.2.263.

Arosio, P., Ingrassia, R., & Cavadini, P. (2009). Ferritins: A family of molecules for iron storage, antioxidation and more. *Biochimica et Biophysica Acta (BBA)—General Subjects*, *1790*(7), 589–599. https://doi.org/10.1016/j.bbagen.2008.09.004.

Barber, B. A., Liyanage, V. R. B., Zachariah, R. M., Olson, C. O., Bailey, M. A. G., & Rastegar, M. (2013). Dynamic expression of MEIS1 homeoprotein in E14.5 forebrain and differentiated forebrain-derived neural stem cells. *Annals of Anatomy*, *195*, 431–440. https://doi.org/10.1016/j.aanat.2013.04.005.

Bartzokis, G., Cummings, J., Perlman, S., Hance, D. B., & Mintz, J. (1999). Increased basal ganglia iron levels in Huntington disease. *Archives of Neurology*, *56*, 569–574. https://doi.org/10.1001/archneur.56.5.569.

Bartzokis, G., Tishler, T. A., Lu, P. H., Villablanca, P., Altshuler, L. L., Carter, M., et al. (2007). Brain ferritin iron may influence age- and gender-related risks of neurodegeneration. *Neurobiology of Aging*, *28*(3), 414–423. https://doi.org/10.1016/j.neurobiolaging.2006.02.005.

Bazzett, T. J., & Becker, J. B. (1994). Sex differences in the rapid and acute effects of estrogen on striatal D2 dopamine receptor binding. *Brain Research*, *637*, 163–172. https://doi.org/10.1016/0006-8993(94)91229-7.

Beard, J. L., & Connor, J. R. (2003). Iron status and neural functioning. *Annual Review of Nutrition*, *23*(1), 41–58. https://doi.org/10.1146/annurev.nutr.23.020102.075739.

Beard, J. L., Dawson, H., & Piñero, D. J. (1996). Iron metabolism: A comprehensive review. *Nutrition Reviews*, *54*(10), 295–317. Retrieved from http://www.ncbi.nlm.nih.gov/pubmed/9063021.

Berger, K., & Kurth, T. (2007). RLS epidemiology—Frequencies, risk factors and methods in population studies. *Movement Disorders*, *22*, S420–S423. https://doi.org/10.1002/mds.21589.

Berger, K., Luedemann, J., Trenkwalder, C., John, U., & Kessler, C. (2004). Sex and the risk of restless legs syndrome in the general population. *Archives of Internal Medicine*, *164*, 196–202. https://doi.org/10.1001/archinte.164.2.196.

Bradbury, M. W. (1997). Transport of iron in the blood-brain-cerebrospinal fluid system. *Journal of Neurochemistry*, *69*, 443–454. https://doi.org/10.1046/j.1471-4159.1997.69020443.x.

Brightman, M. W., & Reese, T. S. (1969). Junctions between intimately apposed cell membranes in the vertebrate brain. *The Journal of Cell Biology*, *40*, 648–677. https://doi.org/10.1083/jcb.40.3.648.

Burdo, J. R., Menzies, S. L., Simpson, I. A., Garrick, L. M., Garrick, M. D., Dolan, K. G., et al. (2001). Distribution of divalent metal transporter 1 and metal transport protein 1 in the normal and Belgrade rat. *Journal of Neuroscience Research*, *66*(6), 1198–1207. https://doi.org/10.1002/jnr.1256.

Catoire, H., Dion, P. A., Xiong, L., Amari, M., Gaudet, R., Girard, S. L., et al. (2011). Restless legs syndrome-associated MEIS1 risk variant influences iron homeostasis. *Annals of Neurology, 70*, 170–175. https://doi.org/10.1002/ana.22435.

Chen, T. T., Li, L., Chung, D.-H., Allen, C. D. C., Torti, S. V., Torti, F. M., et al. (2005). TIM-2 is expressed on B cells and in liver and kidney and is a receptor for H-ferritin endocytosis. *The Journal of Experimental Medicine, 202*(7), 955–965. https://doi.org/10.1084/jem.20042433.

Chiou, B., & Connor, J. (2018). Emerging and dynamic biomedical uses of ferritin. *Pharmaceuticals, 11*(4), 124. https://doi.org/10.3390/ph11040124.

Chiou, B., Neal, E. H., Bowman, A. B., Lippmann, E. S., Simpson, I. A., & Connor, J. R. (2018a). Endothelial cells are critical regulators of iron transport in a model of the human blood–brain barrier. *Journal of Cerebral Blood Flow & Metabolism*. https://doi.org/10.1177/0271678X18783372.

Chiou, B., Neal, E. H., Bowman, A. B., Lippmann, E. S., Simpson, I. A., & Connor, J. R. (2018b). Pharmaceutical iron formulations do not cross a model of the human blood-brain barrier. *PLoS One, 13*(6), e0198775. https://doi.org/10.1371/journal.pone.0198775.

Clardy, S. L., Earley, C. J., Allen, R. P., Beard, J. L., & Connor, J. R. (2006). Ferritin subunits in CSF are decreased in restless legs syndrome. *Journal of Laboratory and Clinical Medicine, 147*(2), 67–73. https://doi.org/10.1016/j.lab.2005.06.011.

Clardy, S. L., Wang, X., Boyer, P. J., Earley, C. J., Allen, R. P., & Connor, J. R. (2006). Is ferroportin-hepcidin signaling altered in restless legs syndrome? *Journal of the Neurological Sciences, 247*, 173–179. https://doi.org/10.1016/j.jns.2006.04.008.

Cohen, L. A., Gutierrez, L., Weiss, A., Leichtmann-Bardoogo, Y., Zhang, D.-L., Crooks, D. R., et al. (2010). Serum ferritin is derived primarily from macrophages through a nonclassical secretory pathway. *Blood, 116*(9), 1574–1584. https://doi.org/10.1182/blood-2009-11-253815.

Connor, J. R., Boyer, P. J., Menzies, S. L., Dellinger, B., Allen, R. P., Ondo, W. G., et al. (2003). Neuropathological examination suggests impaired brain iron acquisition in restless legs syndrome. *Neurology, 61*, 304–309. https://doi.org/10.1212/01.WNL.0000078887.16593.12.

Connor, J. R., & Menzies, S. L. (1995). Cellular management of iron in the brain. *Journal of the Neurological Sciences, 134*, 33–44. https://doi.org/10.1016/0022-510X(95)00206-H.

Connor, J. R., & Menzies, S. L. (1996). Relationship of iron to oligodendrocytes and myelination. *Glia, 17*(2), 83–93. https://doi.org/10.1002/(SICI)1098-1136(199606)17:2<83::AID-GLIA1>3.0.CO;2–7.

Connor, J. R., Milward, E. A., Moalem, S., Sampietro, M., Boyer, P., Percy, M. E., et al. (2001). Is hemochromatosis a risk factor for Alzheimer's disease? *Journal of Alzheimer's Disease, 3*, 471–477. https://doi.org/10.3233/JAD-2001-3506.

Connor, J. R., Patton, S. M., Oexle, K., & Allen, R. P. (2017). Iron and restless legs syndrome: Treatment, genetics and pathophysiology. *Sleep Medicine, 31*, 61–70. https://doi.org/10.1016/j.sleep.2016.07.028.

Connor, J. R., Ponnuru, P., Lee, B. Y., Podskalny, G. D., Alam, S., Allen, R. P., et al. (2011). Postmortem and imaging based analyses reveal CNS decreased myelination in restless legs syndrome. *Sleep Medicine, 12*, 614–619. https://doi.org/10.1016/j.sleep.2010.10.009.

Connor, J. R., Ponnuru, P., Wang, X.-S., Patton, S. M., Allen, R. P., Earley, C. J., et al. (2011). Profile of altered brain iron acquisition in restless legs syndrome. *Brain, 134*, 959–968. https://doi.org/10.1093/brain/awr012.

Connor, J. R., Snyder, B. S., Beard, J. L., Fine, R. E., & Mufson, E. J. (1992). Regional distribution of iron and iron-regulatory proteins in the brain in aging and Alzheimer's disease. *Journal of Neuroscience Research*, *31*, 327–335. https://doi.org/10.1002/jnr.490310214.

Connor, J. R., Zhang, X., Nixon, A. M., Webb, B., & Perno, J. R. (2015). Comparative evaluation of nephrotoxicity and management by macrophages of intravenous pharmaceutical iron formulations. *PLoS One*, *10*(5), e0125272. https://doi.org/10.1371/journal.pone.0125272.

Das, A., Nag, S., Mason, A. B., & Barroso, M. M. (2016). Endosome–mitochondria interactions are modulated by iron release from transferrin. *The Journal of Cell Biology*, *214*(7), 831–845. https://doi.org/10.1083/jcb.201602069.

Dexter, D. T., Wells, F. R., Lee, A. J., Agid, F., Agid, Y., Jenner, P., et al. (1989). Increased nigral iron content and alterations in other metal ions occurring in brain in Parkinson's disease. *Journal of Neurochemistry*, *52*, 1830–1836. https://doi.org/10.1111/j.1471-4159.1989.tb07264.x.

Duck, K. A., Neely, E. B., Simpson, I. A., & Connor, J. R. (2018). A role for sex and a common HFE gene variant in brain iron uptake. *Journal of Cerebral Blood Flow & Metabolism*, *38*(3), 540–548. https://doi.org/10.1177/0271678X17701949.

Duck, K. A., Simpson, I. A., & Connor, J. R. (2017). Regulatory mechanisms for iron transport across the blood-brain barrier. *Biochemical and Biophysical Research Communications*, *494*(1–2), 70–75. https://doi.org/10.1016/j.bbrc.2017.10.083.

Earle, K. M. (1968). Studies on Parkinson's disease including X-ray fluorescent spectroscopy of formalin fixed brain tissue. *Journal of Neuropathology and Experimental Neurology*, *27*, 1–14. https://doi.org/10.1097/00005072-196801000-00001.

Earley, C. J., Connor, J. R., Beard, J. L., Malecki, E. A., Epstein, D. K., & Allen, R. P. (2000). Abnormalities in CSF concentrations of ferritin and transferrin in restless legs syndrome. *Neurology*, *54*, 1698–1700. https://doi.org/10.1212/WNL.54.8.1698.

Ekbom, K. A. (1960). Restless legs syndrome. *Neurology*, *10*(9), 868 LP–868. Retrieved from http://n.neurology.org/content/10/9/868.abstract.

Enerson, B. E., & Drewes, L. R. (2006). The rat blood-brain barrier transcriptome. *Journal of Cerebral Blood Flow and Metabolism*, *26*, 959–973. https://doi.org/10.1038/sj.jcbfm.9600249.

Fiandra, L., Mazzucchelli, S., Truffi, M., Bellini, M., Sorrentino, L., & Corsi, F. (2016). In vitro permeation of FITC-loaded ferritins across a rat blood-brain barrier: A model to study the delivery of nanoformulated molecules. *Journal of Visualized Experiments*, (114), 1–9. https://doi.org/10.3791/54279.

Fisher, J., Devraj, K., Ingram, J., Slagle-Webb, B., Madhankumar, A. B., Liu, X., et al. (2007). Ferritin: A novel mechanism for delivery of iron to the brain and other organs. *American Journal of Physiology. Cell Physiology*, *293*(2), C641–C649. https://doi.org/10.1152/ajpcell.00599.2006.

Fishman, J. B., Rubin, J. B., Handrahan, J. V., Connor, J. R., & Fine, R. E. (1987). Receptor-mediated transcytosis of transferrin across the blood-brain barrier. *Journal of Neuroscience Research*, *18*(2), 299–304. https://doi.org/10.1002/jnr.490180206.

Fleming, D. J., Jacques, P. F., Massaro, J. M., D'Agostino, S., Wilson, P. W. F., & Wood, R. J. (2001). Aspirin intake and the use of serum ferritin as a measure of iron status. *The American Journal of Clinical Nutrition*, *74*, 219–226. https://doi.org/10.1093/ajcn/74.2.219.

Garrick, L. M., Dolan, K. G., Romano, M. A., & Garrick, M. D. (1999). Non-transferrin-bound iron uptake in Belgrade and normal rat erythroid cells. *Journal of Cellular Physiology*, *178*, 349–358. https://doi.org/10.1002/(SICI)1097-4652(199903)178:3 < 349::AID-JCP9 > 3.0.CO;2-R.

Gunshin, H., Mackenzie, B., Berger, U. V., Gunshin, Y., Romero, M. F., Boron, W. F., et al. (1997). Cloning and characterization of a mammalian proton-coupled metal-ion transporter. *Nature*, *388*, 482–488. https://doi.org/10.1038/41343.

Hagemeier, J., Dwyer, M. G., Bergsland, N., Schweser, F., Magnano, C. R., Heininen-Brown, M., et al. (2013). Effect of age on MRI phase behavior in the subcortical deep gray matter of healthy individuals. *American Journal of Neuroradiology*, *34*(11), 2144–2151. https://doi.org/10.3174/ajnr.A3569.

Hahn, P., Song, Y., Ying, G. s., He, X., Beard, J., & Dunaief, J. L. (2009). Age-dependent and gender-specific changes in mouse tissue iron by strain. *Experimental Gerontology*, *44*, 594–600. https://doi.org/10.1016/j.exger.2009.06.006.

Hallgren, B., & Sourander, P. (1958). The effect of age on the non-haemin iron in the human brain. *Journal of Neurochemistry*, *3*(1), 41–51. https://doi.org/10.1111/j.1471-4159.1958.tb12607.x.

Han, J., Seaman, W. E., Di, X., Wang, W., Willingham, M., Torti, F. M., et al. (2011). Iron uptake mediated by binding of H-ferritin to the TIM-2 receptor in mouse cells. *PLoS One*, *6*(8), 1–9. https://doi.org/10.1371/journal.pone.0023800.

Hilditch-Maguire, P., Trettel, F., Passani, L. A., Auerbach, A., Persichetti, F., & MacDonald, M. E. (2000). Huntingtin: An iron-regulated protein essential for normal nuclear and perinuclear organelles. *Human Molecular Genetics*, *9*, 2789–2797.

Hill, J. M., & Switzer, R. C. (1984). The regional distribution and cellular localization of iron in the rat brain. *Neuroscience*, *11*, 595–603. https://doi.org/10.1016/0306-4522(84)90046-0.

Hisa, T., Spence, S. E., Rachel, R. A., Fujita, M., Nakamura, T., Ward, J. M., et al. (2004). Hematopoietic, angiogenic and eye defects in Meis1 mutant animals. *The EMBO Journal*, *23*, 450–459. https://doi.org/10.1038/sj.emboj.7600038.

Ikeda, Y., & Long, D. M. (1990). The molecular basis of brain injury and brain edema: The role of oxygen free radicals. *Neurosurgery*, *27*, 1–11. https://doi.org/10.1227/00006123-199007000-00001.

Kell, D. B., & Pretorius, E. (2014). Serum ferritin is an important inflammatory disease marker, as it is mainly a leakage product from damaged cells. *Metallomics*, *6*(4), 748. https://doi.org/10.1039/c3mt00347g.

Kim, M., Rho, Y., Jin, K. S., Ahn, B., Jung, S., Kim, H., et al. (2011). pH-dependent structures of ferritin and apoferritin in solution: Disassembly and reassembly. *Biomacromolecules*, *12*(5), 1629–1640. https://doi.org/10.1021/bm200026v.

Knutson, M. D. (2018). Non-transferrin-bound iron transporters. *Free Radical Biology & Medicine*, *133*, 101–111. https://doi.org/10.1016/j.freeradbiomed.2018.10.413.

Lee, K. A., Zaffke, M. E., & Baratte-Beebe, K. (2001). Restless legs syndrome and sleep disturbance during pregnancy: The role of folate and iron. *Journal of Women's Health & Gender-Based Medicine*, *10*, 335–341. https://doi.org/10.1089/152460901750269652.

Li, L., Fang, C. J., Ryan, J. C., Niemi, E. C., Lebrón, J. A., Björkman, P. J., et al. (2010). Binding and uptake of H-ferritin are mediated by human transferrin receptor-1. *Proceedings of the National Academy of Sciences of the United States of America*, *107*(8), 3505–3510. https://doi.org/10.1073/pnas.0913192107.

Li, R., Luo, C., Mines, M., Zhang, J., & Fan, G.-H. (2006). Chemokine CXCL12 induces binding of ferritin heavy chain to the chemokine receptor CXCR4, alters CXCR4 signaling, and induces phosphorylation and nuclear translocation of ferritin heavy chain. *Journal of Biological Chemistry*, *281*(49), 37616–37627. https://doi.org/10.1074/jbc.M607266200.

Li, J. Y., Paragas, N., Ned, R. M., Qiu, A., Viltard, M., Leete, T., et al. (2009). Scara5 is a ferritin receptor mediating non-transferrin iron delivery. *Developmental Cell*, *16*(1), 35–46. https://doi.org/10.1016/j.devcel.2008.12.002.

Liuzzi, J. P., Aydemir, F., Nam, H., Knutson, M. D., & Cousins, R. J. (2006). Zip14 (Slc39a14) mediates non-transferrin-bound iron uptake into cells. *Proceedings of the National Academy of Sciences of the United States of America*, *103*, 13612–13617. https://doi.org/10.1109/21.21602.

Mazzucchelli, S., Bellini, M., Fiandra, L., Truffi, M., Rizzuto, M. A., Sorrentino, L., et al. (2016). Nanometronomic treatment of 4T1 breast cancer with nanocaged doxorubicin prevents drug resistance and circumvents cardiotoxicity. *Oncotarget*, *8*(5), 8383–8396. https://doi.org/10.18632/oncotarget.14204.
Mazzucchelli, S., Truffi, M., Baccarini, F., Beretta, M., Sorrentino, L., Bellini, M., et al. (2017). H-ferritin-nanocaged olaparib: A promising choice for both BRCA-mutated and sporadic triple negative breast cancer. *Scientific Reports*, 7(1), 7505. https://doi.org/10.1038/s41598-017-07617-7.
McCarthy, R. C., & Kosman, D. J. (2012). Mechanistic analysis of iron accumulation by endothelial cells of the BBB. *Biometals*, *25*, 665–675. https://doi.org/10.1007/s10534-012-9538-6.
McCarthy, R. C., & Kosman, D. J. (2014). Glial cell ceruloplasmin and hepcidin differentially regulate iron efflux from brain microvascular endothelial cells. *PLoS One*, *9*, e89003. https://doi.org/10.1371/journal.pone.0089003.
McCarthy, R. C., & Kosman, D. J. (2015a). Iron transport across the blood-brain barrier: Development, neurovascular regulation and cerebral amyloid angiopathy. *Cellular and Molecular Life Sciences*, *72*, 709–727. https://doi.org/10.1007/s00018-014-1771-4.
McCarthy, R. C., & Kosman, D. J. (2015b). Mechanisms and regulation of iron trafficking across the capillary endothelial cells of the blood-brain barrier. *Frontiers in Molecular Neuroscience*, *8*, 31. https://doi.org/10.3389/fnmol.2015.00031.
McDermott, J. L., Liu, B., & Dluzen, D. E. (1994). Sex differences and effects of estrogen on dopamine and dopac release from the striatum of male and female cd-1 mice. *Experimental Neurology*, *125*, 306–311. https://doi.org/10.1006/exnr.1994.1034.
Meadowcroft, M. D., Wang, J., Purnell, C. J., Peters, D. G., Eslinger, P. J., Neely, E. B., et al. (2016). Reduced white matter MRI transverse relaxation rate in cognitively normal H63D-HFE human carriers and H67D-HFE mice. *Brain Imaging and Behavior*, *10*, 1231–1242. https://doi.org/10.1007/s11682-015-9494-1.
Merryweather-Clarke, A. T., Pointon, J. J., Jouanolle, A. M., Rochette, J., & Robson, K. J. (2000). Geography of HFE C282Y and H63D mutations. *Genetic Testing*, *4*(2), 183–198. https://doi.org/10.1089/10906570050114902.
Merryweather-Clarke, A. T., Pointon, J. J., Shearman, J. D., & Robson, K. J. (1997). Global prevalence of putative haemochromatosis mutations. *Journal of Medical Genetics*, *34*, 275–278. https://doi.org/10.1136/jmg.34.4.275.
Meyron-Holtz, E. G., Moshe-Belizowski, S., & Cohen, L. A. (2011). A possible role for secreted ferritin in tissue iron distribution. *Journal of Neural Transmission*, *118*(3), 337–347. https://doi.org/10.1007/s00702-011-0582-0.
Mizuno, S., Mihara, T., Miyaoka, T., Inagaki, T., & Horiguchi, J. (2005). CSF iron, ferritin and transferrin levels in restless legs syndrome. *Journal of Sleep Research*, *14*(1), 43–47. https://doi.org/10.1111/j.1365-2869.2004.00403.x.
Moos, T., & Morgan, E. H. (2003). The significance of the mutated divalent metal transporter (DMT1) on iron transport into the Belgrade rat brain. *Journal of Neurochemistry*, *88*, 233–245. https://doi.org/10.1046/j.1471-4159.2003.02142.x.
Moos, T., Nielsen, T. R., Skjørringe, T., & Morgan, E. H. (2007). Iron trafficking inside the brain. *Journal of Neurochemistry*, *103*, 1730–1740. https://doi.org/10.1111/j.1471-4159.2007.04976.x.
Moos, T., Skjoerringe, T., Gosk, S., & Morgan, E. H. (2006). Brain capillary endothelial cells mediate iron transport into the brain by segregating iron from transferrin without the involvement of divalent metal transporter 1. *Journal of Neurochemistry*, *98*, 1946–1958. https://doi.org/10.1111/j.1471-4159.2006.04023.x.
Mrowczynski, O. D., Madhankumar, A. B., Slagle-Webb, B., Lee, S. Y., Zacharia, B. E., & Connor, J. R. (2017). HFE genotype affects exosome phenotype in cancer. *Biochimica et Biophysica Acta (BBA)—General Subjects*, *1861*(8), 1921–1928. https://doi.org/10.1016/j.bbagen.2017.05.014.

Munro, C. A., McCaul, M. E., Wong, D. F., Oswald, L. M., Zhou, Y., Brasic, J., et al. (2006). Sex differences in striatal dopamine release in healthy adults. *Biological Psychiatry, 59*, 966–974. https://doi.org/10.1016/j.biopsych.2006.01.008.

Nandar, W., & Connor, J. R. (2011). HFE gene variants affect iron in the brain. *The Journal of Nutrition, 141*(4), 729S–739S. https://doi.org/10.3945/jn.110.130351.

Nandar, W., Neely, E. B., Unger, E., & Connor, J. R. (2013). A mutation in the HFE gene is associated with altered brain iron profiles and increased oxidative stress in mice. *Biochimica et Biophysica Acta, 1832*(6), 729–741. https://doi.org/10.1016/j.bbadis.2013.02.009.

Norlander, N. B. (1953). Therapy in restless legs. *Acta Medica Scandinavica, 145*(6), 455–457. https://doi.org/10.1111/j.0954-6820.1953.tb07042.x.

Oexle, K., Schormair, B., Ried, J. S., Czamara, D., Heim, K., Frauscher, B., et al. (2013). Dilution of candidates: The case of iron-related genes in restless legs syndrome. *European Journal of Human Genetics, 21*(4), 410–414. https://doi.org/10.1038/ejhg.2012.193.

O'keeffe, S. T., Gavin, K., & Lavan, J. N. (1994). Iron status and restless legs syndrome in the elderly. *Age and Ageing, 23*, 200–203. https://doi.org/10.1093/ageing/23.3.200.

Owa, T., Taya, S., Miyashita, S., Yamashita, M., Adachi, T., Yamada, K., et al. (2018). Meis1 coordinates cerebellar granule cell development by regulating Pax6 transcription, BMP signaling and Atoh1 degradation. *The Journal of Neuroscience, 38*(5), 1277–1294. https://doi.org/10.1523/JNEUROSCI.1545-17.2017.

Patton, S. M., Wang, Q., Hulgan, T., Connor, J. R., Jia, P., Zhao, Z., et al. (2017). Cerebrospinal fluid (CSF) biomarkers of iron status are associated with CSF viral load, antiretroviral therapy, and demographic factors in HIV-infected adults. *Fluids and Barriers of the CNS, 14*(1), 11. https://doi.org/10.1186/s12987-017-0058-1.

Persson, N., Wu, J., Zhang, Q., Liu, T., Shen, J., Bao, R., et al. (2015). Age and sex related differences in subcortical brain iron concentrations among healthy adults. *NeuroImage, 122*, 385–398. https://doi.org/10.1016/j.neuroimage.2015.07.050.

Piñero, D., Jones, B., & Beard, J. (2000). Variations in dietary iron alter behavior in developing rats. *The Journal of Nutrition, 131*(2), 311–318. https://doi.org/10.1057/9780230210752_8.

Ponpuak, M., Mandell, M. A., Kimura, T., Chauhan, S., Cleyrat, C., & Deretic, V. (2015). Secretory autophagy. *Current Opinion in Cell Biology, 35*, 106–116. https://doi.org/10.1016/j.ceb.2015.04.016.

Rajan, K. S., Colburn, R. W., & Davis, J. M. (1976). Distribution of metal ions in the subcellular fractions of several rat brain areas. *Life Sciences, 18*, 423–431. https://doi.org/10.1016/0024-3205(76)90220-4.

Roberts, R. L., Fine, R. E., & Sandra, A. (1993). Receptor-mediated endocytosis of transferrin at the blood-brain barrier. *Journal of Cell Science, 104*, 521–532.

Siddappa, A. J. M., Rao, R. B., Wobken, J. D., Leibold, E. A., Connor, J. R., & Georgieff, M. K. (2002). Developmental changes in the expression of iron regulatory proteins and iron transport proteins in the perinatal rat brain. *Journal of Neuroscience Research, 68*, 761–775. https://doi.org/10.1002/jnr.10246.

Simpson, I. A., Ponnuru, P., Klinger, M. E., Myers, R. L., Devraj, K., Coe, C. L., et al. (2015). A novel model for brain iron uptake: Introducing the concept of regulation. *Journal of Cerebral Blood Flow and Metabolism, 35*, 48–57. https://doi.org/10.1038/jcbfm.2014.168.

Skjørringe, T., Burkhart, A., Johnsen, K. B., & Moos, T. (2015). Divalent metal transporter 1 (DMT1) in the brain: Implications for a role in iron transport at the blood-brain barrier, and neuronal and glial pathology. *Frontiers in Molecular Neuroscience, 8*, 19. https://doi.org/10.3389/fnmol.2015.00019.

Snyder, A. M., & Connor, J. R. (2009). Iron, the substantia nigra and related neurological disorders. *Biochimica et Biophysica Acta—General Subjects, 1790*(7), 606–614. https://doi.org/10.1016/j.bbagen.2008.08.005.

Sofic, E., Riederer, P., Heinsen, H., Beckmann, H., Reynolds, G. P., Hebenstreit, G., et al. (1988). Increased iron (III) and total iron content in post mortem substantia nigra of parkinsonian brain. *Journal of Neural Transmission*, *74*, 199–205. https://doi.org/10.1007/BF01244786.

Spieler, D., Kaffe, M., Knauf, F., Bessa, J., Tena, J. J., Giesert, F., et al. (2014). Restless legs syndrome-associated intronic common variant in Meis1 alters enhancer function in the developing telencephalon. *Genome Research*, *24*, 592–603. https://doi.org/10.1101/gr.166751.113.

Tanzi, R. E., & Hyman, B. T. (1991). Alzheimer's mutation [8]. *Nature*, *350*, 564. https://doi.org/10.1038/350564a0.

Tishler, T. A., Raven, E. P., Lu, P. H., Altshuler, L. L., & Bartzokis, G. (2012). Premenopausal hysterectomy is associated with increased brain ferritin iron. *Neurobiology of Aging*, *33*, 1950–1958. https://doi.org/10.1016/j.neurobiolaging.2011.08.002.

Todorich, B., Zhang, X., Slagle-Webb, B., Seaman, W. E., & Connor, J. R. (2008). Tim-2 is the receptor for H-ferritin on oligodendrocytes. *Journal of Neurochemistry*, *107*(6), 1495–1505. https://doi.org/10.1111/j.1471-4159.2008.05678.x.

Tran, T. N., Eubanks, S. K., Schaffer, K. J., Zhou, C. Y. J., & Linder, M. C. (1997). Secretion of ferritin by rat hepatoma cells and its regulation by inflammatory cytokines and iron. *Blood*, *90*(12), 4979–4986. https://doi.org/10.1145/36206.36201.

Trenkwalder, C., Hening, W. A., Walters, A. S., Campbell, S. S., Rahman, K., & Chokroverty, S. (1999). Circadian rhythm of periodic limb movements and sensory symptoms of restless legs syndrome. *Movement Disorders*, *14*, 102–110. https://doi.org/10.1002/1531-8257(199901)14:1<102::AID-MDS1017>3.0.CO;2-E.

Trotti, L. M., Bhadriraju, S., & Becker, L. A. (2009). Iron for restless legs syndrome. *Cochrane Database of Systematic Reviews*, (2), CD007834. https://doi.org/10.1016/S1571-0661(05)80190-2.

Truman-Rosentsvit, M., Berenbaum, D., Spektor, L., Cohen, L. A., Belizowsky-Moshe, S., Lifshitz, L., et al. (2018). Ferritin is secreted via 2 distinct nonclassical vesicular pathways. *Blood*, *131*(3), 342–352. https://doi.org/10.1182/blood-2017-02-768580.

Uchino, E., Tsuzuki, T., & Inoue, K. (1990). The effects of age and sex on seven elements in Sprague-Dawley rat organs. *Laboratory Animals*, *24*, 253–264. https://doi.org/10.1258/002367790780866182.

Wang, C. Y., Jenkitkasemwong, S., Duarte, S., Sparkman, B. K., Shawki, A., Mackenzie, B., et al. (2012). ZIP8 is an iron and zinc transporter whose cell-surface expression is up-regulated by cellular iron loading. *The Journal of Biological Chemistry*, *287*, 34032–34043. https://doi.org/10.1074/jbc.M112.367284.

Whitfield, J. B., Treloar, S., Zhu, G., Powell, L. W., & Martin, N. G. (2003). Relative importance of female-specific and non-female-specific effects on variation in iron stores between women. *British Journal of Haematology*, *120*, 860–866. https://doi.org/10.1046/j.1365-2141.2003.04224.x.

Winkelmann, J., Schormair, B., Lichtner, P., Ripke, S., Xiong, L., Jalilzadeh, S., et al. (2007). Genome-wide association study of restless legs syndrome identifies common variants in three genomic regions. *Nature Genetics*, *39*, 1000–1006. https://doi.org/10.1038/ng2099.

Xiong, L., Catoire, H., Dion, P., Gaspar, C., Lafrenière, R. G., Girard, S. L., et al. (2009). MEIS1 intronic risk haplotype associated with restless legs syndrome affects its mRNA and protein expression levels. *Human Molecular Genetics*, *18*(6), 1065–1074. https://doi.org/10.1093/hmg/ddn443.

Xu, J., & Ling, E. a. (1994). Studies of the ultrastructure and permeability of the blood-brain barrier in the developing corpus callosum in postnatal rat brain using electron dense tracers. *Journal of Anatomy*, *184*(Pt 2), 227–237.

Xu, X., Wang, Q., & Zhang, M. (2008). Age, gender, and hemispheric differences in iron deposition in the human brain: An in vivo MRI study. *NeuroImage*, *40*(1), 35–42. https://doi.org/10.1016/j.neuroimage.2007.11.017.

Youdim, M. B., Ben-Shachar, D., Ashkenazi, R., & Yehuda, S. (1983). Brain iron and dopamine receptor function. *Advances in Biochemical Psychopharmacology*, *37*, 309–321. https://doi.org/6138953.

Yu, Y. J., Atwal, J. K., Zhang, Y., Tong, R. K., Wildsmith, K. R., Tan, C., et al. (2014). Therapeutic bispecific antibodies cross the blood-brain barrier in nonhuman primates. *Science Translational Medicine*, *6*(261), 1–10. https://doi.org/10.1126/scitranslmed.3009835.

Zuchero, Y. J. Y., Chen, X., Bien-Ly, N., Bumbaca, D., Tong, R. K., Gao, X., et al. (2016). Discovery of novel blood-brain barrier targets to enhance brain uptake of therapeutic antibodies. *Neuron*, *89*(1), 70–82. https://doi.org/10.1016/j.neuron.2015.11.024.

Further reading

Chiou, B., Lucassen, E., Sather, M., Kallianpur, A., & Connor, J. (2018). Semaphorin4A and H-ferritin utilize Tim-1 on human oligodendrocytes: A novel neuro-immune axis. *Glia*, *66*(7), 1317–1330. https://doi.org/10.1002/glia.23313.

CHAPTER SEVEN

Caenorhabditis elegans and its applicability to studies on restless legs syndrome

Pan Chen[a], Omamuyovwi Meashack Ijomone[a,b], Kun He Lee[a], Michael Aschner[a,*]

[a]Department of Molecular Pharmacology, Albert Einstein College of Medicine, Bronx, NY, United States
[b]Department of Human Anatomy, Federal University of Technology, Akure, Nigeria
*Corresponding author: e-mail address: michael.aschner@einstein.yu.edu

Contents

Abstract

Restless legs syndrome (RLS) is a common neurological disorder in the United States. This disorder is characterized by an irresistible urge to move the legs, although the symptoms vary in a wide range. The pathobiology of RLS has been linked to iron (Fe) deficiency and dopaminergic (DAergic) dysfunction. Several genetic factors have been reported to increase the risk of RLS. *Caenorhabditis elegans* (*C. elegans*) is a well-established animal model with a fully sequenced genome, which is highly conserved with mammals. Given the detailed knowledge of its genomic architecture, ease of genetic manipulation and conserved biosynthetic and metabolic pathways, as well as its small size, ease of maintenance, speedy generation time and large brood size,

Advances in Pharmacology, Volume 84
ISSN 1054-3589
https://doi.org/10.1016/bs.apha.2018.12.003
© 2019 Elsevier Inc.
All rights reserved.

C. elegans provides numerous advantages in studying RLS-associated gene-environment interactions. Here we will review current knowledge about RLS symptoms, pathology and treatments, and discuss the application of *C. elegans* in RLS study, including the worm homologous genes and methods that could be performed to advance the pathophysiology RLS.

Abbreviations

AD Alzheimer's disease
ADHD attention-deficit/hyperactivity disorder
C. elegans *Caenorhabditis elegans*
CNS central nervous system
DA dopamine
DAergic dopaminergic
Fe iron
GFP green fluorescent protein
GWAS genome-wide association studies
HD Huntington's disease
HPLC high-performance liquid chromatography
ICP-MS inductively coupled plasma mass spectrometry
Mn manganese
MRI magnetic resonance imaging
PD Parkinson's disease
RLS restless legs syndrome
SNPs single-nucleotide polymorphisms
TEM transmission electronic microscopy
TH tyrosine hydroxylase

1. Introduction

Restless legs syndrome (RLS) is a neurological disorder affecting ~10% of people in the United States, and ~2.5% of the population exhibit symptoms serious enough to seek medical attention (Allen, Bharmal, & Calloway, 2011). RLS is often neglected or misdiagnosed especially when the symptoms are intermittent or mild. The primary symptom of RLS is an irresistible urge to move one's legs to relieve discomfort, with four common accompanying clinical features: (1) sensations starting at rest (e.g., creeping, crawling, burning, tingling, painful or indescribable); (2) symptoms worsen later during the day or at night; (3) partial or temporary relief with motor activity; and (4) leg twitching at night. ~80% of RLS patients have involuntary twitching leg movements either when asleep or awake that recurs on a semi-regular basis (Periodic Limb Movements, PLMs) (Allen et al., 2003). These symptoms often result in sleep deprivation, which can seriously impact life quality to a degree similar to osteoarthritis, hypertension or diabetes (Allen et al., 2005). Patients may ceaselessly walk at night with job tardiness, lost work productivity, unemployment, anxiety, depression and attention-deficit/hyperactivity disorder (ADHD) symptoms (Allen et al., 2011; Wagner, Walters, & Fisher, 2004). Finally, RLS may portend more serious consequences, including hypertension, heart disease and stroke (Li et al., 2012; Pennestri, Montplaisir, Colombo, Lavigne, & Lanfranchi, 2007; Siddiqui et al., 2007; Walters & Rye, 2009).

RLS is associated with structural and biochemical changes in the brain. Iron (Fe) deficiency and altered dopaminergic (DAergic) system have been closely related to RLS. All studies to date support a role for diminished brain Fe in RLS, even when blood Fe stores appear to be normal (Connor et al., 2008). Fe is a cofactor of tyrosine hydroxylase (TH), the rate-limiting step in dopamine (DA) synthesis, and required for DA production. Fe deficiency causes DA receptor dysfunction (Beard, Erikson, & Jones, 2003). Autopsy studies have shown up-regulation of TH and decreased DA D2 receptors in the basal ganglia of RLS patients (Connor et al., 2009). Magnetic resonance imaging (MRI) studies have shown mild presynaptic and postsynaptic deficits in nigrostriatal DAergic pathways in RLS patients (Tan, 2006; Wetter, Eisensehr, & Trenkwalder, 2004). The DAergic agonists, pramipexole and ropinirole, have been approved to treat moderate to severe RLS. RLS exhibits both familial and non-familiar (idiopathic) forms, with ~60% of cases having a family history of the disease (Lazzarini et al., 1999; Montplaisir et al., 1997; Trenkwalder, Seidel, Gasser, & Oertel, 1996; Walters et al., 1996; Winkelmann, Stautner, Samtleben, & Trenkwalder, 2002). Independent genome-wide association studies (GWAS) reported single-nucleotide polymorphisms (SNPs) in four genes that impart increased risk of having RLS. These genes (and SNPs) are *MEIS1* (rs2300478), *BTBD9* (rs9357271), *MAP2K5* (rs1026732), and *PTPRD* (Kemlink et al., 2009; Schormair et al., 2008; Stefansson et al., 2007; Winkelmann et al., 2007; Yang, Li, Chen, et al., 2011; Yang, Li, Yang, et al., 2011).

Caenorhabditis elegans (*C. elegans*) offers a rubust model for dissecting neuropathological mechanisms of RLS, given the simplicity of this model organism. First of all, *C. elegans* has ~20,000 genes, with up to 80% of corresponding human homologs, including many genetic risk factors of human diseases (Titus & Michael, 2006). Second, the small size, short generation time, large brood size and ease of maintenance allow for a nearly limitless worm supply for cellular, molecular and genetic analysis. The adult nematode is only ~1 mm long and it takes 3 days from a fresh embryo to a reproductive adult, which can lay ~300 eggs when self-inseminated. The worm feed on bacterium-*Escherichia coli* (*E. coli*), and a large population (millions) of worms can be harvested on a 100 mm petri-dish within couple days. Third, the transparency of worms, when combined with fluorescent proteins, allows in vivo study of various cellular and intracellular activities, such as gene transcription, protein function, endocytosis, fat metabolism, axon guidance and neurodegeneration, etc. Fourth, many tools are available for various studies. The genome, cell lineage and 3D anatomy of *C. elegans* have been mapped out. A large pool of mutants, covering majority of the genome, can be directly ordered from *C. elegans* genetic center (CGC) or the national bioresource project (NBRP). Genome editing by CRISPR-Cas9 technology and conventional transgenic techniques can be readily performed (Mello, Kramer, Stinchcomb, & Ambros, 1991; Schwartz & Jorgensen, 2016). Over 90% of genes can be easily knocked down by bacteria feeding using the RNA interference (RNAi) library (Kamath et al., 2003). Fifth, the worm is sensitive to biometals and a wide-range of neuroactive drugs and xenobiotics, which facilitates the discovery of pharmaceutic compounds (Avery & Horvitz, 1990; Jayanthi et al., 1998; Lewis, 1980; Morgan, Sedensky, Meneely, & Cascorbi, 1988). Last but not the least, *C. elegans* has a simple and well-characterized nervous system. An adult hermaphrodite has a total of 302 neurons and ~8000 synapses, yet their neurotransmitters, Fe channels and synaptic components are highly conversed with human (Hobert, 2013). Regarding the DAergic system, *C. elegans* hermaphrodites possess eight identifiable DAergic neurons (Sulston, Dew, & Brenner, 1975). All genes responsible for DA biosynthesis, packaging, reuptake and degradation have recognizable orthologues in the worm genome, including tyrosine hydroxylase (TH/*cat-2*), GTP cyclohydrolase I (GTPCH/*cat-4*), aromatic amino acid decarboxylase (AADC/*bas-1*), monoamine oxidase (MAO/*amx-1,2,3*), catechol-*O*-methyl transferase (COMT/*comt-1,2,3,4,5*), vesicular monoamine transporter (VMAT/*cat-1*) and DA transporter (DAT/*dat-1*) (Hobert, 2013; Jayanthi et al., 1998). These eight neurons are more sensitive to environmental toxins than other neurons in worms (Benedetto, Au, Avila, Milatovic, & Aschner, 2010). Given these features, *C. elegans* has been widely used to decipher genetic and environmental aspects of neurological disorders, such as Alzheimer's disease (AD), Parkinson's disease (PD), Huntington's disease (HD), to name a few. In this review, we will address the symptoms, causes and treatment of RLS, and explore the potential techniques and methods to study the pathology of RLS in *C. elegans*.

2. RLS symptoms, potential causes and treatments

2.1 Symptoms

The main characteristics of RLS are symptoms of neurosensation. These include robust feelings of restiveness and distressful prickling-like sensations in the legs (Garcia-Borreguero & Cano-Pumarega, 2017). These are accompanied by an irresistible longing to move the body, particularly the legs, to relieve the unbearable sensations. Patients often describe these feelings of restiveness and distressful sensations as tingling, crawling tingling, creeping, pulling or painful within one or both lower limbs (Trenkwalder, Paulus, & Walters, 2005). RLS also affects other parts of the body as well. It is known that the longer the condition persists, the more likely the arms or the other regions of the body become symptomatic. These symptoms are said to typically become evident when patients are at rest, with a higher possibility of symptoms occurring during a relaxed or cosy state (Garcia-Borreguero & Cano-Pumarega, 2017; Trenkwalder et al., 2005). RLS symptoms commonly show a circadian rhythm, with symptoms being worse in the evenings, followed by short lessening after waking up in the morning (Garcia-Borreguero & Cano-Pumarega, 2017). Consequently, patient's sleep is affected. The lack of proper sleep (insomnia) that accompanies RLS is the main reason behind a patient looking for medical consultation. Struggle to initiate sleep is the most common insomnia-related issues associated with RLS.

RLS symptoms differ substantially in regularity from barely once a month or year to daily. Also, symptoms show varying degree of severity from slightly disturbing to incapacitating, and symptoms may also attenuate for varying periods (Allen et al., 2014). Patient's health-related quality of life (HRQoL) is affected depending on the severity of symptoms. In patients with mild RLS, the symptoms happen relatively less frequent, show reduced severity and only slightly influence sleep. Patients with severe RLS symptoms show obvious deficits in general health, vitality, physicality, emotional and social stability among other features (Trenkwalder et al., 2005). Mostly, these patients complain of having trouble in normal life schedules almost on daily basis, including poor performance on their jobs and social functions. Diagnosis of RLS is based on symptoms reported by patients. Current diagnostic criteria for RLS are highlighted in Table 1.

Table 1 Diagnostic criteria for RLS.

Essential diagnostic criteria (all must be met)

- An urge to move the legs usually but not always accompanied by or felt to be caused by uncomfortable and unpleasant sensations in the legs.
- The urge to move the legs and any accompanying unpleasant sensations begin or worsen during periods of rest or inactivity such as lying down or sitting.
- The urge to move the legs and any accompanying unpleasant sensations are partially or
- Totally relieved by movement, such as walking or stretching, at least as long as the activity continues.
- The urge to move the legs and any accompanying unpleasant sensations during rest or inactivity only occur or are worse in the evening or night than during the day.
- The occurrence of the above features is not solely accounted for as symptoms primary to another medical or a behavioral condition (e.g., myalgia, venous stasis, leg oedema, arthritis, leg cramps, positional discomfort, habitual foot tapping).

Specifiers for Clinical Course of RLS

- Chronic-persistent RLS: symptoms left untreated would occur on average at least two times a week for the past year.
- Intermittent RLS: symptoms left untreated treated would occur on average less than two times in a week for the past year, with at least five lifetime events.

Specifier for Clinical Significance of RLS

- RLS symptoms cause significant distress or impairment in social, occupational, educational or other important areas of functioning by the impact on sleep, energy/vitality, daily activities, behavior, cognition or mood.

2012 Revised International Restless Legs Syndrome Study Group (IRLSSG) Diagnostic Criteria for RLS. http://irlssg.org/diagnostic-criteria/

2.2 Causes

The pathology of RLS remains unclear. However, current research has identified several genetic risk factors, as well as anomalies in iron metabolism and DAergic neurotransmission. Additionally, other systems, including opiates, adenosine, orexin and glutamate may be involved in RLS pathogenesis.

RLS has been found to associate with both genetic and environmental risk factors. Several studies have reported robust association between onset of RLS and predisposing genetics. Genome-wide association studies (GWAS) have demonstrated several single-nucleotide polymorphisms associated with RLS, including BTBD9 (on chromosome6p21.2), MEIS1 (on chromosome 2p14), MAP2K5/SCOR1 (on chromosome 15q23), PTPRD (on chromosome 9p24.1-p23), and chromosome 16q12.1 (Garcia-Borreguero & Cano-Pumarega, 2017). Deficiency in Fe has been repeatedly demonstrated to involve in RLS pathogenesis. Particularly Fe stores in the central nervous system (CNS) have been depleted in RLS patients, even when systemic Fe levels are normal. However, low serum Fe and/or ferritin levels have also been linked with several cases of RLS (Ward, Zucca, Duyn, Crichton, & Zecca, 2014). The severity of RLS has been correlated with a reduction in brain Fe levels. MRI studies have shown that Fe levels decrease in the substantia nigra and putamen of RLS patients, particularly in severe cases (Moon et al., 2014). These brain regions are the major sites of CNS dopaminergic neurotransmission, hence there is likely an association between low Fe in these regions and dopaminergic dysfunction in RLS. Fe is a cofactor for tyrosine hydroxylase (the rate-limiting enzyme in dopamine production), hence Fe deficiency may affect dopaminergic systems in the brain. However, this potential link largely remains unclear (Bogan & Cheray, 2013; Dauvilliers & Winkelmann, 2013).

The case for DAergic dysfunction in pathogenesis of RLS is mostly due to effects seen upon administration of drugs that modulates DAergic neurotransmission. DAergic medications have been reported to relieve RLS symptoms whereas antagonists of dopamine worsen the symptoms. Interestingly, the need for DAergic medications to be able to cross the blood brain barrier as a determinant for a positive effect on RLS demonstrates that DA actions in the central nervous system but not the peripheral nervous system is involved in RLS (Bogan & Cheray, 2013; Galbiati et al., 2015; Garcia-Borreguero et al., 2013; Garcia-Borreguero & Williams, 2014). The number of DA transporters may be decreased in RLS, as shown by a PET study (Earley et al., 2011). Additionally, lesion of the area where DAergic pathway projects to spinal cord (area A11) led to overactivity in a rodent model, although this could not be corroborated in autopsy study of RLS patients (Garcia-Borreguero & Cano-Pumarega, 2017).

2.3 Treatments

Treatment for RLS can be grouped into non-pharmacological and pharmacological approaches. Use of pharmacological substance should be started when patient's quality of life, social functioning, daytime activities and sleep becomes impaired as a result of RLS symptoms. Non-pharmacological options should be used before drug options are considered. Non-pharmacological options may be adequate in cases of mild or rare occurrence of RLS symptoms, though there is dearth of evidence regarding their efficacy and practicability in management of RLS (Symvoulakis, Anyfantakis, & Lionis, 2010; Trenkwalder et al., 2005).

Non-pharmacological options are commonly targeted toward improving patient's sleep quality primarily via activities that attain healthier sleeping habits (Symvoulakis et al., 2010). These usually require modifying patients' overall lifestyle. Patients are encouraged to develop structured sleep routines, with consistent times for beginning sleep and waking up. Activities that could hinder particularly preceding sleeping times should be avoided, and sleeping environments should be made relaxed and quiet to encourage ease of sleep (Symvoulakis et al., 2010). Other lifestyle modifications may include reducing or avoiding intake of alcohol, nicotine or caffeine as these are known to intensify RLS symptoms. Additionally, medications that worsen RLS symptoms, such as antidepressants, antihistamines, DA antagonists, should be discontinued. Furthermore moderate levels of exercise daily, massages and use of hot baths may also result in respite from RLS symptoms (Symvoulakis et al., 2010).

Oral Fe supplementations and in some cases, intravenous Fe administration can be used, particularly in patients with low serum ferritin (Trenkwalder, Winkelmann, Inoue, & Paulus, 2015). However, DAergic agents are considered the first line of pharmacological treatments for RLS (Garcia-Borreguero & Cano-Pumarega, 2017). These drugs which have dopamine increasing effects have been demonstrated to attenuate RLS symptoms, particularly when taken at bedtime. Pramipexole, ropinirole and rotigotine are FDA approved medications for the treatment of moderate to severe RLS. A combination of levodopa and carbidopa has been shown to be effective following intermittent use (Garcia-Borreguero & Cano-Pumarega, 2017). These agents, while well tolerated, have their side effects. Common side effects include gastrointestinal complaints, nausea, daytime sleepiness and other short-time side effects. Additionally, long-term use of these agents may result in exacerbation of RLS symptoms (Garcia-Borreguero & Cano-Pumarega, 2017). Furthermore, some patients on these DAergic agonists may develop compulsive behaviors such as pathological gambling, eating, shopping or hypersexuality (Garcia-Borreguero & Cano-Pumarega, 2017; Trenkwalder et al., 2015). Besides, antiseizure agents are becoming a better choice of treatment for RLS. Gabapentin enacarbil has been approved by FDA for treatment of moderate to severe RLS. This drug is as effective as the DAergic agonists and with no reports of exacerbation of symptoms (Garcia-Borreguero & Cano-Pumarega, 2017).

Another class of medications used for RLS treatment includes opioids and benzodiazepines. Opioids, such as oxycodone, are used in individuals with more severe RLS symptoms which do not get improved following other medications. There are several side effects associated with these agents as well as the risk of addiction. Benzodiazepines can be useful to obtain a more relaxing sleep; however, they may cause or worsen sleep apnea. These agents are mostly used as last line of therapy, particularly during severe augmentation (Garcia-Borreguero & Cano-Pumarega, 2017; Trenkwalder et al., 2005, 2015).

3. RLS genetics

RLS exhibits both familial and non-familiar (idiopathic) forms, with ~60% of cases having a family history of the disease (Lazzarini et al., 1999; Montplaisir et al., 1997; Trenkwalder et al., 1996; Walters et al., 1996; Winkelmann et al., 2002). In a familial study in a French-Canadian population, siblings of an RLS patient had 3.6 times the risk of themselves having RLS, and an offspring, 1.8 times (Xiong et al., 2010). For early-onset RLS patients, Allen et al. also reported a greater risk for RLS among the patients' first-degree relatives compared to the first-degree relatives of late-onset RLS patients (23.6% vs 10.1%). The same study found that first-degree and second-degree relatives of RLS patients generally had higher risk of developing RLS than did the relatives of non-RLS suffering individuals (Allen, La Buda, Becker, & Earley, 2002). Twin studies also have revealed the genetic nature of RLS. Ondo et al. showed a concordance rate of 83.3% between monozygotic twins for RLS, despite varying symptom descriptions and ages of onset. They also showed evidence for genetic anticipation—patients' having earlier onset of symptoms if they have family history of RLS (Ondo, Vuong, & Wang, 2000). Higher concordance rate was observed in monozygotic twins than dizygotic twins (Xiong et al., 2007). Female sex has been linked to increased risk of RLS as well. Even among both monozygotic and dizygotic twins, female predominance of RLS patients has been shown (Xiong et al., 2007). In fact, in a Turkish family, all affected individuals were women (Akpinar, Turker, Aygun, & Aytac, 2017).

Genome-wide association studies (GWAS) have reported single-nucleotide polymorphisms (SNPs) in several genes that impart increased risk

Table 2 Genetic risk factors of RLS.

RLS genetic risk factors	Proposed functions in the nervous system	Predicted *C. elegans* orthologs[a]
MEIS1	Neurogenesis	UNC-62
BTBD9	Long-term memory potentiation, Fe homeostasis	HPO-9
PTPRD	Axonal guidance/myelination, neural development	PTP-3
MAP2K5	Neurogenesis	MEK-2
TOX3	Neural protection in CNS injury, neurogenesis	HMG-6

[a]The orthologs are predicted based on their amino acid sequence similarity, but have not been individually verified.

of having RLS (Table 2). In German and French-Canadian RLS cases, three loci were identified: MEIS1, a homeobox gene, BTBD9 containing a BTB domain, and MAP2K5, a mitogen-activated protein kinase (Winkelmann et al., 2007). TOX3, which contains a high mobility group (HMG) box, and PTPRD, encoding for protein tyrosine phosphatase receptor type D, have also been shown to be associated with RLS (Moore et al., 2014). MEIS1, BTBD9, MAP2K5, and TOX3 polymorphisms and their association with RLS have been shown in other ethnic populations around the world as well (Haba-Rubio et al., 2016; Li et al., 2017; Vilarino-Guell, Farrer, & Lin, 2008; Yang, Li, Chen, et al., 2011). Stefansson et al. showed that BTBD9 is associated with Fe depletion, which is consistent with currently accepted pathogenesis of RLS (Stefansson et al., 2007). MEIS1 has been shown to be associated with defective Fe homeostasis as well (Vilarino-Guell et al., 2009).

Genes associated with common risk factors and treatment of RLS have been studied in association with RLS. Garcia-Martin et al. showed that allelic variants of heme oxygenases-1 and 2, enzymes which degrade the heme protein and commonly associated with Parkinson's disease, were lower in patients with RLS (Garcia-Martin et al., 2015). Given improvement on RLS symptoms with GABAergic medications, Jimenez-Jimenez et al. showed that the frequencies of GABA receptor gene rho three allelic variant rs832032T was significantly higher in RLS patients than in controls (Jimenez-Jimenez et al., 2018).

4. *C. elegans* homologs of RLS and their function

C. elegans is a free-living nematode that was established as a model organism for the study of human disease pathophysiology by Sydney Brenner in middle of 20th century (Corsi, Wightman, & Chalfie, 2015). Since then, *C. elegans* has been studied extensively to shed light on processes such as establishing genetic bases of programmed cell death and stress-induced sleep (Ellis & Horvitz, 1986; Nelson et al., 2014). *C. elegans* has many advantages as a genetic tool, including inexpensive cost of maintenance, rapid lifecycle, and fully sequenced genome (Corsi et al., 2015).

Previous studies have revealed the function of several RLS genes in *C. elegans* and other animal models. Myeloid ectopic viral integration site 1, or MEIS1, is a homeoprotein belonging to a subfamily of three amino acid loop extension (TALE) homeoproteins, which are important in embryonic survival and development, including hematopoiesis and angiogenesis (Azcoitia, Aracil, Martinez, & Torres, 2005; Barber et al., 2013). As a transcription factor, MEIS1 has also been implicated in the pathogenesis of malignancies (Zhu et al., 2017). In the nervous system, MEIS1 was shown to be critical in neurogenesis, and its inactivation leads to sudden cardiac deaths in mice secondary to altered sympathetic innervation of the heart (Barber & Rastegar, 2010; Bouilloux et al., 2016). The importance of MEIS1 in *C. elegans* has also been observed. Arata et al. confirmed that a Meis-related gene, *psa-3*, is essential in determining the fate of hypodermal cells, and Van Auken et al. showed mutation in *unc-62*, an ortholog of MEIS1, causes early embryonic arrest or death (Arata et al., 2006; Van Auken et al., 2002). In *C. elegans*, UNC-62::GFP is expressed in a variety of tissues in the hermaphrodite, including the hypodermis, the intestine and the nervous system (Fig. 1) (Van Nostrand, Sánchez-Blanco, Wu, Nguyen, & Kim, 2013). Interestingly, UNC-62 is expressed in DAergic neurons (Fig. 1), which facilitates study of its function in DAergic system. Using RNA interference, Catoire et al. showed that decreased expression of UNC-62 was associated with increased the expression of ferritin in *C. elegans*, supporting the derangement of Fe homeostasis in the pathophysiology of RLS (Catoire et al., 2011).

BTB domain containing 9, or BTBD9, gene encodes for a protein with two domains: at the N-terminus is a bric-a-brac, tramtrack (BTB), broad complex/pox virus and zinc finger domain, which has been associated with regulation of transcription, and at the C-terminus is a BTB and Kelch, associated with ubiquination (DeAndrade, Zhang, et al., 2012). The overall

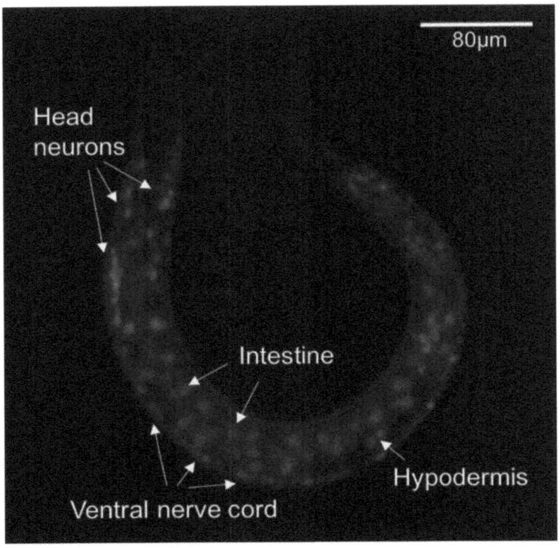

Fig. 1 The expression pattern of UNC-62 in *C. elegans*. Strain SD1897 carries a translational GFP fusion UNC-62:GFP. At Larva 1 stage, GFP is seen in the intestine, hypodermis, head neurons and the ventral nerve cord. *Image was taken using Zeiss LSM5 Live Duo Scan.*

function of BTBD9, however, is currently not established (Li, Doroodchi, Yang, & DeAndrade, 2011). In mice, BTBD9 deficiency has been shown to impair pre-synaptic activity and enhance long-term memory potentiation (DeAndrade, Zhang, et al., 2012). Btbd9 knock-out mice also have been established as a murine model for RLS, given their motor restlessness, resting-phase sensory alterations, altered Fe homeostasis, and symptomatic resolution upon administration of ropinirole, a dopaminergic agonist commonly used for the treatment of RLS (DeAndrade, Johnson, et al., 2012). HPO-9, the *C. elegans* ortholog of BTBD9, has been shown to be involved in embryonic and larval development and response to bacterial infection (Kao et al., 2011; McKay et al., 2003; Simmer et al., 2003). However, its role in the nervous system remains to be investigated. *C. elegans* model of RLS based on *hpo-9* knockout showed alterations in egg-laying behavior and locomotion, but the nematode model has not been fully characterized (Li et al., 2011). In addition, KEL-8, a BTB-Kelch containing protein, has been shown to regulate synaptic transmission via its association with GLR-1, a glutamate receptor. Specifically, mutants for *kel-8* have increased GLR-1 levels in neurons and a higher frequency of spontaneous reversals of body bends (Schaefer & Rongo, 2006).

Protein tyrosine phosphatase, receptor type D (PTPRD), a member of the leukocyte common antigen-related subfamily of receptor protein tyrosine phosphatases, has been implicated in multiple disease processes, including non-alcoholic fatty liver disease, laryngeal squamous cell carcinoma, diabetes mellitus, and hypertension (Chen, Xu, et al., 2016; Gong et al., 2015; Li et al., 2015; Nakajima et al., 2018; Szaumkessel et al., 2017. In the CNS, PTPRD has been shown to play a role in axonal guidance and neuronal development. In mice, Shishikura et al. showed through immunohistochemistry that PTPRD is localized to olfactory bulb, cerebral cortex, hippocampus, cerebellum, and several brainstem nuclei. At the cellular level, PTPRD was shown to be expressed not only in the axons, but also in dendrites (Shishikura et al., 2016). Zhu et al. demonstrated time and spatial variations in the expression of PTPRD in the embryonic and post-natal CNS of mice, and that PTPRD mutants had a defective axonal myelination process (Zhu et al., 2015). In *C. elegans*, PTP-3 is the only known ortholog of PTPRD, and it also has been implicated in similar processes in the nervous system (Ackley et al., 2005). Nakamura et al. showed that PTP-3 in *C. elegans* plays a role in cortical dendritic growth and axonal guidance (Nakamura et al., 2017). Ackley et al. demonstrated that two isomers of PTP-3, PTP-3A and PTP-3B, may play a different role. PTP-3A was shown to localize specifically at neuronal synapses, while, PTP-3B, extrasynaptically. Furthermore, PTP-3B rescued axon guidance defect caused by *ptp-3* mutation, whereas PTP-3A could not. Still, mutation in PTP-3A caused altered synaptic morphology (Ackley et al., 2005).

Mitogen-activated protein kinase kinase 5, or MAP2K5, belongs to the MAP kinase kinase family, and thus it plays a critical role in cellular signal transduction pathways (Zhou, Bao, & Dixon, 1995). In humans, MAP2K5 activity is associated with many disease states, including colorectal cancer, obesity, RLS, and prostate cancer (Diao et al., 2016; Li et al., 2017; Mehta et al., 2003; Rask-Andersen et al., 2012). In mice, Map2k5 has been implicated in cellular differentiation, apoptosis, sarcomere hypertrophy, among other processes (Kaneshiro, Otsuki, Yoshida, Yoshikawa, & Higuchi, 2015; Nicol et al., 2001; Sohn, Lewis, & Winoto, 2008). Knock-out of Map2k5 has been shown to enhance adult neurogenesis in the olfactory bulb on mice as well (Wang et al., 2015). The closest *C. elegans* ortholog of MAP2K5 is MEK-2, a MAP kinase kinase that has been shown to be associated in viability of larvae, development of the vulva, egg-laying, and immune system

(Hsu, Zobel, Lambie, Schedl, & Kornfeld, 2002; Nicholas & Hodgkin, 2004; Wu, Han, & Guan, 1995). MEK-2's role in the nervous system of the nematode has not been well-studied, however.

Along with its association with RLS, TOX high mobility group box family member 3, or TOX3, has been associated with breast cancer, Parkinson's disease, and polycystic ovarian syndrome in humans (Li et al., 2018; Mohtashami et al., 2018; Ning, Jiayi, Jian, & Wanli, 2017). In the CNS of mice, Tox3 has been shown to be expressed mainly in the developing embryonic brain in the neural stem cells (Sahu et al., 2016). There is evidence that shows increased expression of Tox3 leads to neural protection and facilitates recovery in spinal cord injury in mice via protection of oligodendrocytes (Bastien et al., 2015). The closest predicted ortholog of TOX3 in *C. elegans* is HMG-6, which has been shown to be expressed in neurons and sperm (Blazie et al., 2017; Lockhead et al., 2016; Spencer et al., 2011). However, there has not been any evidence establishing its function in the nematode so far.

5. *C. elegans* methods for RLS study

Given the above features, *C. elegans* provides a robust model in delineating the pathogenesis, and progression of RLS, as well as testing therapeutic measures particularly aspects requiring genetic modifications. Below we present a few areas where this model organism is suitable to research into RLS.

5.1 Circadian rhythms

It is well established that RLS symptoms demonstrate a circadian pattern, with several symptoms worsening at bedtime. Understanding how circadian rhythms influence RLS symptoms is thus an essential to unraveling the disorder. Organisms demonstrate circadian rhythmicity in physiology and behavior that is timed to an approximately 24 h period, and this rhythm appears to be strongly conserved. Circadian rhythm in organisms appears to be driven by clock-controlled feedback loop of transcriptional and translational processes and/or through post-transcription or post-translation alterations. In this feedback loop, transcription factors drive expression of clock genes such as *tim* (timeless) and *per* (period) that then induces negative regulation of their own transcription, thus generating an oscillatory rhythms of gene expression within the approximately 24 h period. These biological rhythms are synchronized by two major external cues (zeitgebers); light and temperature (Goya, Romanowski, Caldart, Bénard, & Golombek, 2016).

Several studies have examined circadian patterns in *C. elegans*. Though a true circadian rhythm is yet to be fully elucidated in this model, circadian rhythms have been demonstrated in several behavioral and physiological functions. These include defecation, swimming behaviors and general locomotor activity, as well as response to osmotic stress. Additionally, circadian patterns have been demonstrated in several other metabolic activities such as pharyngeal contractions, food and oxygen consumption (Migliori et al., 2012). Gene expression profiling studies afford a powerful tool to characterize clock genes under circadian transcriptional regulation as such profiling is not influenced by known assumptions of specific physiological and behavioral outcomes. A study using genome-wide expression profiling identified light and temperature controlled transcriptional rhythms in *C. elegans* and demonstrated that subsets of such transcripts are controlled in a circadian pattern. The study also showed that expression of many genes in this organism is globally driven by these two zeitgebers, thus suggesting that *C. elegans* show systemic responses to light and temperature (van der Linden et al., 2010). A recent study applied an in vivo bioluminescence assay to demonstrate major features of the *C. elegans* circadian system. The study demonstrated that *C. elegans* expresses approximately 24-h rhythms that are entrained by temperature and light/dark cycles in both single-nematode and population-based assays. The study also demonstrated that light and temperature detection involve the use of photoreceptors GUR-3 and LITE, as well as TAX-2 cyclic nucleotide-gated channel subunit. Importantly, this bioluminescence assay is extremely sensitive, non-invasive and has immediate resolution (Goya et al., 2016). Therefore, *C. elegans* can be optimized to elucidate the molecular mechanisms behind the circadian patterns of RLS symptoms using those characterized behavioral and physiological activities controlled by circadian rhythms in *C. elegans*. Genetic modifications of RLS genes in *C. elegans* can be elucidated using simple behavioral assessment of several activities that show circadian rhythmic patterns (Migliori et al., 2012) in *C. elegans*. Such behavioral assessment can include:

Pharyngeal pumping actions: These actions are controlled by several mechanisms in *C. elegans*. The pharynx contracts rhythmically to aid feeding in worms. Rate of this activity commonly referred to as pharyngeal pumping can be measured manually counting pumps per minute under a dissecting microscope. A study reported that pharyngeal pumps in *C. elegans* show daily variations that are influenced by light/dark cycles (Migliori et al., 2012).

General locomotor activities: Rate of movement (locomotion) in *C. elegans* can be assessed by quantifying (counting) body bends over a specified period of time. A body bend is described as change in the direction of the pharynx's posterior bulb. Simply, it is counted every time the part of the worm just behind the pharynx reaches a maximum bend in the opposite direction from the bend last counted. Such assays can either be carried out on nematode growth media (NGM) or in water. Body bends can be assessed manually under dissecting microscope or with use of several available programs such as Worm Tracker, OptoTracker, Nemo, etc., on videotaped sessions (Chen, Chen, Jiang, Chen, & Pan, 2013).

5.2 DAergic function

DAergic dysfunction is implicated in the pathogenesis of RLS; however, specific molecular mechanisms are still unclear (Garcia-Borreguero & Cano-Pumarega, 2017; Garcia-Borreguero & Williams, 2014). *C. elegans* has a very simple nervous system. The DAergic system in *C. elegans* is particularly well studied. The *C. elegans* model can be harnessed to elucidate the role of DAergic neurotransmission in development of RLS symptoms. Structural and functional integrity of the DAergic system in *C. elegans* can be assessed using several tools described below.

5.2.1 Assessing DA neuronal morphology

Worms are transparent, thus allowing for easy in vivo imaging and visualization of fluorescently tagged neurons. Interestingly, the *C. elegans* hermaphrodites have only eight dopaminergic neurons, all of which can be visualized in vivo. Soma and processes of neurons can be visualized via expression of fluorescent proteins. Morphological changes including blebs, puncta, neuronal shrinkage, breaks or complete loss of neuronal processes, as well as vacuolation have been characterized as a phenotypic readout of neurodegenerative processes (Chen et al., 2013), which have been confirmed by transmission electronic microscopy (TEM) previously (Nass, Hall, Miller, & Blakely, 2002). Several worm strains are available for visualization of DA-producing neurons in *C. elegans*. These include but not limited to BY200 (dat-1:GFP (vtIs1) V.) and OH7193 (otIs181 [dat-1::mCherry + ttx-3::mCherry]) III) which expresses green fluorescent protein (GFP) and mCherry, respectively, in their dopaminergic neurons (Caito & Aschner, 2016; Ijomone, Miah, Peres, Nwoha, & Aschner, 2016). Homologs of RLS genes can be modified in these worms to understand the effect of RLS genes in dopaminergic morphology.

5.2.2 Assessing DAergic functions

Several behavioral paradigms are available to test DAergic functions using the *C. elegans* model. These can be used to unravel dopamine functions in *C. elegans* mutation of RLS homolog genes. These include:

Basal slowing response: This is assay assessed bacterial mechanosensation as measure of DAergic functions (Sawin, Ranganathan, & Horvitz, 2000). DAergic neurotransmission causes worms to slow locomotor rate in the presence of food. *C. elegans* feed on bacterial. This assay is performed by counting number of body bends (to quantify locomotor rate) in a 20 s interval in the presence or absence of food. Worms with normal or intact DA systems down locomotion when they encounter food as opposed to worms with defective DA systems which do not slow down. Worms with deficient tyrosine hydroxylase homolog, *cat-2*, are used as positive control as they show defective bacterial mechanosensation (Caito & Aschner, 2016; Ijomone et al., 2016).

Dauer spontaneous movement: In the absence of food and enabling environment, *C. elegans* morph into a developmental stage called dauer, after the larva-1 stage. Dauer worms are in a period of hibernation marked by almost complete inactivity. During this assay, dauers are considered to be moving if they make more than one body bend backward or forward within 1 min. Increased dauer movement is reported to be a response to decreased DA levels (Chen et al., 2015).

Area restricted searching (ARS): Wildtype *C. elegans* will expand search for food to neighboring areas when food source in immediate vicinity is depleted. This behavior is scored by reduction in regularity of high-angled turns when food in immediate vicinity is depleted and worms begin to explore farther areas. This behavior which is referred to as area restricted searching (ARS) is DAergic dependent (Chen et al., 2013).

Habituation task/tap withdrawer response: *C. elegans* growing on a plate respond to tapping of the plate by increasing forward or backward movement. Continuous tapping results in habituation and decrease in number of reversals. All worms respond to this stimulus by reducing rate of reversals, however, the lag time in response is DA-dependent, as worms with defective DA systems habituate faster (Chen et al., 2013).

5.3 Measurement of neurotransmitters

Levels of neurotransmitters such as DA can be determined in worm extract using high-performance liquid chromatography (HPLC). This requires use of many worms (about several hundred thousands of Larva 1 stage worms), and they must be properly washed off bacteria (Chen et al., 2013).

5.4 Metal toxicity

Fe deficiency is implicated in RLS pathogenesis (Bogan & Cheray, 2013). Studies in several models, including mouse, fly and worm, have demonstrated a functional interaction between homologs of RLS gene BTBD9 and Fe biology and DAergic activity (Catoire et al., 2011; DeAndrade, Johnson, et al., 2012; DeAndrade, Zhang, et al., 2012). An association between RLS and PD has been proposed. MRI studies demonstrated slight presynaptic and postsynaptic deficits in nigrostriatal dopaminergic pathways in RLS patients without PD. Increased prevalence of PD is noted in RLS, and vice versa (Gao, Schwarzschild, O'Reilly, Wang, & Ascherio, 2010; Peeraully & Tan, 2012).

Metals, particularly manganese (Mn) have been indicated as risk factors for PD (Chen et al., 2015). Mn and Fe have similar characteristics and share several homeostatic and transport pathways. Furthermore, Fe depletion, a key feature of RLS is associated with higher deposition of Mn in the brain. There is an established *C. elegans* model of Mn neurotoxicity (Chen et al., 2015; Ijomone et al., 2016; Peres et al., 2018; Ruszkiewicz et al., 2018). Given the association between Mn and Fe, this model can be harnessed to evaluate whether neuronal and/or systemic alteration in Mn may contribute to the pathophysiology of RLS. Potential modulation of neurotoxic impact of metals due to modifications of RLS genes in *C. elegans* can be assessed using several techniques including:

Survival assay: This assay is used to determine lethal dose of a substance on *C. elegans* and how much toxicity is imparted by that substance. Specifically, survival assay could determine if modifications of RLS genes improve or worsen toxicity following exposures to heavy metals such as Mn. In performing this assay, a specific number of worms treated with Mn, for example, are transferred onto NGM with food. The number of worms alive after 24 or 48 h are counted and scored as percentage of initially transferred worms. Dose-response curves are generated to determine if any genetic modifications influence survival of worms (Caito & Aschner, 2016; Ijomone et al., 2016).

Lifespan assay: This assay particularly takes advantage of the short life span of the *C. elegans* (about 2–3 weeks). During this assay, a specified number of worms are grown to L4 stage (seen as day 0) and transferred to NGM plates. Number of surviving worms are scored every 24 or 48 h till all worms are dead. To prevent confusion with progeny, the initial worms are transferred every 2 days or NGM plates are constituted with fluorodeoxyuridine (FUDR) to prevent eggs from hatching (Chen et al., 2015). The impact of modification of RLS genes in *C. elegans* on lifespan can be evaluated in the absence or presence of cofounders such as Mn toxicity.

Inductively coupled plasma mass spectrometry (ICP-MS) analysis: ICP-MS can be used to quantify metal content in *C. elegans*. This may require several thousands of worms (Peres et al., 2018). This method could be used to elucidate the influence of RLS gene modifications in *C. elegans* on levels of metals implicated in DAergic perturbations such as Fe and Mn.

6. Conclusion

RLS is common neurological disorder in the United States. Although it is not a life-threatening disease, RLS can seriously impair life quality. The consequences include sleep deprivation, low work productivity, anxiety, depression and attention-deficit/hyperactivity disorder (ADHD) symptoms (Allen et al., 2011; Wagner et al., 2004). Finally, RLS may portend more serious consequences, including hypertension, heart disease and stroke (Li et al., 2012; Pennestri et al., 2007; Siddiqui et al., 2007; Walters & Rye, 2009). It is undoubtedly that both environmental and genetic factors are involved, given the varied severity of symptoms. Although current research has revealed that brain Fe deficiency and DAergic dysfunction play important roles, it is far from drawing a conclusive understanding of the pathology of RLS. Biometals such as Fe, copper, zinc, Mn, usually share the transporters and complete for their influx and efflux of cells. It is very likely that Fe deficiency in the brain disrupts other metal homeostasis. Among these metals, Mn is the most similar one of Fe, given their biochemical property, metabolism and physiological functions in human. For example, Fe and Mn use the divalent metals transporter 1 (DMT1) and transferrin/transferrin receptor as the primary route of influx, and use ferroportin as the major efflux route (Chen, Bornhorst, & Aschner, 2018; Chen, Bornhorst, Diana Neely, & Avila, 2018; Chen, Parmalee, & Aschner, 2014). Low levels of Fe in the brain may activate expression of influx transporters in order to compensate for Fe deficiency; however, this also brings the risk of transporting more Mn in the brain. The accumulation of Mn has been reported to impair DAergic system and may cause neurological disorders such as Parkinson's disease and dystonia (Chen et al., 2015; Chen, Chakraborty, Peres, Bowman, & Aschner, 2014; Chen, Culbreth, & Aschner, 2016; Chen, Miah, & Aschner, 2016). Therefore, it is necessary to investigate the levels of Mn and other metals in the brain of RLS patients to clarify whether Fe deficiency or high levels of other metals might play a role in the etiology of RLS.

The identified genetic risk factors are of great research value to elucidate the molecular mechanism of RLS, especially when combined with a suitable model organism. *C. elegans* provides numerous advantages in studying RLS-associated gene-environment interactions. These include its small size, short lifespan, a quick lifecycle and a simple nervous system. Additionally, the worm's small and well-characterized genome is ideal for genetic manipulation. It contains all homologs of currently known RLS genetic risk factors (Table 2), as well as all genes necessary for DA biosynthesis, packaging and reuptake (Brenner, 1974; Sulston et al., 1975; White, Southgate, Thomson, & Brenner, 1976). More specifically, the circadian pattern of RLS symptoms can be studied in *C. elegans* via pharyngeal pumping actions and general locomotor activities, which are controlled by the worm circadian system. DAergic function can be accessed by studying individual neuronal morphology, behaviors regulated by DAergic neurons and measurement of neurotransmitters. Last, but not the least, the nematode is sensitive to metals and a wide-range of neuroactive drugs and xenobiotics, thus it can be applied to investigate the effect of Fe and other biometals, as well as to discover novel pharmaceutical compounds beneficial for RLS patients. Despite these advantages, very limited research on RLS has been reported in *C. elegans*. Therefore, we anticipate the involvement of *C. elegans* in RLS study will shed new light on the etiology and molecular mechanism of RLS, as well as identify novel drugs for treatment of RLS patients in the next decade.

Acknowledgements

The manuscript was supported by NIH grant NIEHS R01 10563, NIEHS R01 07331 and NIEHS R01 020852.

Conflict of interest

The authors declare no known or perceived conflict of interest.

References

Ackley, B. D., Harrington, R. J., Hudson, M. L., Williams, L., Kenyon, C. J., Chisholm, A. D., et al. (2005). The two isoforms of the *Caenorhabditis elegans* leukocyte-common antigen related receptor tyrosine phosphatase PTP-3 function independently in axon guidance and synapse formation. *The Journal of Neuroscience*, *25*(33), 7517–7528. https://doi.org/10.1523/jneurosci.2010-05.2005.

Akpinar, C. K., Turker, H., Aygun, D., & Aytac, E. (2017). Familial restless legs syndrome: A family with all female patients. *Archives of Iranian Medicine*, *20*(2), 105–107. 0172002/aim.009 (web archive link).

Allen, R. P., Bharmal, M., & Calloway, M. (2011). Prevalence and disease burden of primary restless legs syndrome: Results of a general population survey in the United States. *Movement Disorders*, *26*(1), 114–120. https://doi.org/10.1002/mds.23430.

Allen, R. P., La Buda, M. C., Becker, P., & Earley, C. J. (2002). Family history study of the restless legs syndrome. *Sleep Medicine*, *3*(Suppl), S3–S7.

Allen, R. P., Picchietti, D. L., Garcia-Borreguero, D., Ondo, W. G., Walters, A. S., Winkelman, J. W., et al. (2014). Restless legs syndrome/Willis-Ekbom disease diagnostic criteria: Updated International Restless Legs Syndrome Study Group (IRLSSG) consensus criteria—History, rationale, description, and significance. *Sleep Medicine*, *15*(8), 860–873. https://doi.org/10.1016/j.sleep.2014.03.025.

Allen, R. P., Picchietti, D., Hening, W. A., Trenkwalder, C., Walters, A. S., & Montplaisi, J. (2003). Restless legs syndrome: Diagnostic criteria, special considerations, and epidemiology. A report from the restless legs syndrome diagnosis and epidemiology workshop at the National Institutes of Health. *Sleep Medicine*, *4*(2), 101–119. doi:S1389945703000108 [pii].

Allen, R. P., Walters, A. S., Montplaisir, J., Hening, W., Myers, A., Bell, T. J., et al. (2005). Restless legs syndrome prevalence and impact: REST general population study. *Archives of Internal Medicine*, *165*(11), 1286–1292. 165/11/1286 [pii]. https://doi.org/10.1001/archinte.165.11.1286.

Arata, Y., Kouike, H., Zhang, Y., Herman, M. A., Okano, H., & Sawa, H. (2006). Wnt signaling and a Hox protein cooperatively regulate psa-3/Meis to determine daughter cell fate after asymmetric cell division in C. elegans. *Developmental Cell*, *11*(1), 105–115. https://doi.org/10.1016/j.devcel.2006.04.020.

Avery, L., & Horvitz, H. R. (1990). Effects of starvation and neuroactive drugs on feeding in Caenorhabditis elegans. *The Journal of Experimental Zoology*, *253*(3), 263–270. https://doi.org/10.1002/jez.1402530305.

Azcoitia, V., Aracil, M., Martinez, A. C., & Torres, M. (2005). The homeodomain protein Meis1 is essential for definitive hematopoiesis and vascular patterning in the mouse embryo. *Developmental Biology*, *280*(2), 307–320. https://doi.org/10.1016/j.ydbio.2005.01.004.

Barber, B. A., Liyanage, V. R., Zachariah, R. M., Olson, C. O., Bailey, M. A., & Rastegar, M. (2013). Dynamic expression of MEIS1 homeoprotein in E14.5 forebrain and differentiated forebrain-derived neural stem cells. *Annals of Anatomy*, *195*(5), 431–440. https://doi.org/10.1016/j.aanat.2013.04.005.

Barber, B. A., & Rastegar, M. (2010). Epigenetic control of Hox genes during neurogenesis, development, and disease. *Annals of Anatomy*, *192*(5), 261–274. https://doi.org/10.1016/j.aanat.2010.07.009.

Bastien, D., Bellver Landete, V., Lessard, M., Vallieres, N., Champagne, M., Takashima, A., et al. (2015). IL-1alpha gene deletion protects oligodendrocytes after spinal cord injury through upregulation of the survival factor Tox3. *The Journal of Neuroscience*, *35*(30), 10715–10730. https://doi.org/10.1523/jneurosci.0498-15.2015.

Beard, J., Erikson, K. M., & Jones, B. C. (2003). Neonatal iron deficiency results in irreversible changes in dopamine function in rats. *Journal of Nutrition*, *133*(4), 1174–1179.

Benedetto, A., Au, C., Avila, D. S., Milatovic, D., & Aschner, M. (2010). Extracellular dopamine potentiates Mn-induced oxidative stress, lifespan reduction, and dopaminergic neurodegeneration in a BLI-3-dependent manner in *Caenorhabditis elegans*. *PLoS Genetics*, *6*(8), e1001084.

Blazie, S. M., Geissel, H. C., Wilky, H., Joshi, R., Newbern, J., & Mangone, M. (2017). Alternative polyadenylation directs tissue-specific miRNA targeting in *Caenorhabditis elegans* somatic tissues. *Genetics*, *206*(2), 757–774. https://doi.org/10.1534/genetics.116.196774.

Bogan, R. K., & Cheray, J. A. (2013). Restless legs syndrome: A review of diagnosis and management in primary care. *Postgraduate Medicine*, *125*(3), 99–111. https://doi.org/10.3810/pgm.2013.05.2636.

Bouilloux, F., Thireau, J., Venteo, S., Farah, C., Karam, S., Dauvilliers, Y., et al. (2016). Loss of the transcription factor Meis1 prevents sympathetic neurons target-field innervation and increases susceptibility to sudden cardiac death. *eLife*, *5*, e11627. https://doi.org/10.7554/eLife.11627.

Brenner, S. (1974). The genetics of Caenorhabditis elegans. *Genetics*, 77(1), 71–94.

Caito, S. W., & Aschner, M. (2016). NAD+ supplementation attenuates methylmercury dopaminergic and mitochondrial toxicity in *Caenorhabditis elegans*. *Toxicological Sciences*, *151*(1), 139–149. https://doi.org/10.1093/toxsci/kfw030.

Catoire, H., Dion, P. A., Xiong, L., Amari, M., Gaudet, R., Girard, S. L., et al. (2011). Restless legs syndrome-associated MEIS1 risk variant influences iron homeostasis. *Annals of Neurology*, *70*(1), 170–175. https://doi.org/10.1002/ana.22435.

Chen, P., Bornhorst, J., & Aschner, M. (2018). Manganese metabolism in humans. *Frontiers in Bioscience (Landmark Edition)*, *23*, 1655–1679.

Chen, P., Bornhorst, J., Diana Neely, M., & Avila, D. S. (2018). Mechanisms and disease pathogenesis underlying metal-induced oxidative stress. *Oxidative Medicine and Cellular Longevity*, *2018*, 7612172. https://doi.org/10.1155/2018/7612172.

Chen, P., Chakraborty, S., Mukhopadhyay, S., Lee, E., Paoliello, M. M. B., Bowman, A. B., et al. (2015). Manganese homeostasis in the nervous system. *Journal of Neurochemistry*, *134*(4), 601–610. https://doi.org/10.1111/jnc.13170.

Chen, P., Chakraborty, S., Peres, T. V., Bowman, A. B., & Aschner, M. (2014). Manganese-induced neurotoxicity: From *C. elegans* to humans. *Toxicology Research*, *4*, 191–202. https://doi.org/10.1039/C4TX00127C.

Chen, C. H., Chen, Y. C., Jiang, H. C., Chen, C. K., & Pan, C. L. (2013). Neuronal aging: Learning from *C. elegans*. *Journal of Molecular Signaling*, *8*(1), 14. https://doi.org/10.1186/1750-2187-8-14.

Chen, P., Culbreth, M., & Aschner, M. (2016). Exposure, epidemiology, and mechanism of the environmental toxicant manganese. *Environmental Science and Pollution Research*, *23*(14), 13802–13810. https://doi.org/10.1007/s11356-016-6687-0.

Chen, P., Miah, M. R., & Aschner, M. (2016). Metals and neurodegeneration. *F1000Research*, *5*, 366 (F1000 Faculty Rev). https://doi.org/10.12688/f1000research.7431.1.

Chen, P., Parmalee, N., & Aschner, M. (2014). Genetic factors and manganese-induced neurotoxicity. *Frontiers in Genetics*, *5*, 265. https://doi.org/10.3389/fgene.2014.00265.

Chen, T., Xu, J., Liu, G., Liu, H., Chen, M., Qin, Y., et al. (2016). Genetic variants in PTPRD and risk of gestational diabetes mellitus. *Oncotarget*, 7(46), 76101–76107. https://doi.org/10.18632/oncotarget.12599.

Connor, J. R., Wang, X. S., Allen, R. P., Beard, J. L., Wiesinger, J. A., Felt, B. T., et al. (2009). Altered dopaminergic profile in the putamen and substantia nigra in restless leg syndrome. *Brain*, *132*(Pt 9), 2403–2412. https://doi.org/10.1093/brain/awp125. awp125 [pii].

Connor, J. R., Wang, X. S., Neely, E. B., Ponnuru, P., Morita, H., & Beard, J. (2008). Comparative study of the influence of Thy1 deficiency and dietary iron deficiency on dopaminergic profiles in the mouse striatum. *Journal of Neuroscience Research*, *86*(14), 3194–3202. https://doi.org/10.1002/jnr.21758.

Corsi, A. K., Wightman, B., & Chalfie, M. (2015). A transparent window into biology: A primer on *Caenorhabditis elegans*. *Genetics*, *200*(2), 387–407. https://doi.org/10.1534/genetics.115.176099.

Dauvilliers, Y., & Winkelmann, J. (2013). Restless legs syndrome: Update on pathogenesis. *Current Opinion in Pulmonary Medicine*, *19*(6), 594–600. https://doi.org/10.1097/MCP.0b013e328365ab07.

DeAndrade, M. P., Johnson, R. L., Jr., Unger, E. L., Zhang, L., van Groen, T., Gamble, K. L., et al. (2012). Motor restlessness, sleep disturbances, thermal sensory alterations and elevated serum iron levels in Btbd9 mutant mice. *Human Molecular Genetics*, *21*(18), 3984–3992. https://doi.org/10.1093/hmg/dds221.

DeAndrade, M. P., Zhang, L., Doroodchi, A., Yokoi, F., Cheetham, C. C., Chen, H. X., et al. (2012). Enhanced hippocampal long-term potentiation and fear memory in Btbd9 mutant mice. *PLoS One*, 7(4), e35518. https://doi.org/10.1371/journal.pone.0035518.

Diao, D., Wang, L., Wan, J., Chen, Z., Peng, J., Liu, H., et al. (2016). MEK5 overexpression is associated with the occurrence and development of colorectal cancer. *BMC Cancer*, *16*, 302. https://doi.org/10.1186/s12885-016-2327-9.

Earley, C. J., Kuwabara, H., Wong, D. F., Gamaldo, C., Salas, R., Brasic, J., et al. (2011). The dopamine transporter is decreased in the striatum of subjects with restless legs syndrome. *Sleep*, *34*(3), 341–347.

Ellis, H. M., & Horvitz, H. R. (1986). Genetic control of programmed cell death in the nematode *C. elegans*. *Cell*, *44*(6), 817–829.

Galbiati, A., Marelli, S., Giora, E., Zucconi, M., Oldani, A., & Ferini-Strambi, L. (2015). Neurocognitive function in patients with idiopathic restless legs syndrome before and after treatment with dopamine-agonist. *International Journal of Psychophysiology*, *95*(3), 304–319. https://doi.org/10.1016/j.ijpsycho.2014.12.005.

Gao, X., Schwarzschild, M. A., O'Reilly, E. J., Wang, H., & Ascherio, A. (2010). Restless legs syndrome and erectile dysfunction. *Sleep*, *33*(1), 75–79.

Garcia-Borreguero, D., & Cano-Pumarega, I. (2017). New concepts in the management of restless legs syndrome. *BMJ*, *356*, j104. https://doi.org/10.1136/bmj.j104.

Garcia-Martin, E., Jimenez-Jimenez, F. J., Alonso-Navarro, H., Martinez, C., Zurdo, M., Turpin-Fenoll, L., et al. (2015). Heme oxygenase-1 and 2 common genetic variants and risk for restless legs syndrome. *Medicine (Baltimore)*, *94*(34), e1448. https://doi.org/10.1097/md.0000000000001448.

Garcia-Borreguero, D., Kohnen, R., Silber, M. H., Winkelman, J. W., Earley, C. J., Högl, B., et al. (2013). The long-term treatment of restless legs syndrome/Willis-Ekbom disease: Evidence-based guidelines and clinical consensus best practice guidance: A report from the International Restless Legs Syndrome Study Group. *Sleep Medicine*, *14*(7), 675–684. https://doi.org/10.1016/j.sleep.2013.05.016.

Garcia-Borreguero, D., & Williams, A. M. (2014). An update on restless legs syndrome (Willis-Ekbom disease): Clinical features, pathogenesis and treatment. *Current Opinion in Neurology*, *27*(4), 493–501. https://doi.org/10.1097/WCO.0000000000000117.

Gong, Y., McDonough, C. W., Beitelshees, A. L., El Rouby, N., Hiltunen, T. P., O'Connell, J. R., et al. (2015). PTPRD gene associated with blood pressure response to atenolol and resistant hypertension. *Journal of Hypertension*, *33*(11), 2278–2285. https://doi.org/10.1097/hjh.0000000000000714.

Goya, M. E., Romanowski, A., Caldart, C. S., Bénard, C. Y., & Golombek, D. A. (2016). Circadian rhythms identified in Caenorhabditis elegans by in vivo long-term monitoring of a bioluminescent reporter. *Proceedings of the National Academy of Sciences of the United States of America*, *113*(48), E7837–E7845.

Haba-Rubio, J., Marti-Soler, H., Marques-Vidal, P., Tobback, N., Andries, D., Preisig, M., et al. (2016). Prevalence and determinants of periodic limb movements in the general population. *Annals of Neurology*, *79*(3), 464–474. https://doi.org/10.1002/ana.24593.

Hobert, O. (2013). The neuronal genome of *Caenorhabditis elegans*. *WormBook*, 1–106. https://doi.org/10.1895/wormbook.1.161.1.

Hsu, V., Zobel, C. L., Lambie, E. J., Schedl, T., & Kornfeld, K. (2002). *Caenorhabditis elegans* lin-45 raf is essential for larval viability, fertility and the induction of vulval cell fates. *Genetics*, *160*(2), 481–492.

Ijomone, O. M., Miah, M. R., Peres, T. V., Nwoha, P. U., & Aschner, M. (2016). Null allele mutants of trt-1, the catalytic subunit of telomerase in *Caenorhabditis elegans*, are less sensitive to Mn-induced toxicity and DAergic degeneration. *Neurotoxicology*, *57*, 54–60. https://doi.org/10.1016/j.neuro.2016.08.016.

Jayanthi, L. D., Apparsundaram, S., Malone, M. D., Ward, E., Miller, D. M., Eppler, M., et al. (1998). The Caenorhabditis elegans gene T23G5.5 encodes an antidepressant- and cocaine-sensitive dopamine transporter. *Molecular Pharmacology*, *54*(4), 601–609.

Jimenez-Jimenez, F. J., Esguevillas, G., Alonso-Navarro, H., Zurdo, M., Turpin-Fenoll, L., Millan-Pascual, J., et al. (2018). Gamma-aminobutyric acid (GABA) receptors genes polymorphisms and risk for restless legs syndrome. *The Pharmacogenomics Journal*, *18*, 565–577. https://doi.org/10.1038/s41397-018-0023-7.

Kamath, R. S., Fraser, A. G., Dong, Y., Poulin, G., Durbin, R., Gotta, M., et al. (2003). Systematic functional analysis of the *Caenorhabditis elegans* genome using RNAi. *Nature*, *421*(6920), 231–237. http://www.nature.com/nature/journal/v421/n6920/suppinfo/nature01278_S1.html.

Kaneshiro, S., Otsuki, D., Yoshida, K., Yoshikawa, H., & Higuchi, C. (2015). MEK5 suppresses osteoblastic differentiation. *Biochemical and Biophysical Research Communications*, *463*(3), 241–247. https://doi.org/10.1016/j.bbrc.2015.05.035.

Kao, C. Y., Los, F. C., Huffman, D. L., Wachi, S., Kloft, N., Husmann, M., et al. (2011). Global functional analyses of cellular responses to pore-forming toxins. *PLoS Pathogens*, 7(3), e1001314. https://doi.org/10.1371/journal.ppat.1001314.

Kemlink, D., Polo, O., Frauscher, B., Gschliesser, V., Hogl, B., Poewe, W., et al. (2009). Replication of restless legs syndrome loci in three European populations. *Journal of Medical Genetics*, *46*(5), 315–318. jmg.2008.062992 [pii]. https://doi.org/10.1136/jmg.2008.062992.

Lazzarini, A., Walters, A. S., Hickey, K., Coccagna, G., Lugaresi, E., Ehrenberg, B. L., et al. (1999). Studies of penetrance and anticipation in five autosomal-dominant restless legs syndrome pedigrees. *Movement Disorders*, *14*(1), 111–116.

Lewis, J. A. (1980). On the uses of small nematode worms. *Neuroscience*, *5*(6), 961–966. doi:0306-4522(80)90179-7 [pii].

Li, Y., Doroodchi, A., Yang, Y., & DeAndrade, M. P. (2011). Characterization of BTBD9 homolog knockout in *C. elegans*. *Sleep Medicine*, *12*, S1–S130.

Li, L., Guo, G., Wang, F., Lv, P., Zhu, M., Gu, Y., et al. (2018). TOX high mobility group box family member 3 rs3803662 and breast cancer risk: A meta-analysis. *Journal of Cancer Research and Therapeutics*, *14*(Suppl), S208–s212. https://doi.org/10.4103/0973-1482.167611.

Li, G., Tang, H., Wang, C., Qi, X., Chen, J., Chen, S., et al. (2017). Association of BTBD9 and MAP2K5/SKOR1 with restless legs syndrome in Chinese population. *Sleep*, *40*(4). https://doi.org/10.1093/sleep/zsx028.

Li, Y., Walters, A. S., Chiuve, S. E., Rimm, E. B., Winkelman, J. W., & Gao, X. (2012). Prospective study of restless legs syndrome and coronary heart disease among women. *Circulation*, *126*(14), 1689–1694. https://doi.org/10.1161/CIRCULATIONAHA.112.112698. CIRCULATIONAHA.112.112698 [pii].

Li, Y., Zhang, P., Choi, T. Y., Park, S. K., Park, H., Lee, E. J., et al. (2015). Splicing-dependent trans-synaptic SALM3-LAR-RPTP interactions regulate excitatory synapse development and locomotion. *Cell Reports*, *12*(10), 1618–1630. https://doi.org/10.1016/j.celrep.2015.08.002.

Lockhead, D., Schwarz, E. M., O'Hagan, R., Bellotti, S., Krieg, M., Barr, M. M., et al. (2016). The tubulin repertoire of *C. elegans* sensory neurons and its context-dependent role in process outgrowth. *Molecular Biology of the Cell*, *27*, 3717–3728. https://doi.org/10.1091/mbc.E16-06-0473.

McKay, S. J., Johnsen, R., Khattra, J., Asano, J., Baillie, D. L., Chan, S., et al. (2003). Gene expression profiling of cells, tissues, and developmental stages of the nematode C. elegans. *Cold Spring Harbor Symposia on Quantitative Biology*, *68*, 159–169.

Mehta, P. B., Jenkins, B. L., McCarthy, L., Thilak, L., Robson, C. N., Neal, D. E., et al. (2003). MEK5 overexpression is associated with metastatic prostate cancer, and stimulates proliferation, MMP-9 expression and invasion. *Oncogene*, *22*(9), 1381–1389. https://doi.org/10.1038/sj.onc.1206154.

Mello, C. C., Kramer, J. M., Stinchcomb, D. T., & Ambros, V. R. (1991). Efficient gene transfer in *C. elegans*: Extrachromosomal maintenance and integration of transforming sequences. *EMBO Journal*, *10*, 3959–3970. Doi:Citeulike-article-id:3275905.

Migliori, M. L., Romanowski, A., Simonetta, S. H., Valdez, D., Guido, M., & Golombek, D. A. (2012). Daily variation in melatonin synthesis and arylalkylamine N-acetyltransferase activity in the nematode *Caenorhabditis elegans*. *Journal of Pineal Research*, *53*(1), 38–46. https://doi.org/10.1111/j.1600-079X.2011.00969.x.

Mohtashami, S., He, Q., Ruskey, J. A., Zhou, S., Dion, P. A., Allen, R. P., et al. (2018). TOX3 variants are involved in restless legs syndrome and Parkinson's disease with opposite effects. *Journal of Molecular Neuroscience*, *64*(3), 341–345. https://doi.org/10.1007/s12031-018-1031-4.

Montplaisir, J., Boucher, S., Poirier, G., Lavigne, G., Lapierre, O., & Lesperance, P. (1997). Clinical, polysomnographic, and genetic characteristics of restless legs syndrome: A study of 133 patients diagnosed with new standard criteria. *Movement Disorders*, *12*(1), 61–65. https://doi.org/10.1002/mds.870120111.

Moon, H. J., Chang, Y., Lee, Y. S., Song, H. J., Chang, H. W., Ku, J., et al. (2014). T2 relaxometry using 3.0-tesla magnetic resonance imaging of the brain in early- and late-onset restless legs syndrome. *Journal of Clinical Neurology*, *10*(3), 197–202. https://doi.org/10.3988/jcn.2014.10.3.197.

Moore, H. t., Winkelmann, J., Lin, L., Finn, L., Peppard, P., & Mignot, E. (2014). Periodic leg movements during sleep are associated with polymorphisms in BTBD9, TOX3/BC034767, MEIS1, MAP2K5/SKOR1, and PTPRD. *Sleep*, *37*(9), 1535–1542. https://doi.org/10.5665/sleep.4006.

Morgan, P. G., Sedensky, M. M., Meneely, P. M., & Cascorbi, H. F. (1988). The effect of two genes on anesthetic response in the nematode Caenorhabditis elegans. *Anesthesiology*, *69*(2), 246–251.

Nakajima, S., Tanaka, H., Sawada, K., Hayashi, H., Hasebe, T., Abe, M., et al. (2018). Polymorphism of receptor-type tyrosine-protein phosphatase delta gene in the development of non-alcoholic fatty liver disease. *Journal of Gastroenterology and Hepatology*, *33*(1), 283–290. https://doi.org/10.1111/jgh.13820.

Nakamura, F., Okada, T., Shishikura, M., Uetani, N., Taniguchi, M., Yagi, T., et al. (2017). Protein tyrosine phosphatase delta mediates the Sema3A-induced cortical basal dendritic arborization through the activation of Fyn tyrosine kinase. *The Journal of Neuroscience*, *37*(30), 7125–7139. https://doi.org/10.1523/jneurosci.2519-16.2017.

Nass, R., Hall, D. H., Miller, D. M., 3rd, & Blakely, R. D. (2002). Neurotoxin-induced degeneration of dopamine neurons in Caenorhabditis elegans. *Proceedings of the National Academy of Sciences of the United States of America*, *99*(5), 3264–3269. https://doi.org/10.1073/pnas.042497999. 042497999 [pii].

Nelson, M. D., Lee, K. H., Churgin, M. A., Hill, A. J., Van Buskirk, C., Fang-Yen, C., et al. (2014). FMRFamide-like FLP-13 neuropeptides promote quiescence following heat stress in *Caenorhabditis elegans*. *Current Biology*, *24*(20), 2406–2410. https://doi.org/10.1016/j.cub.2014.08.037.

Nicholas, H. R., & Hodgkin, J. (2004). The ERK MAP kinase cascade mediates tail swelling and a protective response to rectal infection in C. elegans. *Current Biology*, *14*(14), 1256–1261. https://doi.org/10.1016/j.cub.2004.07.022.

Nicol, R. L., Frey, N., Pearson, G., Cobb, M., Richardson, J., & Olson, E. N. (2001). Activated MEK5 induces serial assembly of sarcomeres and eccentric cardiac hypertrophy. *The EMBO Journal*, *20*(11), 2757–2767. https://doi.org/10.1093/emboj/20.11.2757.

Ning, Z., Jiayi, L., Jian, R., & Wanli, X. (2017). Relationship between abnormal TOX3 gene methylation and polycystic ovarian syndrome. *European Review for Medical and Pharmacological Sciences*, *21*(9), 2034–2038.

Ondo, W. G., Vuong, K. D., & Wang, Q. (2000). Restless legs syndrome in monozygotic twins: Clinical correlates. *Neurology*, *55*(9), 1404–1406.

Peeraully, T., & Tan, E. K. (2012). Linking restless legs syndrome with Parkinson's disease: Clinical, imaging and genetic evidence. *Translational Neurodegeneration*, *1*(1), 6. https://doi.org/10.1186/2047-9158-1-6.

Pennestri, M. H., Montplaisir, J., Colombo, R., Lavigne, G., & Lanfranchi, P. A. (2007). Nocturnal blood pressure changes in patients with restless legs syndrome. *Neurology*, *68*(15), 1213–1218. 68/15/1213 [pii]. https://doi.org/10.1212/01.wnl.0000259036.89411.52.

Peres, T. V., Arantes, L. P., Miah, M. R., Bornhorst, J., Schwerdtle, T., Bowman, A. B., et al. (2018). Role of Caenorhabditis elegans AKT-1/2 and SGK-1 in manganese toxicity. *Neurotoxicity Research*, *34*(3), 584–596. https://doi.org/10.1007/s12640-018-9915-1.

Rask-Andersen, M., Jacobsson, J. A., Moschonis, G., Ek, A. E., Chrousos, G. P., Marcus, C., et al. (2012). The MAP2K5-linked SNP rs2241423 is associated with BMI and obesity in two cohorts of Swedish and Greek children. *BMC Medical Genetics*, *13*, 36. https://doi.org/10.1186/1471-2350-13-36.

Ruszkiewicz, J. A., Pinkas, A., Miah, M. R., Weitz, R. L., Lawes, M. J. A., Akinyemi, A. J., et al. (2018). *C. elegans* as a model in developmental neurotoxicology. *Toxicology and Applied Pharmacology*, *354*, 126–135. https://doi.org/10.1016/j.taap.2018.03.016.

Sahu, S. K., Fritz, A., Tiwari, N., Kovacs, Z., Pouya, A., Wullner, V., et al. (2016). TOX3 regulates neural progenitor identity. *Biochimica et Biophysica Acta*, *1859*(7), 833–840. https://doi.org/10.1016/j.bbagrm.2016.04.005.

Sawin, E. R., Ranganathan, R., & Horvitz, H. R. (2000). *C. elegans* locomotory rate is modulated by the environment through a dopaminergic pathway and by experience through a serotonergic pathway. *Neuron*, *26*(3), 619–631.

Schaefer, H., & Rongo, C. (2006). KEL-8 is a substrate receptor for CUL3-dependent ubiquitin ligase that regulates synaptic glutamate receptor turnover. *Molecular Biology of the Cell*, *17*(3), 1250–1260. https://doi.org/10.1091/mbc.e05-08-0794.

Schormair, B., Kemlink, D., Roeske, D., Eckstein, G., Xiong, L., Lichtner, P., et al. (2008). PTPRD (protein tyrosine phosphatase receptor type delta) is associated with restless legs syndrome. *Nature Genetics*, *40*(8), 946–948. ng.190 [pii]. https://doi.org/10.1038/ng.190.

Schwartz, M. L., & Jorgensen, E. M. (2016). SapTrap, a toolkit for high-throughput CRISPR/Cas9 gene modification in *Caenorhabditis elegans*. *Genetics*, *202*(4), 1277–1288. https://doi.org/10.1534/genetics.115.184275.

Shishikura, M., Nakamura, F., Yamashita, N., Uetani, N., Iwakura, Y., & Goshima, Y. (2016). Expression of receptor protein tyrosine phosphatase delta, PTPdelta, in mouse central nervous system. *Brain Research*, *1642*, 244–254. https://doi.org/10.1016/j.brainres.2016.03.030.

Siddiqui, F., Strus, J., Ming, X., Lee, I. A., Chokroverty, S., & Walters, A. S. (2007). Rise of blood pressure with periodic limb movements in sleep and wakefulness. *Clinical Neurophysiology*, *118*(9), 1923–1930. S1388-2457(07)00199-X [pii]. https://doi.org/10.1016/j.clinph.2007.05.006.

Simmer, F., Moorman, C., van der Linden, A. M., Kuijk, E., van den Berghe, P. V., Kamath, R. S., et al. (2003). Genome-wide RNAi of C. elegans using the hypersensitive rrf-3 strain reveals novel gene functions. *PLoS Biology*, *1*(1), E12. https://doi.org/10.1371/journal.pbio.0000012.

Sohn, S. J., Lewis, G. M., & Winoto, A. (2008). Non-redundant function of the MEK5-ERK5 pathway in thymocyte apoptosis. *The EMBO Journal*, *27*(13), 1896–1906. https://doi.org/10.1038/emboj.2008.114.

Spencer, W. C., Zeller, G., Watson, J. D., Henz, S. R., Watkins, K. L., McWhirter, R. D., et al. (2011). A spatial and temporal map of *C. elegans* gene expression. *Genome Research*, *21*(2), 325–341. https://doi.org/10.1101/gr.114595.110.

Stefansson, H., Rye, D. B., Hicks, A., Petursson, H., Ingason, A., Thorgeirsson, T. E., et al. (2007). A genetic risk factor for periodic limb movements in sleep. *New England Journal of Medicine*, *357*(7), 639–647. NEJMoa072743 [pii]. https://doi.org/10.1056/NEJMoa072743.

Sulston, J., Dew, M., & Brenner, S. (1975). Dopaminergic neurons in the nematode Caenorhabditis elegans. *The Journal of Comparative Neurology*, *163*(2), 215–226. https://doi.org/10.1002/cne.901630207.

Szaumkessel, M., Wojciechowska, S., Janiszewska, J., Zemke, N., Byzia, E., Kiwerska, K., et al. (2017). Recurrent epigenetic silencing of the PTPRD tumor suppressor in laryngeal squamous cell carcinoma. *Tumour Biology*, *39*(3). https://doi.org/10.1177/1010428317691427. 1010428317691427.

Tan, E. K. (2006). Restless legs syndrome and Parkinson's disease: Is there an etiologic link? *Journal of Neurology*, *253*(Suppl. 7), VII33–37. https://doi.org/10.1007/s00415-006-7008-1.

Titus, K., & Michael, O. H. (2006). Finding function in novel targets: *C. elegans* as a model organism. *Nature Reviews Drug Discovery*, *5*(5), 387–399. https://doi.org/10.1038/nrd2031.

Trenkwalder, C., Paulus, W., & Walters, A. S. (2005). The restless legs syndrome. *Lancet Neurology*, *4*(8), 465–475.

Trenkwalder, C., Seidel, V. C., Gasser, T., & Oertel, W. H. (1996). Clinical symptoms and possible anticipation in a large kindred of familial restless legs syndrome. *Movement Disorders*, *11*(4), 389–394. https://doi.org/10.1002/mds.870110407.

Trenkwalder, C., Winkelmann, J., Inoue, Y., & Paulus, W. (2015). Restless legs syndrome-current therapies and management of augmentation. *Nature Reviews Neurology*, *11*(8), 434–445. https://doi.org/10.1038/nrneurol.2015.122.

Van Auken, K., Weaver, D., Robertson, B., Sundaram, M., Saldi, T., Edgar, L., et al. (2002). Roles of the Homothorax/Meis/Prep homolog UNC-62 and the Exd/Pbx homologs CEH-20 and CEH-40 in *C. elegans* embryogenesis. *Development*, *129*(22), 5255–5268.

van der Linden, A. M., Beverly, M., Kadener, S., Rodriguez, J., Wasserman, S., Rosbash, M., & Sengupta, P. (2010). Genome-wide analysis of light- and temperature-entrained circadian transcripts in *Caenorhabditis elegans*. *PLoS Biology*, *8*(10), e1000503. https://doi.org/10.1371/journal.pbio.1000503.

Van Nostrand, E. L., Sánchez-Blanco, A., Wu, B., Nguyen, A., & Kim, S. K. (2013). Roles of the developmental regulator unc-62/Homothorax in limiting longevity in Caenorhabditis elegans. *PLoS Genetics*, *9*(2), e1003325.

Vilarino-Guell, C., Chai, H., Keeling, B. H., Young, J. E., Rajput, A., Lynch, T., et al. (2009). MEIS1 p.R272H in familial restless legs syndrome. *Neurology*, *73*(3), 243–245. https://doi.org/10.1212/WNL.0b013e3181ae7c79.

Vilarino-Guell, C., Farrer, M. J., & Lin, S. C. (2008). A genetic risk factor for periodic limb movements in sleep. *The New England Journal of Medicine*, *358*(4), 425–427. https://doi.org/10.1056/NEJMc072518.

Wagner, M. L., Walters, A. S., & Fisher, B. C. (2004). Symptoms of attention-deficit/hyperactivity disorder in adults with restless legs syndrome. *Sleep*, *27*(8), 1499–1504.

Walters, A. S., Hickey, K., Maltzman, J., Verrico, T., Joseph, D., Hening, W., et al. (1996). A questionnaire study of 138 patients with restless legs syndrome: The 'Night-Walkers' survey. *Neurology*, *46*(1), 92–95.

Walters, A. S., & Rye, D. B. (2009). Review of the relationship of restless legs syndrome and periodic limb movements in sleep to hypertension, heart disease, and stroke. *Sleep*, *32*(5), 589–597.

Wang, W., Lu, S., Li, T., Pan, Y.-W., Zou, J., Abel, G. M., et al. (2015). Inducible activation of ERK5 MAP kinase enhances adult neurogenesis in the olfactory bulb and improves olfactory function. *The Journal of Neuroscience*, *35*(20), 7833–7849. https://doi.org/10.1523/JNEUROSCI.3745-14.2015.

Ward, R. J., Zucca, F. A., Duyn, J. H., Crichton, R. R., & Zecca, L. (2014). The role of iron in brain ageing and neurodegenerative disorders. *Lancet Neurology*, *13*(10), 1045–1060. https://doi.org/10.1016/S1474-4422(14)70117-6.

Wetter, T. C., Eisensehr, I., & Trenkwalder, C. (2004). Functional neuroimaging studies in restless legs syndrome. *Sleep Medicine*, *5*(4), 401–406. https://doi.org/10.1016/j.sleep.2004.01.009. S1389945704000218 [pii].

White, J. G., Southgate, E., Thomson, J. N., & Brenner, S. (1976). The structure of the ventral nerve cord of Caenorhabditis elegans. *Philosophical Transactions of the Royal Society of London, Series B*, *275*(938), 327–348.

Winkelmann, J., Schormair, B., Lichtner, P., Ripke, S., Xiong, L., Jalilzadeh, S., et al. (2007). Genome-wide association study of restless legs syndrome identifies common variants in three genomic regions. *Nature Genetics*, *39*(8), 1000–1006. ng2099 [pii]. https://doi.org/10.1038/ng2099.

Winkelmann, J., Stautner, A., Samtleben, W., & Trenkwalder, C. (2002). Long-term course of restless legs syndrome in dialysis patients after kidney transplantation. *Movement Disorders*, *17*(5), 1072–1076. https://doi.org/10.1002/mds.10231.

Wu, Y., Han, M., & Guan, K. L. (1995). MEK-2, a *Caenorhabditis elegans* MAP kinase kinase, functions in Ras-mediated vulval induction and other developmental events. *Genes & Development*, *9*(6), 742–755.

Xiong, L., Jang, K., Montplaisir, J., Levchenko, A., Thibodeau, P., Gaspar, C., et al. (2007). Canadian restless legs syndrome twin study. *Neurology*, *68*(19), 1631–1633. https://doi.org/10.1212/01.wnl.0000261016.90374.fd.

Xiong, L., Montplaisir, J., Desautels, A., Barhdadi, A., Turecki, G., Levchenko, A., et al. (2010). Family study of restless legs syndrome in Quebec, Canada: Clinical characterization of 671 familial cases. *Archives of Neurology*, *67*(5), 617–622. https://doi.org/10.1001/archneurol.2010.67.

Yang, Q., Li, L., Chen, Q., Foldvary-Schaefer, N., Ondo, W. G., & Wang, Q. K. (2011). Association studies of variants in MEIS1, BTBD9, and MAP2K5/SKOR1 with restless legs syndrome in a US population. *Sleep Medicine*, *12*(8), 800–804. S1389-9457(11)00228-0 [pii]. https://doi.org/10.1016/j.sleep.2011.06.006.

Yang, Q., Li, L., Yang, R., Shen, G. Q., Chen, Q., Foldvary-Schaefer, N., et al. (2011). Family-based and population-based association studies validate PTPRD as a risk factor for restless legs syndrome. *Movement Disorders*, *26*(3), 516–519. https://doi.org/10.1002/mds.23459.

Zhou, G., Bao, Z. Q., & Dixon, J. E. (1995). Components of a new human protein kinase signal transduction pathway. *The Journal of Biological Chemistry*, *270*(21), 12665–12669.

Zhu, J., Cui, L., Xu, A., Yin, X., Li, F., & Gao, J. (2017). MEIS1 inhibits clear cell renal cell carcinoma cells proliferation and in vitro invasion or migration. *BMC Cancer*, *17*(1), 176. https://doi.org/10.1186/s12885-017-3155-2.

Zhu, Q., Tan, Z., Zhao, S., Huang, H., Zhao, X., Hu, X., et al. (2015). Developmental expression and function analysis of protein tyrosine phosphatase receptor type D in oligodendrocyte myelination. *Neuroscience*, *308*, 106–114. https://doi.org/10.1016/j.neuroscience.2015.08.062.

CHAPTER EIGHT

Role of MEIS1 in restless legs syndrome: From GWAS to functional studies in mice

Aaro V. Salminen[a,b], Daniel D. Lam[a,c], Juliane Winkelmann[a,c,d,*]

[a]Institute of Neurogenomics, Helmholtz Zentrum München, Neuherberg, Germany
[b]Department of Neurology, Klinikum Rechts der Isar, Technische Universität München, Munich, Germany
[c]Lehrstuhl für Neurogenetik und Institut für Humangenetik, School of Medicine, Klinikum Rechts der Isar, Technische Universität München, Munich, Germany
[d]Munich Cluster for Systems Neurology (SyNergy), Munich, Germany
*Corresponding author: e-mail address: juliane.winkelmann@tum.de

Contents

Abstract

MEIS1 is a transcription factor playing an important role in the development of several organs, including central and peripheral nervous systems. A genetic locus spanning the *MEIS1* coding region has been associated with the risk of RLS in genome-wide association studies, with increasing evidence that *MEIS1* is the causal RLS gene. The RLS-linked genetic signal has been mapped to an intronic regulatory element within *MEIS1*. This element plays a role in the ganglionic eminences of the developing forebrain, with the RLS risk allele related to a reduced activation of the enhancer. This suggests that the ganglionic eminences play an important role in the development of genetic susceptibility to RLS. In addition, rare variants within MEIS1 have been shown to contribute to the disease risk. These variants were identified first in RLS families and later found in further RLS cases by targeted sequencing. Some of these variants alone are sufficient to suppress MEIS1 function in neural development, providing further evidence of the importance of neurodevelopmental processes in the pathological mechanism of MEIS1 in RLS. Heterozygous *Meis1* inactivation in mice causes hyperactivity at the onset of the inactive period, consistent with human RLS. In addition, these mice revealed an effect of MEIS1 on the dopaminergic system at both the spinal and supraspinal level.

Advances in Pharmacology, Volume 84
ISSN 1054-3589
https://doi.org/10.1016/bs.apha.2019.03.003
© 2019 Elsevier Inc.
All rights reserved.

More studies are needed in human genetics to determine the exact role of *MEIS1* variants in the risk of RLS, as well as in functional genetics and animal studies to further elucidate the pathological mechanism of MEIS1 in RLS.

Abbreviations

EEG electroencephalography
GWAS genome-wide association study
MEIS myeloid ecotropic virus integration site
NREM non-rapid eye movement (sleep stage)
PLMS periodic leg movements during sleep
SNP single nucleotide polymorphism
REM rapid eye movement (sleep stage)
RLS restless legs syndrome

1. Introduction

MEIS1 is a gene encoding the MEIS1 transcription factor, which contains a DNA-binding homeodomain. MEIS1 forms complexes with other homeodomain transcription factors, including PBX and HOX proteins, in order to regulate gene expression. MEIS1, a homolog of the invertebrate homothorax gene, plays central roles in diverse developmental processes, including development of the limbs, cardiovascular system, and blood (Azcoitia, Aracil, Martínez-A, & Torres, 2005; Hisa et al., 2004; Mercader et al., 1999; Stankunas et al., 2008). In addition, MEIS1 is a significant regulator of nervous system development, with important roles demonstrated in development of the sympathetic nervous system (Bouilloux et al., 2016), eye (Hisa et al., 2004), and cerebellar granule cells (Owa et al., 2018). *MEIS1* is also strongly expressed in the developing spinal cord, hindbrain, midbrain, and forebrain, but as yet its role in development of these regions remains to be clarified. In adult tissues, *MEIS1* is strongly expressed in various types of neurons and glia in a wide range of brain areas, including the cerebellum, hindbrain, midbrain, forebrain, and olfactory bulb in both mice (Saunders et al., 2018; Zeisel et al., 2018) and humans (Aguet et al., 2017). However, its role there similarly remains unclear.

MEIS1 has a close homolog, *MEIS2*, which is expressed in many of the same tissues as *MEIS1*, including the developing forebrain, in a partially overlapping pattern. This redundancy underlines the critical importance of MEIS proteins in regulating developmental processes.

MEIS1 was first described as a myeloid ecotropic virus integration site (hence its name), whereby virus integration caused overexpression of MEIS1 contributing to leukemogenesis (Moskow, Bullrich, Huebner, Daar, & Buchberg, 1995; Wong et al., 2007). Through genome-wide association studies, different *MEIS1* genetic variants have also been associated with RLS (Schormair et al., 2017), periodic leg movements during sleep (Moore et al., 2014), symptoms of insomnia (Hammerschlag et al., 2017; Lane et al., 2016), circadian rhythmicity (Ferguson et al., 2018), PR interval (Butler et al., 2012) and waist-to-hip ratio (Shungin et al., 2015).

In this chapter, we review the literature on the association between *MEIS1* and RLS, ranging from the genetic association in humans to animal models and what is known about the functional role of MEIS1 in disease etiology.

2. The genetic association between MEIS1 and RLS

Genetic associations with human phenotypes, such as a particular disease, can be studied with different methods depending on the population frequency and type of genetic variants of interest. When studying common genetic variants (minor allele frequency >5%), genome-wide association studies (GWAS) using genotyping arrays are the preferred approach. When studying rare genetic variants, exome sequencing or next-generation sequencing is used. RLS is a complex genetic disorder where both rare and common variants may contribute to the disease risk, and therefore requires the application of both approaches.

In the GWAS performed in RLS, the genetic locus tagged by the single nucleotide polymorphism (SNP) rs113851554 in intron 8 of *MEIS1* has consistently been the highest effect-size association (Schormair et al., 2017; Winkelmann et al., 2011, 2007). These studies have assessed the genetic associations with RLS diagnosed either by a physician or by a self-reported questionnaire. The association of RLS with the *MEIS1* locus also is detected when motor symptoms often associated with RLS, such as periodic leg movements during sleep (PLMS), are used as the phenotype (Moore et al., 2014). The association remained when corrected for the presence of RLS, indicating an independent effect of *MEIS1* on PLMS.

In the most recent meta-GWAS, combining three large population datasets, the SNP tagging the *MEIS1* locus showed an odds ratio of up to 2.16, exceptionally high for a common genetic variant (Schormair et al., 2017). This effect size was largest in the EU-RLS cohort where the disease had been diagnosed by an experienced physician. The locus does not contain alternative genes within the linkage disequilibrium block, increasing the chances that *MEIS1* is the causal gene in that specific locus. A second independent signal tagged by the SNP rs1820989 was observed near *MEIS1*, 1.3Mb downstream of the highest-confidence *MEIS1* SNP (Schormair et al., 2017) and also located in a conserved region potentially regulating the expression of the *MEIS1* gene. This second association further underlines the importance of *MEIS1* in RLS. Recently, the *MEIS1* locus has also been associated with symptoms of insomnia (Hammerschlag et al., 2017; Lane et al., 2016) and circadian rhythmicity measured by actigraphy (Ferguson et al., 2018). The association with insomnia was only partly explained by possible inclusion of RLS patients in the insomnia group (Hammerschlag et al., 2017). Therefore, it remains possible that in addition to the overlap in the traits, *MEIS1* functions in RLS, insomnia and circadian rhythmicity independent of each other.

In addition to common genetic variants detected in GWAS, rare variants also contribute to the heritability of RLS. A variant screening study showed an enrichment of loss-of-function variants within the coding region of the *MEIS1* gene in RLS patients compared to the general population (Schulte et al., 2014). Among the variants detected in this screening study is G815A, a missense variant encoding the amino acid change Arg272His, located in the DNA-binding homeodomain of MEIS1. This variant has previously been detected in two independent RLS families (Schulte et al., 2011; Vilariño-Güell et al., 2009), although with limited penetrance, making it the best documented RLS-associated rare variant.

3. The functional role of MEIS1 in RLS

Human genetic studies have shown that intronic variants in the *MEIS1* gene influence the susceptibility of an individual to develop RLS. However, intronic variants do not necessarily regulate their host gene, but may regulate other, more linearly distant genes (Smemo et al., 2014). To confirm a causal role of *MEIS1* in RLS, and to explore the potential mechanisms through which these variants affects the development of RLS, a series of functional studies in mice and zebrafish have been undertaken.

The RLS-linked GWAS signal located in an intron of *MEIS1* was mapped to a candidate causal variant (rs12469063) in a putative *MEIS1*-regulating enhancer element through high-resolution melting curve analysis (Spieler et al., 2014). In order to track the spatiotemporal activity pattern of this regulatory element, the sequence was coupled to a reporter gene in transgenic mouse and zebrafish assays. The regulatory element was observed to have highly specific activation pattern in the ganglionic eminences of the developing forebrain. The RLS risk allele of the candidate causal variant reduced the activity of the enhancer, as confirmed in both zebrafish and mouse experiments. In addition, the RLS risk allele modified the binding of CREB1, an upstream transcription factor, to the regulatory element. Taken together, these results strongly suggest that the RLS-linked regulatory element is involved in the development of the forebrain, implicating this process as a potential mechanism behind the genetic susceptibility to develop RLS (Spieler et al., 2014).

Homozygosity of the RLS risk allele is also associated with decreased expression of the MEIS1 transcript and protein in the thalamus, as indicated by a postmortem study on patients diagnosed with RLS (Xiong et al., 2009). Decreased expression was also detected in lymphoblastoid cells of homozygous RLS risk haplotype carriers, but not in the pons. Because MEIS1 is a transcription factor, changes in MEIS1 expression are expected to modify the expression of its target genes. Interestingly, the RLS-linked risk variant in *MEIS1* has also been associated with reduced expression of another RLS candidate gene, *SKOR1*, in lymphoblastoid cells and thalamus (Catoire et al., 2018). The effect of the RLS risk allele on *MEIS1* expression supports impaired MEIS1 function as a possible mechanism driving the disease predisposition, possibly through its effect on the iron storage and transport (Catoire et al., 2011). In addition, these data provide support for the hypothesis that *MEIS1* is indeed the gene affected by the genetic variants in that locus.

In another approach, rare variants within the *MEIS1* coding region were tested for their effect on MEIS1 function in a zebrafish neurodevelopmental assay (Schulte et al., 2014). Out of the 17 potentially RLS-linked nonsynonymous genetic variants tested, 6 were classified as null variants, indistinguishable from the complete suppression of MEIS1 by a splice-blocking morpholino. Among these deleterious variants was the Arg272His variant, previously detected in RLS families. The six null variants were significantly enriched in RLS patients compared to population controls. The complete suppression of MEIS1 function by the RLS-linked coding variants adds further support for impaired MEIS1 function in the developing nervous system as the pathological mechanism behind the MEIS1-related genetic susceptibility to develop RLS.

Taken together, the experimental data show that *MEIS1* is likely the causal gene mediating the genetic association of the intronic variants with RLS. In addition, there is good evidence that a neurodevelopmental mechanism of *MEIS1* might be the basis for disease susceptibility in humans.

4. MEIS1-based animal models

While the evidence for impaired MEIS1 function in RLS is well established, the consequences of the loss of MEIS1 in mouse models have not been explored until recently. Moreover, studying RLS-like behavior in mice has proven challenging due to the subjective nature of the disease in humans. In recent years, a heterozygous *Meis1* knock-out mouse line (Azcoitia et al., 2005) has enabled the investigation of the effects of reduced *Meis1* function on RLS-related phenotypes in mice.

The best characterized effect of loss of *Meis1* function in mice is the increased motor activity, confirmed in several independent cohorts in a novel environment (Salminen et al., 2017; Spieler et al., 2014) as well as in a 7-day activity recording where the mouse can acclimatize to the new environment (Meneely et al., 2018). When observing an aged cohort in a voluntary running wheel experiment, hyperactivity specific to the beginning of the inactive period was observed (Salminen et al., 2017). Motor coordination and grip strength in these mice is normal. The diurnal activity profile mirrors the appearance of the RLS symptoms in humans, suggesting the involvement of loss of MEIS1 function in generating this diurnal movement pattern.

MEIS1 deficiency also affects sensory function in these mice. The *Meis1* heterozygous null mice show a highly reproducible deficiency in sensorimotor gating, as indicated by decreased auditory prepulse inhibition (Salminen et al., 2017). This appears despite normal reflexes in the hotplate test (Salminen et al., 2017) and Hargreaves' test (Meneely et al., 2018), suggesting that nociceptive spinal circuits in these mice are functional, but supraspinal gating of sensory stimuli is impaired.

Another aspect that is heavily impacted by human RLS is sleep. Thus, fragmentation or reduction of sleep could be expected from an RLS mouse model. However, most sleep parameters in these mice are normal (Salminen et al., 2018). *Meis1* deficiency does not affect sleep latency, amounts of

NREM or REM sleep, nor sleep bout length. Only a trend toward a lower delta power in the EEG was detected, possibly indicating a lower sleep quality.

Dopamine agonists are the most commonly used medication in human RLS, and a dopaminergic dysfunction has been proposed as a component of the underlying pathological mechanism of RLS (Ferré, García-Borreguero, Allen, & Earley, 2019). The dopaminergic system has thus also been investigated in *Meis1*-deficient mice through pharmacological challenges. *Meis1*-deficient mice are insensitive to the reduction of prepulse inhibition caused by pramipexole, a D3 receptor preferential dopamine agonist (Salminen et al., 2017). The effect of pramipexole on the withdrawal latency from a thermal stimulus in heterozygous and wildtype mice was comparable (Meneely et al., 2018). This withdrawal latency was, on the other hand, modified by a D1-preferential dopamine receptor agonist in heterozygous mice but not in wildtypes. The differential reactions to D3 and D1 receptor stimulation were supported by the abnormally high spinal expression of the D1 receptor but normal D3 receptor expression (Meneely et al., 2018). Taken together, loss of *Meis1* function has a complex effect on the dopaminergic system, affecting the D3 receptors only in the supraspinal nervous system while increasing the sensory sensitivity to D1 receptor agonists at the spinal level.

While *Meis1*-deficient mice have some of the hallmark behavioral features expected from an RLS animal model (Allen et al., 2017), such as altered motor behavior, they do not show RLS-like sensory or sleep phenotypes. There could be several explanations for this. MEIS1 has multiple functions in different tissues and different developmental stages, and a global knockout model may be too unspecific to generate a clear RLS phenotype. On the other hand, in humans, RLS often requires an environmental trigger before the disease manifests (Trenkwalder, Allen, Högl, Paulus, & Winkelmann, 2016). Therefore, environmental challenges on top of genetic modifications may be necessary for a complete RLS phenotype to arise, as already suggested by an iron-deficiency rat model (Lai et al., 2017).

5. Conclusion

Much work remains to be done on how MEIS1 is involved in RLS pathogenesis. In human genetics, it remains inconclusive whether common variants influence the inheritance of RLS in families. As MEIS1 appears to be involved in the development of many parts of the central and peripheral nervous systems, one significant challenge is to prioritize potentially important areas and circuits. Here, guidance from patient genetic association data is particularly valuable, as this can inform which specific regulatory elements are RLS-related. These can then be evaluated in terms of where and when in development they are active (Spieler et al., 2014).

Another hurdle is the pleiotropy of MEIS1. Mice with homozygous null alleles die in mid-gestation due to hematopoietic and angiogenic defects (Azcoitia et al., 2005; Hisa et al., 2004), making it impossible to investigate brain development in the complete absence of functional MEIS1. On the other hand, the redundancy of MEIS1 and MEIS2 pose a different type of challenge, as loss of one allele of either gene has only modest effects (Salminen et al., 2017). Overcoming these challenges will require novel mouse genetic models, such as those with precise RLS-related mutations or conditional null alleles. Finally, disembodied brain organoids would be a valuable model, permitting the investigation of the role of MEIS1 in human brain development, function as well as disease.

Compliance with ethical standards

Conflict of interest statements

Aaro V. Salminen declares no conflict of interest. Daniel D. Lam declares no conflict of interest. Juliane Winkelmann has received speaker honoraria from Bayer and UCB, as well as research grants from Else Kröner Foundation and German Research Foundation (DFG).

Human and animal rights and informed consent

This article does not contain any studies with human or animal subjects performed by any of the authors.

References

Aguet, F., Brown, A. A., Castel, S. E., Davis, J. R., He, Y., Jo, B., et al. (2017). Genetic effects on gene expression across human tissues. *Nature*, *550*(7675), 204–213.

Allen, R. P., Donelson, N. C., Jones, B. C., Li, Y., Manconi, M., Rye, D. B., et al. (2017). Animal models of RLS phenotypes. *Sleep Medicine*, *31*, 23–28.

Azcoitia, V., Aracil, M., Martínez-A, C., & Torres, M. (2005). The homeodomain protein Meis1 is essential for definitive hematopoiesis and vascular patterning in the mouse embryo. *Developmental Biology*, *280*(2), 307–320.

Bouilloux, F., Thireau, J., Ventéo, S., Farah, C., Karam, S., Dauvilliers, Y., et al. (2016). Loss of the transcription factor Meis1 prevents sympathetic neurons target-field innervation and increases susceptibility to sudden cardiac death. *eLife*, *5*, e11627.

Butler, A. M., Yin, X., Evans, D. S., Nalls, M. A., Smith, E. N., Tanaka, T., et al. (2012). Novel loci associated with PR interval in a genome-wide association study of 10 African American cohorts. *Circulation Cardiovascular Genetics*, *5*(6), 639–646.

Catoire, H., Dion, P. A., Xiong, L., Amari, M., Gaudet, R., Girard, S. L., et al. (2011). Restless legs syndrome-associated MEIS1 risk variant influences iron homeostasis. *Annals of Neurology*, *70*(1), 170–175.

Catoire, H., Sarayloo, F., Mourabit Amari, K., Apuzzo, S., Grant, A., Rochefort, D., et al. (2018). A direct interaction between two restless legs syndrome predisposing genes: MEIS1 and SKOR1. *Scientific Reports*, *8*(1), 12173.

Ferguson, A., Lyall, L. M., Ward, J., Strawbridge, R. J., Cullen, B., Graham, N., et al. (2018). Genome-wide association study of circadian rhythmicity in 71,500 UK biobank participants and polygenic association with mood instability. *eBioMedicine*, *35*, 279–287.

Ferré, S., García-Borreguero, D., Allen, R. P., & Earley, C. J. (2019). New insights into the neurobiology of restless legs syndrome. *The Neuroscientist*, *25*, 113–125. https://doi.org/10.1177/1073858418791763.

Hammerschlag, A. R., Stringer, S., de Leeuw, C. A., Sniekers, S., Taskesen, E., Watanabe, K., et al. (2017). Genome-wide association analysis of insomnia complaints identifies risk genes and genetic overlap with psychiatric and metabolic traits. *Nature Genetics*, *49*(11), 1584–1592.

Hisa, T., Spence, S. E., Rachel, R. A., Fujita, M., Nakamura, T., Ward, J. M., et al. (2004). Hematopoietic, angiogenic and eye defects in Meis1 mutant animals. *The EMBO Journal*, *23*(2), 450–459.

Lai, Y.-Y., Cheng, Y.-H., Hsieh, K.-C., Nguyen, D., Chew, K.-T., Ramanathan, L., et al. (2017). Motor hyperactivity of the iron-deficient rat—An animal model of restless legs syndrome. *Movement Disorders*, *32*(12), 1687–1693.

Lane, J. M., Liang, J., Vlasac, I., Anderson, S. G., Bechtold, D. A., Bowden, J., et al. (2016). Genome-wide association analyses of sleep disturbance traits identify new loci and highlight shared genetics with neuropsychiatric and metabolic traits. *Nature Genetics*, *49*(2), 274–281.

Meneely, S., Dinkins, M.-L., Kassai, M., Lyu, S., Liu, Y., Lin, C.-T., et al. (2018). Differential dopamine D1 and D3 receptor modulation and expression in the spinal cord of two mouse models of restless legs syndrome. *Frontiers in Behavioral Neuroscience*, *12*, 199.

Mercader, N., Leonardo, E., Azpiazu, N., Serrano, A., Morata, G., Martínez-A, C., et al. (1999). Conserved regulation of proximodistal limb axis development by Meis1/Hth. *Nature*, *402*(6760), 425–429.

Moore, H., Winkelmann, J., Lin, L., Finn, L., Peppard, P., & Mignot, E. (2014). Periodic leg movements during sleep are associated with polymorphisms in BTBD9, TOX3/BC034767, MEIS1, MAP2K5/SKOR1, and PTPRD. *Sleep*, *37*(9), 1535–1542.

Moskow, J. J., Bullrich, F., Huebner, K., Daar, I. O., & Buchberg, A. M. (1995). Meis1, a PBX1-related homeobox gene involved in myeloid leukemia in BXH-2 mice. *Molecular and Cellular Biology*, *15*(10), 5434–5443.

Owa, T., Taya, S., Miyashita, S., Yamashita, M., Adachi, T., Yamada, K., et al. (2018). Meis1 coordinates cerebellar granule cell development by regulating Pax6 transcription, BMP signaling and Atoh1 degradation. *The Journal of Neuroscience: The Official Journal of the Society for Neuroscience*, *38*(5), 1277–1294.

Salminen, A. V., Garrett, L., Schormair, B., Rozman, J., Giesert, F., Niedermeier, K. M., et al. (2017). *Meis1* : Effects on motor phenotypes and the sensorimotor system in mice. *Disease Models & Mechanisms*, *10*(8), 981–991.

Salminen, A. V., Schormair, B., Flachskamm, C., Torres, M., Müller-Myhsok, B., Kimura, M., et al. (2018). Sleep disturbance by pramipexole is modified by Meis1 in mice. *Journal of Sleep Research*, *27*(4), e12557.

Saunders, A., Macosko, E. Z., Wysoker, A., Goldman, M., Krienen, F. M., de Rivera, H., et al. (2018). Molecular diversity and specializations among the cells of the adult mouse brain. *Cell*, *174*(4), 1015–1030.e16.

Schormair, B., Zhao, C., Bell, S., Tilch, E., Salminen, A. V., Pütz, B., et al. (2017). Identification of novel risk loci for restless legs syndrome in genome-wide association studies in individuals of European ancestry: A meta-analysis. *The Lancet Neurology*, *16*(11), 898–907.

Schulte, E. C., Knauf, F., Kemlink, D., Schormair, B., Lichtner, P., Gieger, C., et al. (2011). Variant screening of the coding regions of MEIS1 in patients with restless legs syndrome. *Neurology*, *76*(12), 1106–1108.

Schulte, E. C., Kousi, M., Tan, P. L., Tilch, E., Knauf, F., Lichtner, P., et al. (2014). Targeted resequencing and systematic in vivo functional testing identifies rare variants in MEIS1 as significant contributors to restless legs syndrome. *American Journal of Human Genetics*, *95*(1), 85–95.

Shungin, D., Winkler, T. W., Croteau-Chonka, D. C., Ferreira, T., Locke, A. E., Mägi, R., et al. (2015). New genetic loci link adipose and insulin biology to body fat distribution. *Nature*, *518*(7538), 187–196.

Smemo, S., Tena, J. J., Kim, K.-H., Gamazon, E. R., Sakabe, N. J., Gómez-Marín, C., et al. (2014). Obesity-associated variants within FTO form long-range functional connections with IRX3. *Nature*, *507*(7492), 371–375.

Spieler, D., Kaffe, M., Knauf, F., Bessa, J., Tena, J. J., Giesert, F., et al. (2014). Restless legs syndrome-associated intronic common variant in Meis1 alters enhancer function in the developing telencephalon. *Genome Research*, *24*(4), 592–603.

Stankunas, K., Shang, C., Twu, K. Y., Kao, S.-C., Jenkins, N. A., Copeland, N. G., et al. (2008). Pbx/Meis deficiencies demonstrate multigenetic origins of congenital heart disease. *Circulation Research*, *103*(7), 702–709.

Trenkwalder, C., Allen, R., Högl, B., Paulus, W., & Winkelmann, J. (2016). Restless legs syndrome associated with major diseases: A systematic review and new concept. *Neurology*, *86*(14), 1336–1343.

Vilariño-Güell, C., Chai, H., Keeling, B. H., Young, J. E., Rajput, A., Lynch, T., et al. (2009). Meis1 p.r272h in familial restless legs syndrome. *Neurology*, *73*(3), 243–245.

Winkelmann, J., Czamara, D., Schormair, B., Knauf, F., Schulte, E. C., Trenkwalder, C., et al. (2011). Genome-wide association study identifies novel restless legs syndrome susceptibility loci on 2p14 and 16q12.1. *PLoS Genetics*, 7(7), 1–10.

Winkelmann, J., Schormair, B., Lichtner, P., Ripke, S., Xiong, L., Jalilzadeh, S., et al. (2007). Genome-wide association study of restless legs syndrome identifies common variants in three genomic regions. *Nature Genetics*, *39*(8), 1000–1006.

Wong, P., Iwasaki, M., Somervaille, T. C. P., So, C. W. E., So, C. W. E., & Cleary, M. L. (2007). Meis1 is an essential and rate-limiting regulator of MLL leukemia stem cell potential. *Genes & Development*, *21*(21), 2762–2774.

Xiong, L., Catoire, H., Dion, P., Gaspar, C., Lafrenière, R. G., Girard, S. L., et al. (2009). MEIS1 intronic risk haplotype associated with restless legs syndrome affects its mRNA and protein expression levels. *Human Molecular Genetics*, *18*(6), 1065–1074.

Zeisel, A., Hochgerner, H., Lönnerberg, P., Johnsson, A., Memic, F., van der Zwan, J., et al. (2018). Molecular architecture of the mouse nervous system. *Cell*, *174*(4), 999–1014.e22.

SECTION III

Treatments and treatment complications

CHAPTER NINE

Non-dopaminergic vs. dopaminergic treatment options in restless legs syndrome

Vivian Wanner[a], Celia Garcia Malo[b], Sofía Romero[b], Irene Cano-Pumarega[b], Diego García-Borreguero[b,*]
[a]Instituto Europeo del Sueño, Santiago, Chile
[b]Sleep Research Institute, Madrid, Spain
*Corresponding author: e-mail address: dgb@iis.es

Contents

Abstract

Two types of drugs have been extensively investigated for the treatment of restless legs syndrome (RLS)/Willis-Ekbom disease (WED): dopamine agonists and α2δ ligands to the α2δ subunit of calcium channels. Comparative studies show that both classes of drugs are similarly effective in treating RLS symptoms over the short- and long-term. While dopamine agonists are more effective in treating periodic limb movements (PLMs), α2δ ligands are more effective in consolidating sleep. However, given the fact that dopamine agonists cause high rates of augmentation of symptoms, recent international guidelines recommend that whenever possible the initial treatment of choice should be an α2δ ligand. In fact, the most effective preventive strategy involves not using dopaminergic agents unless absolutely necessary. Indeed, should dopaminergic treatment be needed to handle the symptoms effectively, then it is recommended that the

Advances in Pharmacology, Volume 84
ISSN 1054-3589
https://doi.org/10.1016/bs.apha.2019.02.003
© 2019 Elsevier Inc.
All rights reserved.

dopaminergic load be reduced by using the lowest effective dose for the shortest possible period of time. However, it must be taken into account that the only α2δ ligand approved for RLS/WED is gabapentin enacarbil, which is not yet available in Europe.

Furthermore, recent studies have also reported on the efficacy of opioids as a second-line treatment of RLS/WED, following treatment failure with dopamine agonists. Recent guidelines have taken these new data into account and highlight that a low dose of an opioid (prolonged-release oxycodone or methadone) may be considered in patients with very severe augmentation of symptoms.

Alternative non-dopaminergic treatment concepts based on glutamatergic and adenosinergic mechanisms are currently in development, and are likely to provide encouraging therapeutic alternatives.

Abbreviations

EURLSSG european restless legs syndrome study group
ICD impulse control disorders.
IRLSSG international restless legs syndrome study group
PLM periodic limb movements
PLMS periodic limb movements of sleep
RLSF restless legs syndrome foundation
WASO wake time after sleep onset

1. Introduction

Although the short-term efficacy of dopaminergic agents is firmly established for the treatment of restless legs syndrome (RLS)/Willis-Ekbom disease (WED) (Garcia-Borreguero et al., 2013) the main long-term complications associated with these drugs include loss of efficacy and augmentation of symptoms (Garcia-Borreguero & Williams, 2010). Loss of efficacy is a reduction of response to dopaminergic treatment in which some degree of response is still preserved (Garcia-Borreguero et al., 2007). In contrast to augmentation, the severity of symptoms is not worse than before treatment initiation. Indeed, during augmentation, symptoms become more severe with dopaminergic treatment than before treatment initiation. Treatment failure is not uncommon under dopaminergic treatment: a number of retrospective evaluations have highlighted that over the long-term, the percentage of patients whose symptoms do not improve, or even worsen despite treatment, is high. Overall, during the first 8–10 years of treatment, studies show that 40–60% of patients worsen or have to discontinue/change their dopaminergic medication (Lipford & Silber, 2012; Mitterling et al., 2015; Silver, Allen, Senerth, & Earley, 2011). Several evidence-based reviews of the literature have examined the degree of therapeutic efficacy and toxicity for different pharmacological agents. Two classes of drugs, namely dopamine agonists and α2δ ligands, have been investigated extensively in placebo-controlled studies lasting 3–6 months.

In the following sections we will perform a critical comparison between the different classes of drugs, paying special attention to the two classes of drugs (dopamine agonists and α2δ ligands) for which comparative studies have been performed. We will also discuss the existing clinical evidence for the use of opioids as a second-line treatment in RLS/WED.

2. Dopamine agonists

Dopaminergic drugs have been widely used over the last decades for the treatment of RLS/WED. The first dopaminergic drug to be used for RLS was levodopa (Akpinar, 1982). Although the first trials were very promising, levodopa has a short half-life that results in early morning rebound of symptoms (Guilleminault, Cetel, & Philip, 1993). This led to dopamine agonists with longer half-lives being studied, these became the first-line treatment for RLS/WED. Following trials that reported on the short-term efficacy of ropinirole, pramipexole, and rotigotine, these dopamine agonists were approved for the treatment of RLS/WED between 2004 and 2009.

3. α2δ Ligands

α2δ Ligands are α2δ subunit ligands of the L-type voltage-regulated calcium channels, and in addition to being approved as anticonvulsants and for the treatment of neuropathic pain, these drugs have also been used for the treatment of RLS since the early 2000s. The main compounds are gabapentin and pregabalin, have yet to receive regulatory approval for RLS/WED. A pro-drug of gabapentin, gabapentin enacarbil, has undergone full clinical development and has received regulatory approval in the United States and Japan. In contrast to dopamine agonists, which exert their effects on dopaminergic receptors, the mechanism of action of α2δ ligands likely consists in a reduction of glutamatergic release (Ferre, Earley, Gulyani, & Garcia-Borreguero, 2017). This type of drug exert a selective, high-affinity binding to the α2δ subtype-1 protein of calcium channels which modulate Ca^{++} influx at nerve terminal in response to depolarization leading to a decrease in excitatory neurotrasmitters (mainly glutamate). Table 1 provides an overview of the half-lives and therapeutic dosages of dopamine agonists and α2δ ligands.

Table 1 Half-lives and therapeutic dosages of dopamine agonists and α2δ ligands.

	Maximum dosage for drugs approved for treating RLS	Half-life (h)
Pramipexole (approved USA, EU, Japan)	0.35 mg, rarely 0.52 mg	8–10
Rotigotine (approved USA, EU, Japan)	3 mg	Acts 24 h during patch application
Ropinirole (approved USA, EU, Japan)	4 mg	6–7
Gabapentin enacarbil (approved USA, Japan)	1200 mg/day[a]	5–6
Pregabalin (not approved)	300 mg/day[b]	6

[a]FDA-approved dose is 600 mg/day.
[b]Not approved by any regulatory agency. If ever used unlabeled, personal recommendation for the maximal dose to be considered based on published data (Allen et al., 2014; Garcia-Borreguero et al., 2010).

4. Short-term efficacy

Dopamine agonists have been shown to be moderately effective for RLS/WED in a number of short-term (up to 7 months) placebo-controlled studies. A meta-analysis (Hornyak, Trenkwalder, Kohnen, & Scholz, 2012) examined 35 placebo-controlled trials including a total of 6954 patients, with a mean treatment duration of 10.3 (standard deviation: 7.3) weeks, with treatment durations up to 7 months. Overall, DAs showed a moderate improvement in the International RLS Severity Scale score (mean difference −5.7 points $P<0.00001$) and the Clinical Global Impression-Improvement response (risk ratio 1.44 $P<0.00001$) compared with placebo.

As for the α2δ ligands, several studies support their efficacy in placebo-controlled studies (Garcia-Borreguero et al., 2013; Winkelman et al., 2016; Winkelmann et al., 2018). While the level of evidence for gabapentin is clearly lower, given the scarcity of controlled studies, both pregabalin and gabapentin enacarbil have been well investigated.

To date, two studies have compared the short-term efficacy of α2δ ligands with dopamine agonists: A first study compared 85 idiopathic RLS patients with sleep disturbance, randomized across 6 treatment sequences comprising three 4-week periods on pregabalin 300 mg/day ($n=75$), pramipexole 0.5 mg/day ($n=76$), or placebo ($n=73$). Although RLS severity was not a primary endpoint, the study showed non-inferiority

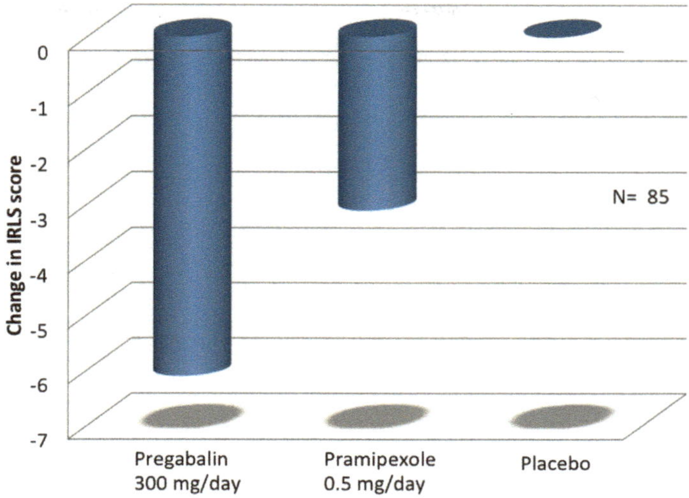

Fig. 1 Change in IRLS score following a 4-week treatment period: pregabalin vs. pramipexole vs. placebo (Garcia-Borreguero et al., 2014).

of 300 mg/day pregabalin compared to 0.5 mg/day pramipexole (Fig. 1) (Garcia-Borreguero et al., 2014).

In another study (Allen et al., 2014), 719 patients were randomized to receive pregabalin 300 mg/day, pramipexole 0.25 mg/day, pramipexole 0.5 mg/day, or placebo. Over a period of 12 weeks, the improvement (reduction) in mean score on the IRLS scale was greater, by 4.5 points, among individuals receiving pregabalin than among those receiving placebo, and the proportion of patients with symptoms that were "very much improved" or "much improved" was also greater with pregabalin than with placebo: 300 mg pregabalin and 0.5 mg pramipexole were both superior to placebo, but not pramipexole 0.25 mg. No differences existed between the therapeutic effects of pregabalin and any of the two doses of pramipexole.

Moreover, in a comprehensive meta-analysis, 58 placebo-controlled, and 4 active-controlled clinical trials, Hornyak et al. found that changes in the IRLS in the substance groups were comparable ($P < 0.78$) across dopaminergics and non-dopaminergic medications, with a mean reduction in the IRLS scale of −5.47 points for dopamine agonists, −5.12 points for anticonvulsants ($\alpha 2\delta$ ligands and levetiracetam), and −4.59 points for iron treatments (Hornyak et al., 2014). Taken together, both comparative studies and meta-analyses suggest that the therapeutic efficacy of 300 mg/day pregabalin and 0.5 mg/day pramipexole is similar.

Table 2 Polysomnography endpoints: comparison between pramipexole, pregabalin and placebo.

	LS mean (SEM)			LS mean difference (95% CI)			
Periodic limb movement	**Pregabalin**	**Pramipexole**	**Placebo**	**Pregabalin vs. placebo**	***P* value**	**Pregabalin vs. pramipexole**	***P* value**
PLMAI, PLMA/h	3.9 (0.7)	2.7 (0.7)	7.6 (0.7)	−3.7 (−5.4 to −1.9)	<0.0001	1.3 (−0.5 to 3.0)	NA
PLMSI, PLMS/h	22.4 (2.5)	8.0 (2.4)	37.0 (2.5)	−14.5 (−20.8 to −8.2)	NA	14.4 (8.2 to 20.7)	NA

Reprinted with permission from Garcia-Borreguero, D., Patrick, J., DuBrava, S., Becker, P. M., Lankford, A., Chen, C., et al. (2014). Pregabalin versus pramipexole: effects on sleep disturbance in restless legs syndrome. *Sleep, 37*(4), 635–643. doi:10.5665/sleep.3558.

5. Periodic limb movements of sleep (PLMS)

Both dopaminergic medications and α2δ ligands have shown superiority over placebo for the treatment of PLMS (Winkelmann et al., 2018). However, in the only comparative trial between both classes of drugs, both 0.5 mg pramipexole and 300 mg pregabalin improved the PLMS-index (Garcia-Borreguero et al., 2014); however, the reduction was lower than with pramipexole. Regarding the periodic limb movement arousal index (PLMAI), the reduction with pregabalin was similar to pramipexole and greater than placebo.

In the above-mentioned meta-analysis, Hornyak et al. (2014) found that PLMSI changes during treatment showed a marked decrease with dopamine agonists (−22.50/h), levodopa (−26.01/h), and oxycodone (−34.46/h) compared with a slight decrease for anticonvulsants (α2δ ligands, levetiracetam; −8.48/h) and iron treatments (−13.10/h). Overall, both classes of drugs are effective for the treatment of PLMS, but dopaminergic agents are more effective in reducing PLMS than α2δ ligands (Table 2 and Fig. 2).

6. Sleep

Both dopamine agonists and α2δ ligands exert an improvement in subjective total sleep time and sleep quality as measured on sleep rating scales (Hornyak et al., 2014, 2012). However, the abovementioned comparative 4-week study between pregabalin 300 mg and pramipexole 0.5 mg showed greater improvements for pregabalin than for pramipexole in subjective total

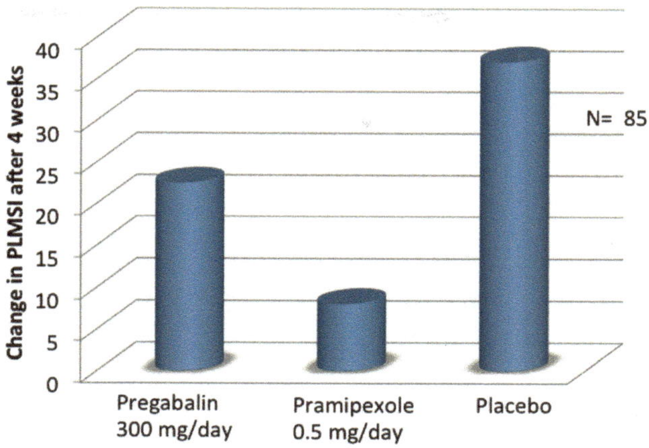

Fig. 2 PLMI following a 4-week treatment period: pregabalin vs. pramipexole vs. placebo (Garcia-Borreguero et al., 2014).

sleep time and sleep maintenance. When measured with polysomnography, pregabalin caused greater increases in slow wave sleep, as well as greater reductions in wake time after sleep onset (WASO) and in the number of awakenings after sleep onset (Garcia-Borreguero et al., 2014). Taken together, α2δ ligands are more effective improving sleep than dopaminergic drugs (Table 3 and Fig. 3).

7. Long-term efficacy

Dopamine agonists have been evaluated in several placebo-controlled trials during periods of up to 6 months (Garcia-Borreguero et al., 2013; Winkelmann et al., 2018). Besides, open long-term evaluations exist for rotigotine, ropinirole, and pramipexole. In all these studies the therapeutic efficacy of these drugs was maintained over the entire duration of the study. Similarly, open-label long-term evaluations exist for gabapentin enacarbil but not for gabapentin.

The only prospective, long-term double-blind study performed so far using two active drugs compared pramipexole (two arms of 0.25 and 0.5 mg) and pregabalin (300 mg) over a period of 52 weeks in 719 patients. The pregabalin group had a mean decrease in IRLS score from baseline that was 3.8 points greater than the decrease in the IRLS score of the 0.25-mg pramipexole group and 3.1 points greater than that of the 0.5-mg pramipexole group) ($P < 0.05$) (Allen et al., 2014). The IRLSSG guidelines on long-term treatment for RLS concluded that pregabalin may be more effective than pramipexole in

Table 3 Sleep parameters: comparison between pramipexole, pregabalin and placebo.

	LS mean (SEM)			LS mean difference (95% CI)			
Sleep maintenance	**Pregabalin**	**Pramipexole**	**Placebo**	**Pregabalin vs. placebo**	***P* value**	**Pregabalin vs. pramipexole**	***P* value**
WASO, min	51.5 (4.2)	78.4 (4.1)	78.6 (4.2)	−27.1 (−35.8 to −18.4)	<0.0001	−26.9 (−35.5 to −18.3)	NA
NAASO, count	18.4 (1.0)	26.3 (1.0)	21.1 (1.0)	−2.7 (−4.6 to −0.7)	NA	−7.9 (−9.8 to −5.9)	<0.0001
TST, min	402.4 (6.0)	376.5 (5.8)	369.7 (6.0)	32.7 (22.0 to 43.4)	NA	25.9 (15.2 to 36.5)	NA
SE, %	83.8 (1.2)	78.6 (1.2)	77.0 (1.2)	6.8 (4.6 to 9.0)	NA	5.2 (3.0 to 7.5)	NA

Reprinted with permission from Garcia-Borreguero, D., Patrick, J., DuBrava, S., Becker, P. M., Lankford, A., Chen, C., et al. (2014). Pregabalin versus pramipexole: effects on sleep disturbance in restless legs syndrome. *Sleep, 37*(4), 635–643. doi:10.5665/sleep.3558.

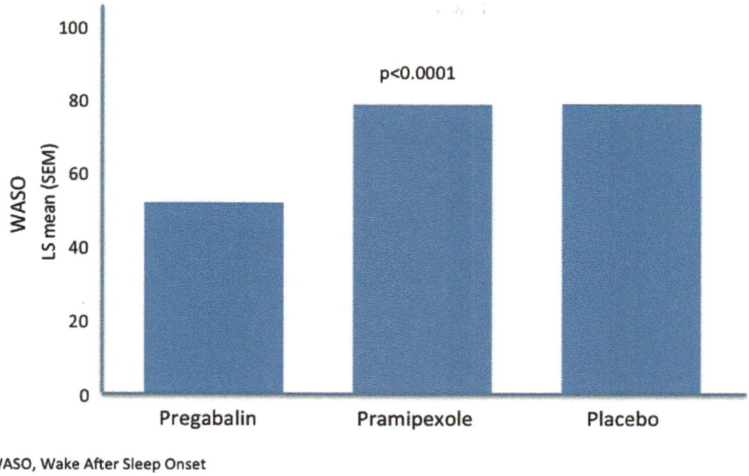

Fig. 3 Effects on wake time after sleep onset: pregabalin vs. pramipexole (Garcia-Borreguero et al., 2014).

treatment of RLS for 1 year. In summary, both types of drugs have shown therapeutic improvement over the long-term, although pregabalin proved to be superior to pramipexole in a double-blind 52-week study.

8. Augmentation

Augmentation is a drug class-specific complication of dopaminergic treatment and was first described in 1996 when it was reported in 73% of RLS/WED patients treated with carbidopa/levodopa (Allen & Earley, 1996). It is defined as a worsening of symptom severity manifested by an earlier onset of symptoms in the afternoon or evening compared to before treatment initiation, a spread of symptoms to the upper arms, a shortening of the latency until onset of symptoms when at rest, and an overall increase in symptom intensity (Garcia-Borreguero, Allen, et al., 2007). Hitherto, augmentation has been reported to occur under all dopaminergic drugs (Garcia-Borreguero & Williams, 2014).

As noted in the most recent IRLSSG guidelines on augmentation (Garcia-Borreguero et al., 2016) it is difficult to evaluate the prevalence of augmentation as it varies according to the drug, its dose, the number of subjects, the duration and type of study, as well as the criteria used to evaluate augmentation (see Table 4). Nevertheless, reported augmentation rates increase with study duration: in short-term studies augmentation rates

Table 4 Overview of tools used to assess augmentation in RLS/WED trials.

Method	Description
Allen Earley criteria (Allen & Earley, 1996)	First description of RLS/WED: augmentation was characterized as an earlier onset of symptoms in the afternoon, a shorter latency to onset of symptoms when at rest, a spreading of symptoms to the upper limbs and the trunk, an overall increase in the intensity of symptoms and a shorter effect of the medication
NIH criteria (Allen et al., 2003)	Clinical criteria based on consensus. The primary features of augmentation were identified as a drug-induced shifting of symptoms to a period of time 2 h earlier than was the typical time of daily onset prior to pharmacological intervention OR increased leg movements, decreased duration of treatment benefit, spread of the symptoms to other body parts, decreased amount of time that it is possible to stay at rest without symptoms, and paradoxical response to dose increase
Max Planck Institute (MPI) criteria for diagnosing RLS augmentation (Garcia-Borreguero, Allen, et al., 2007)	Criteria developed based on empirical information from clinical studies with levodopa and short-acting dopamine agonists, not longer duration dopamine agents. The main criteria outlined in this definition are a 4-h time advance of symptoms, or a smaller (2–4 h) advance of symptoms expressed along with other required clinical indications, such as a shorter latency of symptoms at rest, a spread of symptoms to other body parts in addition to the lower limbs, or a greater intensity of symptoms. A paradoxical response to treatment—an increase in severity with increasing dose of medication, and an improvement following decrease in medication—was considered an alternative key feature for diagnosis. The greater emphasis on time shift of symptoms may benefit longer-acting dopamine agonists, and this may explain the lower rate of augmentation found for these drugs
Augmentation severity rating scale (ASRS)	Three items are used to assess the severity of augmentation: earlier onset of symptoms, shorter latency to symptom occurrence at rest, and spreading to other body parts. Augmentation severity is represented in a total score

Reprinted with permission from Garcia-Borreguero, D., Patrick, J., DuBrava, S., Becker, P. M., Lankford, A., Chen, C., et al. (2014). Pregabalin versus pramipexole: effects on sleep disturbance in restless legs syndrome. *Sleep, 37*(4), 635–643. doi:10.5665/sleep.3558.

of <10% have been reported, (Allen et al., 2014; Ferini-Strambi, 2002; Garcia-Borreguero et al., 2012, 2007; Högl et al., 2011) while in studies lasting 2–3 years augmentation rates are higher at 30% (Allen et al., 2011; Ondo, Romanyshyn, Vuong, & Lai, 2004; Silber, Girish, & Izurieta, 2003; Silber, Shepard, & Wisbey, 1997; Winkelman & Johnston, 2004) and in two very long-term studies (approx. 10 years) augmentation has been reported to be 42–68% (Lipford & Silber, 2012; Silver et al., 2011).

Augmentation manifests as a frequently fluctuating but slowly progressive increase in symptom severity and as such, it is difficult to differentiate from the symptoms of RLS/WED per se. Due to its progressive nature it does not become evident immediately after treatment initiation. However, its likelihood increases with the duration and dose. All this makes it hard to prevent.

It is also likely that the deterioration of RLS/WED severity taking place during augmentation reduces the response rate to future non-dopaminergic such as $\alpha 2\delta$ ligands, as shown by a recent study (Garcia-Borreguero, Cano, et al., 2018).

The recent IRLSSG/EURLSSG/RLSF guidelines (Garcia-Borreguero et al., 2016) seek to facilitate the identification of augmentation in clinical practice by recommending that physicians consider the presence of augmentation whenever a patient who has been on stable treatment for at least 6 months requests additional medication. Four screening questions, that have yet to be validated, may be used for this purpose in patients currently under treatment with dopaminergic agents. An affirmative answer to any of these four questions should lead the physician to suspect the presence of augmentation:

1. Do RLS/WED symptoms appear earlier than when the drug was first started?
2. Are higher doses of the drug now needed, or do you need to take the medicine earlier, to control the RLS/WED symptoms compared to the original effective dose?
3. Has the intensity of symptoms worsened since starting the medication?
4. Have symptoms spread to other parts of the body (e.g., arms) since starting the medication? (Garcia-Borreguero et al., 2016)

9. General toxicity

Common side effects reported under dopamine agonists include nausea, vomiting, headache, hypotension, excessive daytime sleepiness, weight gain, and impulse control disorders (ICDs). During treatment with

$\alpha2\delta$ ligands, dizziness, somnolence, fatigue, weight gain, and constipation are relatively common (Garcia-Borreguero et al., 2013).

In the above-mentioned 52-week double-blind comparative study between pregabalin and pramipexole (Allen et al., 2014) the overall rate of occurrence of adverse reactions for patients undergoing treatment with pregabalin was 85.2%, and 27.5% of these patients had to discontinue due to adverse effects. In the group of patients treated with the lower dose (0.25 mg) of pramipexole, adverse effects were reported by 79.8% of them, and 18.5 had to discontinue for that reason.

Dizziness and somnolence were far more common during treatment with pregabalin, while headache and nausea were more common under the lower dose of pramipexole (Allen et al., 2014).

10. Impulse control disorders (ICDs)

ICDs—including pathologic gambling, hypersexuality, compulsive eating, compulsive shopping, obsessive-compulsive disorder, or punding—are adverse reactions known to be associated with the use of dopamine-receptor agonists. Published surveys of patients with RLS/WED treated with dopaminergic agents showed rates of ICD up to 17%. These rates of ICDs are presumed to be dose dependent, as noted by Ondo and Lai (2008) who compared ICDs rates in patients with Parkinson's disease and those with RLS/WED. But this has not been a consistent finding in all of studies. Most studies report development or worsening of ICDs with increasing doses of the dopaminergic drug and a decrease in ICDs with decreasing doses (Bayard, Yu, Langenier, Carlander, & Dauvilliers, 2010; Cornelius, Tippmann-Peikert, Slocumb, Frerichs, & Silber, 2010; Dang, Cunnington, & Swieca, 2011; Driver-Dunckley et al., 2007; Evans & Butzkueven, 2007; Kolla, Mansukhani, Barraza, & Bostwick, 2010; Ondo & Lai, 2008; Pourcher, Remillard, & Cohen, 2010; Quickfall & Suchowersky, 2007; Salas, Allen, Earley, & Gamaldo, 2009; Schreglmann, Gantenbein, Eisele, & Baumann, 2012; Tippmann-Peikert, Park, Boeve, Shepard, & Silber, 2007; Voon et al., 2011). ICD behavior resolves when treatment with a dopamine-receptor agonist is stopped. There is some suggestion that ICDs occur more often in women than men, with RLS/WED, and the development of ICDs is also associated with greater psychological stress, depression, sleep disturbance, and a family history of gambling problems.

Studies of patients with RLS/WED who are not on dopamine treatment have not reported an increased incidence of ICDs. It remains somewhat unclear whether or not patients with untreated RLS/WED have an increased risk of developing ICDs. In contrast, there has been limited formal evaluation of the rates of ICDs in patients who are taking non-dopaminergic treatment. Clinical trials have not reported this as an adverse effect for the patients not taking a dopamine-receptor agonist.

11. Opioids

Opioids constitute a third main class of drug being used in RLS. However, this class of drugs is used (and in Europe, also approved) as a second-lines treatment for treatment-resistant cases of RLS/WED. No comparative studies exist between opioids and any of the other classes of drugs (dopaminergics or α2δ ligands).

Two opioids (methadone and oxycodone) have been investigated with more detail than others: one class III study and another class IV study evaluated the use of methadone in the treatment of idiopathic and secondary RLS/WED. Both studies showed sustained therapeutic benefit over a prolonged period, from 2 to 10 years, in patients who had failed treatment with other agents largely due to augmentation. Approximately one-third of the patients were on concomitant therapy. Dropout rates ranged from 13% to 30% and were due to lack of efficacy and side effects (sedation, depression/anxiety, altered consciousness).

A double-blind study on 276 RLS patients who had not responded to dopamine agonists showed that oxycodone extended release-naloxone was efficacious for the short-term treatment of patients with severe RLS/WED inadequately controlled with previous treatment. The study also provided evidence of long-term efficacy of this treatment. Oxycodone extended release-naloxone is approved in Europe for the treatment of patients with severe RLS/WED who have had no benefit with first-line drugs.

12. Recent developments

Based on recent finding about the role of glutamate in RLS/WED, two substances have shown promising results in open studies: First, the selective AMPA-glutamate receptor antagonist perampanel was evaluated in 22 RLS patients over a treatment of 8 weeks (Garcia-Borreguero, Cano, & Granizo, 2017). During the eight-week treatment period the

IRLS score improved from a mean (±S.D.) 23.7 ± 4.2–11.5 ± 5.3. Twelve of 20 patients were full responders (improvement 50% in IRLS total score), and four responded partially. The mean effective dose of perampanel at the end of treatment was 3.8 mg/day. Treatment with perampanel also resulted in an improvement in the mean (±S.D.) PLMI from 27.8 ± 6.9–4.36 ± 2.0.

The use of dipyridamole (Garcia-Borreguero, Guitart, et al., 2018) was based on recent studies showing that brain iron deficiency in an animal model is associated with a hypoadenosinergic state, with striatal down-regulation of adenosine A_1 receptors (A1R) (Quiroz et al., 2016), leading to hypersensitive corticostriatal terminals (Yepes et al., 2017). It was therefore hypothesized that an increase in the tonic A1R activation mediated by endogenous adenosine could represent a new alternative therapeutic strategy for RLS/WED. Since dipyridamole is an inhibitor of adenosine transport, it was thought that it could cause such an increase in extracellular adenosine and thereby exert a therapeutic effect on RLS/WED symptoms. Out of 13 patients who completed the study, IRLS score improved from a mean (±S.D.) of 23.4 ± 4.6 at baseline to 10.7 ± 4.5 at 8 weeks. Six of 13 patients were full responders and four were partial responders. The mean (±S.D.) effective dose of dipyridamole at 8 weeks was 281.8 (±57.5) mg/day. Sleep variables also improved, and the mean (±S.D.) PLMI decreased from 26.7 ± 7.2–4.3 ± 1.9. These results support the hypothesis of adenosine playing a central role in the pathophysiology of RLS/WED, thus mediating the increase in function of dopamine and glutamate in corticostriatal pathways.

13. Conclusion

Two types of drugs have been extensively investigated for the treatment of RLS/WED, dopamine agonists and α2δ ligands. Both have been shown to be clinically effective in treating sensory symptoms (Hornyak et al., 2014) over the short-term, but α2δ are probably more effective over the long-term. Dopamine agonists are more effective in treating PLMs, while α2δ ligands are effective in consolidating sleep. However, given the fact that dopamine agonists cause augmentation of symptoms, the most recent international guidelines recommend that whenever possible the initial treatment of choice should be an α2δ ligand (Garcia-Borreguero et al., 2016). In fact, the most effective preventive strategy involves not using dopaminergic agents unless absolutely necessary. Indeed, should a dopaminergic treatment be needed to handle the symptoms effectively, then it is recommended that the dopaminergic load be reduced by using the lowest effective dose for the shortest possible period of time. However, it must be taken into account that the only α2δ ligand approved for RLS/WED is gabapentin enacarbil, and it has received regulatory approval for the treatment of RLS/WED in Japan, but not in Europe.

Furthermore, recent studies have also reported on the efficacy of opioids for the treatment of RLS/WED, when resistant to dopamine agonists (Silver et al., 2011; Trenkwalder et al., 2015). Recent guidelines have taken these new data into account and highlight that a low dose of an opioid (prolonged-release oxycodone or methadone) may be considered in patients with very severe augmentation (Garcia-Borreguero et al., 2016).

Given the clinical need for new treatments, future research should focus on the development of new—non-dopaminergic substances. Recent pathophysiological models of RLS/WED suggest that hyperactive glutamatergic corticostriatal pathways might be central to the causation of symptoms. Thus, as shown by Ferre, Garcia-Borreguero, Allen, and Earley (2018), animal models show that brain iron deficiency is associated to adenosine—type 1 (A1-R) downregulation in the cortex and striatum, leading ultimately to a hypoadenosinergic state. Moreover, a combination of brain iron deficiency and reduced adenosinergic state might lead to increased glutamate and dopamine, which could explain animal symptoms such as the increased locomotion, hyperarousal, PLMs and disturbed sleep. As previously described, preliminary empirical evidence (Ferre et al., 2018) exists showing that an increase of extracellular adenosine by means of dipyridamole (Garcia-Borreguero, Guitart, et al., 2018) or a reduction of glutamatergic activity by means of AMPA-receptor glutamate antagonism (Garcia-Borreguero et al., 2017) might also improve RLS/WED symptoms in humans. In our opinion, such alternative non-dopaminergic treatment concepts, based on glutamatergic and adenosinergic mechanisms might provide promising therapeutic developments.

Conflict of interest

Vivian Wanner reports no conflicts.

Celia Garcia Malo reports no conflicts.

Sofía Romero reports no conflicts.

Irene Cano reports no conflicts.

Diego García-Borreguero has received research grants for Merck Pharma.

References

Akpinar, S. (1982). Treatment of restless legs syndrome with levodopa plus benserazide. *Archives of Neurology*, *39*(11), 739.

Allen, R. P., Chen, C., Garcia-Borreguero, D., Polo, O., DuBrava, S., Miceli, J., et al. (2014). Comparison of pregabalin with pramipexole for restless legs syndrome. *The New England Journal of Medicine*, *370*(7), 621–631. https://doi.org/10.1056/NEJMoa1303646.

Allen, R. P., & Earley, C. J. (1996). Augmentation of the restless legs syndrome with carbidopa/levodopa. *Sleep*, *19*(3), 205–213.

Allen, R. P., Ondo, W. G., Ball, E., Calloway, M. O., Manjunath, R., Higbie, R. L., et al. (2011). Restless legs syndrome (RLS) augmentation associated with dopamine agonist and levodopa usage in a community sample. *Sleep Medicine*, *12*(5), 431–439. https://doi.org/10.1016/j.sleep.2011.03.003.

Allen, R. P., Picchietti, D., Hening, W. A., Trenkwalder, C., Walters, A. S., & Montplaisir, J. (2003). Restless legs syndrome: Diagnostic criteria, special considerations, and epidemiology. A report from the restless legs syndrome diagnosis and epidemiology workshop at the National Institutes of Health. *Sleep Medicine*, *4*(2), 101–119.

Bayard, S., Yu, H., Langenier, M. C., Carlander, B., & Dauvilliers, Y. (2010). Decision making in restless legs syndrome. *Movement Disorders*, *25*(15), 2634–2640. https://doi.org/10.1002/mds.23326.

Cornelius, J. R., Tippmann-Peikert, M., Slocumb, N. L., Frerichs, C. F., & Silber, M. H. (2010). Impulse control disorders with the use of dopaminergic agents in restless legs syndrome: A case-control study. *Sleep*, *33*(1), 81–87.

Dang, D., Cunnington, D., & Swieca, J. (2011). The emergence of devastating impulse control disorders during dopamine agonist therapy of the restless legs syndrome. *Clinical Neuropharmacology*, *34*(2), 66–70. https://doi.org/10.1097/WNF.0b013e31820d6699.

Driver-Dunckley, E. D., Noble, B. N., Hentz, J. G., Evidente, V. G., Caviness, J. N., Parish, J., et al. (2007). Gambling and increased sexual desire with dopaminergic medications in restless legs syndrome. *Clinical Neuropharmacology*, *30*(5), 249–255. https://doi.org/10.1097/wnf.0b013e31804c780e. 00002826-200709000-00001 [pii].

Evans, A. H., & Butzkueven, H. (2007). Dopamine agonist-induced pathological gambling in restless legs syndrome due to multiple sclerosis. *Movement Disorders*, *22*(4), 590–591.

Ferini-Strambi, L. (2002). Restless legs syndrome augmentation and pramipexole treatment. *Sleep Medicine*, *3*(Suppl), S23–S25.

Ferre, S., Earley, C., Gulyani, S., & Garcia-Borreguero, D. (2017). In search of alternatives to dopaminergic ligands for the treatment of restless legs syndrome: Iron, glutamate, and adenosine. *Sleep Medicine*, *31*, 86–92. https://doi.org/10.1016/j.sleep.2016.08.019.

Ferre, S., Garcia-Borreguero, D., Allen, R. P., & Earley, C. J. (2018). New insights into the neurobiology of restless legs syndrome. *The Neuroscientist*, 1073858418791763. https://doi.org/10.1177/1073858418791763.

Garcia-Borreguero, D., Allen, R. P., Kohnen, R., Högl, B., Trenkwalder, C., Oertel, W., et al. (2007). Diagnostic standards for dopaminergic augmentation of restless legs syndrome: Report from a World Association of Sleep Medicine-International Restless Legs Syndrome Study Group consensus conference at the Max Planck Institute. *Sleep Medicine*, *8*(5), 520–530. https://doi.org/10.1016/j.sleep.2007.03.022.

Garcia-Borreguero, D., Cano, I., & Granizo, J. J. (2017). Treatment of restless legs syndrome with the selective AMPA receptor antagonist perampanel. *Sleep Medicine*, *34*, 105–108. https://doi.org/10.1016/j.sleep.2017.03.012.

Garcia-Borreguero, D., Cano, C., Malo, C. G., Velarde, J. A. C., Granizo, J. J., & Wanner, V. (2018). Reduced response to gabapentin enacarbil in restless legs syndrome following long-term dopaminergic treatment. *Sleep Medicine*, *55*, 74–80.

Garcia-Borreguero, D., Guitart, X., Garcia Malo, C., Cano-Pumarega, I., Granizo, J. J., & Ferre, S. (2018). Treatment of restless legs syndrome/Willis-Ekbom disease with the non-selective ENT1/ENT2 inhibitor dipyridamole: Testing the adenosine hypothesis. *Sleep Medicine*, *45*, 94–97. https://doi.org/10.1016/j.sleep.2018.02.002.

Garcia-Borreguero, D., Hogl, B., Ferini-Strambi, L., Winkelman, J., Hill-Zabala, C., Asgharian, A., et al. (2012). Systematic evaluation of augmentation during treatment with ropinirole in restless legs syndrome (Willis-Ekbom disease): Results from a prospective, multicenter study over 66 weeks. *Movement Disorders*, *27*(2), 277–283. https://doi.org/10.1002/mds.24889.

Garcia-Borreguero, D., Kohnen, R., Hogl, B., Ferini-Strambi, L., Hadjigeorgiou, G. M., Hornyak, M., et al. (2007). Validation of the augmentation severity rating scale (ASRS): A multicentric, prospective study with levodopa on restless legs syndrome. *Sleep Medicine*, *8*(5), 455–463. https://doi.org/10.1016/j.sleep.2007.03.023.

Garcia-Borreguero, D., Kohnen, R., Silber, M. H., Winkelman, J. W., Earley, C. J., Hogl, B., et al. (2013). The long-term treatment of restless legs syndrome/Willis-Ekbom disease: Evidence-based guidelines and clinical consensus best practice guidance: A report from the international restless legs syndrome study group. *Sleep Medicine*, *14*(7), 675–684. https://doi.org/10.1016/j.sleep.2013.05.016.

Garcia-Borreguero, D., Larrosa, O., Williams, A. M., Albares, J., Pascual, M., Palacios, J. C., et al. (2010). Treatment of restless legs syndrome with pregabalin: A double-blind, placebo-controlled study. *Neurology*, *74*(23), 1897–1904. https://doi.org/10.1212/WNL.0b013e3181e1ce73.

Garcia-Borreguero, D., Patrick, J., Dubrava, S., Becker, P. M., Lankford, L., Chen, C., et al. (2014). Pregabalin versus Pramipexole: Effects on sleep disturbance in restless legs syndrome. *Sleep*, *37*(4), 635–643. https://doi.org/10.5665/sleep.3558.

Garcia-Borreguero, D., Silber, M. H., Winkelman, J. W., Högl, B., Bainbridge, J., Buchfuhrer, M., et al. (2016). Guidelines for the first-line treatment of restless legs syndrome/Willis-Ekbom disease, prevention and treatment of dopaminergic augmentation: A combined task force of the IRLSSG, EURLSSG, and the RLS-foundation. *Sleep Medicine*, *21*, 1–11. https://doi.org/10.1016/j.sleep.2016.01.017.

Garcia-Borreguero, D., & Williams, A. M. (2010). Dopaminergic augmentation of restless legs syndrome. *Sleep Medicine Reviews*, *14*(5), 339–346. https://doi.org/10.1016/j.smrv.2009.11.006.

Garcia-Borreguero, D., & Williams, A. M. (2014). An update on restless legs syndrome (Willis-Ekbom disease): Clinical features, pathogenesis and treatment. *Current Opinion in Neurology*, *27*(4), 493–501. https://doi.org/10.1097/WCO.0000000000000117.

Guilleminault, C., Cetel, M., & Philip, P. (1993). Dopaminergic treatment of restless legs and rebound phenomenon. *Neurology*, *43*(2), 445.

Högl, B., Garcia-Borreguero, D., Trenkwalder, C., Ferini-Strambi, L., Hening, W., Poewe, W., et al. (2011). Efficacy and augmentation during 6 months of double-blind pramipexole for restless legs syndrome. *Sleep Medicine*, *12*(4), 351–360. https://doi.org/10.1016/j.sleep.2010.12.007.

Hornyak, M., Scholz, H., Kohnen, R., Bengel, J., Kassubek, J., & Trenkwalder, C. (2014). What treatment works best for restless legs syndrome? Meta-analyses of dopaminergic and non-dopaminergic medications. *Sleep Medicine Reviews*, *18*(2), 153–164. https://doi.org/10.1016/j.smrv.2013.03.004.

Hornyak, M., Trenkwalder, C., Kohnen, R., & Scholz, H. (2012). Efficacy and safety of dopamine agonists in restless legs syndrome. *Sleep Medicine*, *13*(3), 228–236. https://doi.org/10.1016/j.sleep.2011.09.013.

Kolla, B. P., Mansukhani, M. P., Barraza, R., & Bostwick, J. M. (2010). Impact of dopamine agonists on compulsive behaviors: A case series of pramipexole-induced pathological gambling. *Psychosomatics*, *51*(3), 271–273. https://doi.org/10.1176/appi.psy.51.3.271.

Lipford, M. C., & Silber, M. H. (2012). Long-term use of pramipexole in the management of restless legs syndrome. *Sleep Medicine*, *13*(10), 1280–1285. https://doi.org/10.1016/j.sleep.2012.08.004.
Mitterling, T., Heidbreder, A., Stefani, A., Fritz, J., Ulmer, H., Poewe, W., et al. (2015). Natural course of restless legs syndrome/Willis-Ekbom disease: Long-term observation of a large clinical cohort. *Sleep Medicine*, *16*(10), 1252–1258. https://doi.org/10.1016/j.sleep.2015.05.028.
Ondo, W. G., & Lai, D. (2008). Predictors of impulsivity and reward seeking behavior with dopamine agonists. *Parkinsonism & Related Disorders*, *14*(1), 28–32. doi:S1353-8020(07)00078-8 [pii]. https://doi.org/10.1016/j.parkreldis.2007.05.006.
Ondo, W., Romanyshyn, J., Vuong, K. D., & Lai, D. (2004). Long-term treatment of restless legs syndrome with dopamine agonists. *Archives of Neurology*, *61*(9), 1393–1397. https://doi.org/10.1001/archneur.61.9.1393.
Pourcher, E., Remillard, S., & Cohen, H. (2010). Compulsive habits in restless legs syndrome patients under dopaminergic treatment. *Journal of the Neurological Sciences*, *290*(1–2), 52–56. doi:S0022-510X(09)00973-3 [pii]. https://doi.org/10.1016/j.jns.2009.11.010.
Quickfall, J., & Suchowersky, O. (2007). Pathological gambling associated with dopamine agonist use in restless legs syndrome. *Parkinsonism & Related Disorders*, *13*, 535–536.
Quiroz, C., Gulyani, S., Ruiqian, W., Bonaventura, J., Cutler, R., Pearson, V., et al. (2016). Adenosine receptors as markers of brain iron deficiency: Implications for restless legs syndrome. *Neuropharmacology*, *111*, 160–168. https://doi.org/10.1016/j.neuropharm.2016.09.002.
Salas, R. E., Allen, R. P., Earley, C. J., & Gamaldo, C. E. (2009). A case of compulsive behaviors observed in a restless legs syndrome patient treated with a dopamine agonist. *Sleep*, *32*(5), 587–588.
Schreglmann, S. R., Gantenbein, A. R., Eisele, G., & Baumann, C. R. (2012). Transdermal rotigotine causes impulse control disorders in patients with restless legs syndrome. *Parkinsonism & Related Disorders*, *18*(2), 207–209. https://doi.org/10.1016/j.parkreldis.2011.10.010.
Silber, M. H., Girish, M., & Izurieta, R. (2003). Pramipexole in the management of restless legs syndrome: An extended study. *Sleep*, *26*(7), 819–821.
Silber, M. H., Shepard, J. W., Jr., & Wisbey, J. A. (1997). Pergolide in the management of restless legs syndrome: An extended study. *Sleep*, *20*(10), 878–882.
Silver, N., Allen, R. P., Senerth, J., & Earley, C. J. (2011). A 10-year, longitudinal assessment of dopamine agonists and methadone in the treatment of restless legs syndrome. *Sleep Medicine*, *12*(5), 440–444. https://doi.org/10.1016/j.sleep.2010.11.002.
Tippmann-Peikert, M., Park, J. G., Boeve, B. F., Shepard, J. W., & Silber, M. H. (2007). Pathologic gambling in patients with restless legs syndrome treated with dopaminergic agonists. *Neurology*, *68*(4), 301–303.
Trenkwalder, C., Chaudhuri, K. R., Martinez-Martin, P., Rascol, O., Ehret, R., Valis, M., et al. (2015). Prolonged-release oxycodone-naloxone for treatment of severe pain in patients with Parkinson's disease (PANDA): A double-blind, randomised, placebo-controlled trial. *Lancet Neurology*, *14*(12), 1161–1170. https://doi.org/10.1016/S1474-4422(15)00243-4.
Voon, V., Schoerling, A., Wenzel, S., Ekanayake, V., Reiff, J., Trenkwalder, C., et al. (2011). Frequency of impulse control behaviours associated with dopaminergic therapy in restless legs syndrome. *BMC Neurology*, *11*, 117. https://doi.org/10.1186/1471-2377-11-117.
Winkelman, J. W., Armstrong, M. J., Allen, R. P., Chaudhuri, K. R., Ondo, W., Trenkwalder, C., et al. (2016). Practice guideline summary: Treatment of restless legs syndrome in adults: Report of the guideline development, dissemination, and implementation subcommittee of the American Academy of Neurology. *Neurology*, *87*, 2585–2593. https://doi.org/10.1212/WNL.0000000000003388.

Winkelman, J. W., & Johnston, L. (2004). Augmentation and tolerance with long-term pramipexole treatment of restless legs syndrome (RLS). *Sleep Medicine, 5*(1), 9–14.
Winkelmann, J., Allen, R., Högl, B., Inoue, Y., Oertel, W., Salminen, A., et al. (2018). Treatment of restless legs syndrome: An evidence-based review and implications for clinical practice. *Movement Disorders*. https://doi.org/10.1002/mds.27260.
Yepes, G., Guitart, X., Rea, W., Newman, A. H., Allen, R. P., Earley, C. J., et al. (2017). Targeting hypersensitive corticostriatal terminals in restless legs syndrome. *Annals of Neurology, 82*(6), 951–960. https://doi.org/10.1002/ana.25104.

CHAPTER TEN

Idiopathic restless legs syndrome treatment: Progress and pitfalls?

Imad Ghorayeb[a,b,c,*]
[a]Département de Neurophysiologie Clinique, Pôle Neurosciences Cliniques, CHU de Bordeaux, Bordeaux, France
[b]Aquitaine Institute for Cognitive and Integrative Neuroscience, Bordeaux University, CNRS-UMR 5287, Bordeaux, France
[c]CNRS, Institut de Neurosciences Cognitives et Intégratives d'Aquitaine, Bordeaux, France
*Corresponding author: e-mail address: imad.ghorayeb@u-bordeaux.fr

Contents

Advances in Pharmacology, Volume 84
ISSN 1054-3589
https://doi.org/10.1016/bs.apha.2019.01.004
© 2019 Elsevier Inc.
All rights reserved.

Abstract

The pathophysiology of Restless Legs Syndrome (RLS) remains uncertain. Although the dopaminergic and/or the iron breakdown homeostasis hypotheses are still considered to be the mainstay of the RLS underlying mechanism, therapeutic intervention aiming to alleviate RLS syndrome through dopamine agonists use and iron stores recovery failed so far to show short-term remarkable efficacy, and controlled trials to establish sustained long-term efficacy, tolerability and safety are lacking.

Here we review available literature dealing with pharmacological treatment of RLS and consider some rational aspects of RLS pathophysiology that may support the use of available drug classes in treating this condition.

Abbreviations

DA dopamine agonist
D_1R dopamine-1 receptor
D_2R dopamine-2 receptor
D_3R dopamine-3 receptor
D_4R dopamine-4 receptor
D_5R dopamine-5 receptor
DAT dopamine transporter
GABA γ-aminobutyric acid
MOS Medical Outcomes Study
MRI magnetic resonance imaging
PLMS periodic limb movements in sleep
PSG polysomnography
QoL quality of life
RLS Restless Legs Syndrome
SN substantia nigra
5-HT serotonin

1. Introduction

Management of restless legs syndrome (RLS) is primarily pharmacological as nonpharmacological options are, at best, limited and, aside from iron replacement therapy, only symptomatic treatments are empirically used.

Considering the pharmacological management of RLS and since the serendipitous observation by Akpinar in 1982 of the benefit of levodopa for RLS (Akpinar, 1982), dopamine agonists (DA) still remain one of the first-line therapy in de novo patients with moderate to severe RLS (Akpinar, 1982; Kim & Hartzema, 2018b; Limousin, Flamand, Schroder, & Charley Monaca, 2018; Winkelmann et al., 2018), although the use of opiates as a therapy of choice in this condition dates back to the 17th century when

Thomas Willis, an English physician, first documented the disease and believed it to originate in the spinal cord as a product of spinal irritation.

Since that date, and notwithstanding the relatively recent use of $\alpha 2$-δ voltage-gated calcium channels ligands, no convincing breakthrough has been accomplished in RLS treatment strategies. This may be due in part to lack of a definitive broad-based consensus regarding RLS pathophysiology.

The aim of the present review is to recapitulate main pharmacological clinical trials that led to the confirmation of the efficacy of the active drugs used in RLS with an attempt to summarize how current knowledge of the pathophysiology of RLS holds the key for a better understanding of the rational of the use and the mechanism of action of these medications.

2. Dopamine agonists

2.1 Rational

Arguments for a dopaminergic prominent role are to be found in the excellent pharmacological response to low-dose dopaminergic medications (Akpinar, 1982). Evidence of biochemical alterations in the dopaminergic system of patients with RLS has been documented with abnormally high levels of the dopamine metabolite 3-ortho-methyldopa in the cerebrospinal fluid (Allen, Connor, Hyland, & Earley, 2009), decreased striatal dopamine transporter (DAT) and dopamine-2 receptor (D_2R) binding potentials (Earley et al., 2011, 2013), and a significant increase in tyrosine hydroxylase activity in the striatum and substantia nigra (SN) in human tissue (Connor et al., 2009). This would be mostly compatible with a dopaminergic abnormality characterized as an overly activated dopaminergic system at the presynaptic level (Earley et al., 2014) although the widely accepted "enhanced excitability of the spinal cord" in RLS would be best explained by rather a reduced dopaminergic inhibition from the descending diencephalospinal system (Clemens, Rye, & Hochman, 2006; Lanza et al., 2017). How this central dopaminergic dysfunction would clinically translate into the four sensorimotor essential diagnostic criteria is presently unknown.

2.1.1 Ropinirole

Ropinirole is a non-ergot-derived D_2R/D_3R agonist. The ratio of selectivity for D_3R over D_2R was reported to range from 20-fold to only 1.3-fold, raising question about its D_3R selectivity in vivo. In addition to its agonist activity at D_2R subtypes, ropinirole has a very low affinity for D_1R subtypes, 5-HT_{2A} and 5-HT_{2B} receptors, and exerts almost no affinity for β-adrenergic and γ-aminobutyric acid (GABA) receptors (Jost, 2004; Kvernmo, Hartter, & Burger, 2006; Kvernmo, Houben, & Sylte, 2008).

Since the first description of the efficacy of ropinirole in RLS (Ondo, 1999), numerous controlled trials have demonstrated the efficacy of ropinirole in subjectively improving moderate-to-severe RLS symptoms (Allen et al., 2004; Benes et al., 2011; Bliwise et al., 2005; Bogan et al., 2006; Garcia-Borreguero et al., 2012; Giorgi, Asgharian, & Hunter, 2013; Montplaisir, Karrasch, Haan, & Volc, 2006; Ondo, 1999; Trenkwalder et al., 2004; Walters et al., 2004). Long-term efficacy was also demonstrated in a 52-week open-label study, which is very modest period for a chronic disease requiring lifetime treatment (Garcia-Borreguero et al., 2007). Improvement of quality of life was also demonstrated in a short term trial (Cho, Hong, et al., 2013) and of depressive symptoms in a randomized, placebo-controlled study (Benes et al., 2011). Changes in Medical Outcomes Study (MOS) Sleep Scale scores showed significant reductions in sleep disturbance and daytime somnolence, and significant increases in sleep adequacy and sleep quantity, among patients receiving ropinirole compared with those receiving placebo (Allen et al., 2004; Benes et al., 2011; Montplaisir, Karrasch, et al., 2006; Trenkwalder et al., 2004; Walters et al., 2004). The administered ropinirole dose ranged from 0.25 to 4 mg/day, with mean doses of ~ 2 mg/day across trials (Allen et al., 2004; Benes et al., 2011; Bogan et al., 2006; Cho, Hong, et al., 2013; Giorgi et al., 2013; Montplaisir, Karrasch, et al., 2006; Trenkwalder et al., 2004).

In two double-blinded, placebo-controlled studies, ropinirole decreases periodic leg movements in sleep (PLMS) and improves polysomnographic (PSG) sleep parameters in one but not in other study (Allen et al., 2004; Bliwise et al., 2005). The acute and positive effect of ropinirole on PLMS variables was also demonstrated but with however limited number of patients and two small open-label trial showed reduction in PLMS index with ropinirole but contradictory effect on PLMS-arousal index (Happe, Sauter, Klosch, Saletu, & Zeitlhofer, 2003; Saletu et al., 2000). Compared to baseline, objective sleep parameters also worsened following 4 weeks with ropinirole, with reduction of total sleep time, slow wave sleep, REM sleep, sleep efficiency and significant increase in arousals index (Happe et al., 2003).

The adverse events profile for ropinirole was representative of that associated with dopaminergic therapy in general; nausea was the most commonly reported adverse event the majority of which was mild or moderate in severity.

The occurrence of augmentation for ropinirole has been poorly quantified. In one prospective study, the 26-week incidence rate of clinically significant augmentation was 3% for ropinirole versus <1% for placebo (Garcia-Borreguero et al., 2012).

2.1.2 Pramipexole

Pramipexole is a nonergot dopamine agonist with high relative in vitro specificity and full intrinsic activity at the D_2 subfamily of dopamine receptors, binding with higher affinity to D_3R than to D_2R or D_4R subtypes. It has a moderate opioid affinity, a very low affinity for 5-HT_{2A}, 5-HT_{2B} receptors, and D_1R, but no significant α- or β-adrenergic activity (Kvernmo et al., 2006, 2008). The ratio of selectivity for D_3R over D_2R is about 6.5–8, with pramipexole being more selective for the D_3 subtype receptors than ropinirole (Kvernmo et al., 2008).

Pramipexole efficacy has been evaluated in a large number of clinical trials (Allen, 2014; Ferini-Strambi et al., 2008; Hogl et al., 2011; Ma et al., 2012; Montagna et al., 2011; Montplaisir, Nicolas, Denesle, & Gomez-Mancilla, 1999; Oertel et al., 2007; Winkelman et al., 2006; Zhang, Liu, Zheng, Chu, & Yang, 2015) and in four double-blind, placebo-controlled PSG studies (Inoue et al., 2010; Jama et al., 2009; Montplaisir et al., 1999; Partinen et al., 2006). In these trials, ferritin levels were controlled in only three trials and variable ferritin concentrations were considered for patients' exclusion [patients were excluded for serum ferritin ≤20 ng/mL (Montplaisir, Fantini, et al., 2006), ≤30 ng/mL (Hogl et al., 2011) and <11.0 ng/mL (Ma et al., 2012)].

Acute pramipexole intake was also shown to markedly reduce PLMS measures and to slightly improve objective and subjective sleep quality in however a very limited number of patients (Manconi et al., 2007; Saletu, Anderer, Saletu-Zyhlarz, Hauer, & Saletu, 2002). Whether this PLMS reduction is sustained over time was not explored.

By contrast to ropinirole, long-term efficacy and safety of pramipexole has been evaluated and confirmed in numerous studies but over variable periods of time (Ferini-Strambi, 2002; Hogl et al., 2011; Inoue et al., 2010; Lipford & Silber, 2012; Montplaisir, Denesle, & Petit, 2000; Montplaisir, Fantini, et al., 2006; Partinen et al., 2008; Silber, Girish, & Izurieta, 2003; Silver, Allen, Senerth, & Earley, 2011; Takahashi et al., 2017; Trenkwalder et al., 2006; Winkelman & Johnston, 2004).

Accordingly, over years of use, the efficacy of pramipexole would drop with time, with increase in dose and addition of other RLS active drugs.

Tolerance occurred in 46% of patients (Winkelman & Johnston, 2004) and 50% of the patients had discontinued pramipexole by the seventh year after starting it (Silver et al., 2011). Problems included the development of augmentation within the first 4 years of therapy and side effects such as sleepiness increasing with time and the development of impulse control disorder. Similar findings were reported later on with however a small cohort of 50 patients (Lipford & Silber, 2012). In this study, however, two patients had peripheral neuropathy, one has parkinsonism, nine had sleep apnea, two had narcolepsy and nine patients were diagnosed with depression and one with anxiety disorder; all were taking antidepressants. Iron status was assessed in 44 patients with low serum ferritin levels in 11. Coexisting medical, sleep, psychiatric conditions and iron stores should therefore be controlled in future studies before assessing the efficacy of any specific drug in the RLS condition.

The same remark stands when assessing augmentation incidence rates since retrospective studies have reported augmentation rates for pramipexole to range from 8.3% to 42% (Ferini-Strambi, 2002; Hogl et al., 2011; Lipford & Silber, 2012; Silber et al., 2003; Takahashi et al., 2017; Winkelman & Johnston, 2004) but to drop to 5.3% in one randomized controlled trial at 0.25 mg (Allen, 2014). In a 10-year follow-up study of patients with pramipexole, a constant annual rate of augmentation of 7% was shown (Silver et al., 2011). Different assessment methods, variable duration of follow-up and heterogeneity of patient populations, make direct comparison of incidence rates of augmentation between studies impossible.

2.1.3 Rotigotine

Rotigotine is an agonist at all five dopamine receptor subtypes (D_1–D_5) but binds to the D_3R with the highest affinity (Kvernmo et al., 2008). It is also an antagonist at α_2-adrenergic receptors and an agonist at the 5-HT_{1A} receptors. It is formulated as a once-daily transdermal patch, which provides a slow and constant supply of the drug over the course of 24 h.

In RLS, a total of five out of six randomized, double-blind, placebo-controlled trials have demonstrated the efficacy of rotigotine in subjectively improving moderate-to-severe RLS symptoms (Garcia-Borreguero et al., 2016; Hening et al., 2010; Inoue et al., 2013; Oertel et al., 2008; Stiasny-Kolster et al., 2004; Trenkwalder et al., 2008). Rotigotine is generally well tolerated. The most common adverse effects were application-site reactions, nausea and vomiting, more frequently reported in the first period of treatment. In a 5-year open-label extension study, the incidence of application site reactions was 37% of patients during the year 1, 17% in year 2, 14% in year 3, and 5% in years 4 and 5 (Oertel et al., 2011). The majority of patients (67%) recovered without requiring dose reduction or dose decrease.

In two randomized, placebo-controlled PSG studies, mean PLMS index decreased more with rotigotine than with placebo following 4 weeks short-term trial (Bauer et al., 2016; Oertel et al., 2010). In a larger double-blind, placebo-controlled trial with 150 enrolled patients, an attempt to objectively assess the efficacy of rotigotine in daytime symptoms by means of Multiple Suggested Immobilization Test failed to demonstrate the superiority of rotigotine to placebo at end of 4-week maintenance period (Garcia-Borreguero et al., 2016). In this negative trial, rotigotine was not superior to placebo on any of the endpoints, including the International Restless Legs Syndrome Rating Scale and the reduction of PLM during wakefulness.

Maintenance of the efficacy of rotigotine was shown in two open-label studies with a 5-year follow-up. In the first study, of the 295 patients who entered the study, 169 (57%) discontinued treatment before the end of maintenance period, 89 (30%) because of adverse events and 31 (11%) because of lack of efficacy (Oertel et al., 2011). Of the 126 (43%) patients who completed the maintenance period, the mean rotigotine dose at the end of maintenance was 3.09 ± 1.07 mg/24 h and almost half (49%) of patients were on 4 mg/24 h, which is beyond the range approved by the European Medicines Agency (EMA; 1–3 mg/24 h). Clinically significant augmentation was recorded in 5% of patients receiving 1–3 mg/24 h rotigotine and in 8% of those receiving 4 mg/24 h rotigotine (Oertel et al., 2011). In a post hoc analysis of this prospective open-label study, only 45 patients who completed the 5-year period of follow-up were within approved dosage range of rotigotine with sustained efficacy, meaning that rotigotine maintained its efficacy on less than half of the patients (23%) over the 5-year period, when those who discontinued for adverse events (25%) lack of efficacy (3%) or needed higher doses (40%) were eliminated (Dohin et al., 2013).

2.2 Closing thoughts

Although most of the clinical trials concluded to a positive short-term efficacy of DA, these did not keep their initially promising effect over time. Long-term dopaminergic treatment efficacy is hampered by the gradual tolerance and emergence of adverse effects that cause augmentation and impulse control disorder, the latter affecting up to 20.7% of patients with

RLS under DA (Heim et al., 2016). Few case reports of "dopamine agonist withdrawal syndrome" have also been reported in patients with RLS (Dorfman & Nirenberg, 2013; Shimo, Nakajima, & Hattori, 2015). These considerations would in part account for the actual decline observed in DA prescription in RLS (Kim & Hartzema, 2018b).

Long-term studies and more evidence of head-to-head comparisons of DA with other DA, anticonvulsants, and opioids are needed to optimize treatment strategies in RLS.

2.3 Putative mechanism of action of DA in RLS

The precise mechanism of action of DA as a treatment for RLS is unknown but is thought to relate to its ability to stimulate dopamine receptors although other hypothetical mechanism has been proposed (Ferre, Garcia-Borreguero, Allen, & Earley, 2018; von Spiczak et al., 2005).

3. Alpha2-δ ligands

3.1 Rational

Gabapentin and pregabalin were not designed as drugs with α2-δ binding in mind. Rather, they were developed based on the hypothesis that generating analogs of GABA to increase GABA-A receptor activation would lead to the development of novel antiepileptic agents. While these compounds are indeed good anticonvulsants, their activity is surprisingly not due to activity in the GABAergic system as they do not show any significant binding to GABA or benzodiazepine receptors. By purifying the protein to which gabapentin bound, and determining its identity as the α2-δ1 subunit of voltage gated calcium channels, it was possible to make progress in developing new compounds with similar activities to gabapentin, including pregabalin and gabapentin enacarbil. Considered as analgesic compounds, their use to relief the sensorimotor symptoms of RLS is therefore not specific.

3.1.1 Gabapentin

No large multicenter studies that can provide an adequate estimate of the range of benefits and safety issues are available for gabapentin. Since the first documented use of gabapentin for RLS (Mellick & Mellick, 1996) and following two small open-label trials that showed tolerability and efficacy of gabapentin in RLS and in both PLMS index and PLMS-arousal index reduction (Happe et al., 2003; Happe, Klosch, Saletu, & Zeitlhofer, 2001), only one small double-blind, cross-over study showed gabapentin to be superior to placebo in reducing symptoms severity, PLMS index, but not PLMS-arousal index, and in improving sleep architecture on PSG, with however a mean effective dosage at the end of the 6-week treatment period of 1855 mg (Garcia-Borreguero et al., 2002). In this study, 26% of the patients reported malaise while taking gabapentin but none of the cases reached a level of severity that would have requested discontinuation of the study. Although effective in reducing PLMS and PLMS-arousal indexes, gabapentin did not induce any significant changes on sleep efficiency, total sleep time, sleep latency, and duration of slow wave sleep (Happe et al., 2001, 2003). Although these evidences support the use of gabapentin in RLS, its inherent pharmacokinetic deficiencies that may limit its effectiveness make it difficult to predict the dose necessary to achieve an optimal therapeutic effect in a given patient, and the desired treatment response may not be achieved.

3.1.2 Pregabalin

Pregabalin was initially compounded in the late 1980s as an anticonvulsant and has been approved for nociceptive pain conditions such as neuropathic pain and fibromyalgia and in Europe for general anxiety disorders. In RLS, pregabalin was proposed as a new option in the treatment of secondary RLS for patients with neuropathic pain and for idiopathic RLS (Sommer et al., 2007). The short-term efficacy was further documented in few double blind, placebo-controlled studies. In the first 12-week designed study, pregabalin was shown to significantly reduce RLS symptoms' severity at a mean effective dose of 337.5 ± 105.6 mg/day, which is high and could result in sedation and ataxia (Garcia-Borreguero et al., 2010). Improvements were also observed on the MOS sleep scale scores, in the reduction of the mean PLM index and on the marked improvement in sleep architecture, with mean effective dose to improve PLMS index at 300 mg/day (Garcia-Borreguero et al., 2010). The power of the study may have been reduced by the fact that only 43 patients were randomized to either pregabalin ($n=24$) or placebo ($n=19$), which significantly reduced the power of study. The efficacy of pregabalin was further established by a 6-week pregabalin dose-ranging study which used fixed doses from 50 to 450 mg once daily (Allen et al., 2010) and by another 52-week, randomized, double-blind trial with a fixed dose of pregabalin at 330 mg/day (Allen, 2014). In these trials, pregabalin was generally well tolerated. Adverse events were mild but common, and included dizziness, somnolence and headache (Allen et al., 2010; Garcia-Borreguero et al., 2010). Augmentation was reported to affect 2.1% of the patients at 300 mg of pregabalin per day (Allen, 2014).

3.1.3 Gabapentin enacarbil

Gabapentin enacarbil is a transported prodrug of gabapentin that was developed to overcome the pharmacokinetic deficiencies of gabapentin (Cundy et al., 2004). In RLS, its short-term efficacy and safety were demonstrated in numerous randomized clinical trials at daily dose ranging from 600 to 2400 mg (Inoue et al., 2013; Lal et al., 2012; Walters, Ondo, Kushida, et al., 2009; Winkelman et al., 2011). Long-term efficacy of gabapentin enacarbil in up to 13 months of treatment was also reported (Bogan et al., 2010; Ellenbogen et al., 2011; Inoue, Uchimura, Kuroda, Hirata, & Hattori, 2012). In this trial, almost 60% of patients reported sustained improvements in RLS symptoms' severity after 6 months of single-blind treatment with 1200 mg daily gabapentin enacarbil. Gabapentin enacarbil is considered to be generally safe and well tolerated although adverse effects were reported by up to 80.1% of subjects (Ellenbogen et al., 2011), a rate not different from the one reported at 52 weeks for pregabalin at 300 mg/day (85.2%) and pramipexole at 0.5 mg/day (77.8%) (Allen, 2014). The most commonly reported adverse events under gabapentin enacarbil were somnolence and dizziness most of which were rated mild or moderate in intensity.

Objective measures on PSG showed that gabapentin enacarbil at 1200 mg once daily to significantly reduce RLS-associated sleep disturbance and PLMS-arousal index (Winkelman et al., 2011).

3.2 Closing thoughts

The efficacy of α2-δ ligands, pregabalin, gabapentin and gabapentin enacarbil has been documented in many RLS clinical trials. This efficacy is by now considered at least equivalent to therapeutic doses of the DAs (Winkelmann et al., 2018). Although clinical experience with very long-term use of α2-δ ligands in RLS has generally not been documented, it is admitted that they do not have the dopaminergic problems of augmentation, compulsive behaviors, or excessive daytime sleepiness. Since α2-δ ligands can alleviate chronic pain and may be helpful in treating anxiety and insomnia, the presence of any of these comorbidities in RLS may favor their use. Caution must be taken however as evidence also suggests pregabalin and gabapentin to possess potential for abuse. In the general population, a 1.6% prevalence of gabapentinoid abuse was observed, whereas prevalence ranged from 3% to 68% among opioid abusers (Evoy, Morrison, & Saklad, 2017). Prescribers should be aware of high-risk populations and monitor for signs of abuse.

3.3 Putative mechanism of action of α2-δ on RLS

The mechanism of action of α2-δ ligands on symptoms' relief in RLS is non-specific. The binding to the α2-δ subunit of voltage-gated calcium channels in central nervous system tissues, thereby reducing release of excitatory neurotransmitters particularly in circuits involved in pain modulation and sensory information, may account for the α2-δ ligands' effect on RLS, although other hypothetical mechanism has been claimed (Ferre et al., 2018).

4. Opioids

4.1 Rational

Brain imaging as well as post-mortem studies suggested the involvement of the endogenous opiate system in the pathogenesis of RLS (von Spiczak et al., 2005; Walters, Hening, Cote, & Fahn, 1986; Walters, Ondo, Zhu, & Le, 2009). The mechanism by which this dysfunction would generate RLS symptoms is not known.

4.1.1 Prolonged release oxycodone-naloxone

The therapeutic action of opioids was first mentioned by Thomas Willis then in the original description of RLS by Ekbom. This effect was further documented in one small double-blind randomized crossover trial (Walters et al., 1993) and in one large 12-week randomized clinical trial with prolonged release oxycodone-naloxone (Trenkwalder et al., 2013). In this trial, the discontinuation rate was of 37%, but opioids were effective for treating RLS symptoms in the remaining patients and in improving some, but not all, sleep and quality of life (QoL) parameters as reported on the MOS Sleep Scale scores and the RLS-specific QoL questionnaire. The effectiveness of prolonged release oxycodone-naloxone was sustained over the 40 weeks of an open-label extension period (Oertel et al., 2016; Trenkwalder et al., 2013). In a retrospective report on long-term use of opioids in patients with RLS, 55.5% of patients remained on opioid monotherapy for an average of 5 years 11 months (Walters et al., 2001).

Opioids were also shown to be effective in reducing PLMS and while awake, and in increasing total sleep time and sleep efficacy on however a very limited number of patients and therefore without any reported statistical significance (Hening et al., 1986; Walters et al., 2001). Despite reported effectiveness, adverse side effects consistent with the safety profile of opioids such as fatigue, constipation, nausea, headache, somnolence, dizziness, dry mouth and pruritus, may complicate the use of these class drug, particularly in the elderly. Similar to what was reported for gabapentin enacarbil (Ellenbogen et al., 2011), and for pregabalin and pramipexole (Allen, 2014), side effects were reported by up to 84% of the patients on prolonged release oxycodone-naloxone (Trenkwalder et al., 2013). Development of sleep apnea or worsening of preexisting apnea may necessitate regular PSG monitoring (Walters et al., 2001). Opioid-induced hyperalgesia was also described in patient with refractory RLS (Chokroverty, 2015) and augmentation was also reported in cases with tramadol (Earley & Allen, 2006; Vetrugno et al., 2007).

4.1.2 Methadone

Similar to other opioids, methadone was shown to effectively treat severe refractory RLS (Hening et al., 1986; Ondo, 2005). Methadone, a long-acting μ-specific opioid agonist, is most frequently used to treat narcotic addiction, because it has less abuse potential than other narcotics. In a 10-year, longitudinal assessment of DA and methadone in the treatment of RLS, methadone, in contrast to DA, shows neither augmentation nor major problems with continued efficacy after the first year of treatment (Silver et al., 2011).

4.2 Closing thoughts

Only one single randomized clinical trial documented the efficacy of prolonged release oxycodone-naloxone (Trenkwalder et al., 2013). Due to a large number of dropouts before the planned 12 weeks of treatment, this study may have underestimated the occurrence of adverse events (de Oliveira et al., 2016).

As for chronic pain management, evidence of long-term efficacy of opioids for RLS is limited, all the more the risk for abuse and the danger of addiction still limit considerably the clinical use of opioids in this condition.

4.3 Putative mechanism of action of opioids on RLS

The precise mechanism of action of opioids as a treatment for RLS is unknown but is thought to be related to its ability to stimulate opioids receptors within the endogenous opioid system and in circuits involved in pain modulation.

5. Iron

5.1 Rational

A key factor in the development of a hyperdopaminergic state is the altered brain iron homeostasis that is considered so far as the primary pathogenetic mechanism of RLS (Earley et al., 2014). The presence of low serum iron levels in 25% of patients with RLS was first reported by Ekbom (Ekbom, 1960) and several ensuing papers have since pointed to a strong association between the occurrence and severity of RLS and peripheral iron deficiency, with or without anemia (Aul, Davis, & Rodnitzky, 1998; O′Keeffe, Gavin, & Lavan, 1994; Silber & Richardson, 2003; Sun, Chen, Ho, Earley, & Allen, 1998), although this higher prevalence has not been confirmed in population-based survey using the International Restless Legs Syndrome Study Group criteria (Berger et al., 2002; Hogl et al., 2005; Kim et al., 2010). Even in a registry study of 13,448 healthy blood donors in Denmark, the prevalence of restless legs syndrome was not related to plasma ferritin concentrations (Didriksen et al., 2017). Peripheral iron stores do not however mirror brain iron concentration. Indeed, normal levels of iron, ferritin and transferrin were also found in patients' serum with however low CSF-iron and ferritin concentrations and increased CSF-transferrin suggesting brain iron insufficiency (Earley et al., 2000; Mizuno, Mihara, Miyaoka, Inagaki, & Horiguchi, 2005). This brain iron insufficiency was further confirmed by direct magnetic resonance imaging (MRI) assessment of brain regional iron relative concentration in RLS patients that demonstrated a significant decrease in iron stores in the SN and in the putamen, with however conflicting results in the reported iron changes in different brain regions and different RLS phenotypes (Allen, Barker, Wehrl, Song, & Earley, 2001; Astrakas et al., 2008; Earley, B Barker, Horska, & Allen, 2006; Godau, Klose, Di Santo, Schweitzer, & Berg, 2008; Knake et al., 2010; Li et al., 2016; Margariti et al., 2012; Moon et al., 2014; Rizzo et al., 2013). Using a 7-T MRI, no significant difference was found in magnetic susceptibility in the SN between RLS patients and healthy controls (Li et al., 2016). Pathological autopsy studies also showed a decreased iron staining in neuropils consistent with some, but not all, MRI data and with a possible impaired brain iron acquisition in RLS (Connor et al., 2003, 2011, 2004; Pittock et al., 2004).

It is mainly the experimental manipulation of iron in non-human primates and in rodents that highlighted the pivotal role of iron in the modulation of the dopaminergic system, since it reproduces the main alterations in dopaminergic transmission observed in RLS patients. In serum iron-depleted macaques, an increase in nigrostriatal dopaminergic function together with a specific alteration of the serotonin/dopamine interaction in the central nervous system was documented (Hyacinthe et al., 2015). In rats with nutritional iron deficiency, an altered synthesis and functioning of DAT was thought to account for the dramatic increase in dopamine extracellular levels in the caudate-putamen (Beard, Chen, Connor, & Jones, 1994; Bianco, Wiesinger, Earley, Jones, & Beard, 2008; Nelson, Erikson, Pinero, & Beard, 1997) and significant reduction in DAT density was also demonstrated (Erikson, Jones, & Beard, 2000). Iron deficiency also decreases D_1 and D_2R density in the caudate-putamen of rat brains (Ashkenazi, Ben-Shachar, & Youdim, 1982; Ben-Shachar, Finberg, & Youdim, 1985; Erikson, Jones, Hess, Zhang, & Beard, 2001).

5.2 When to use iron?

Consistent with the prevalent opinion, the more the clinical problem the less degree of iron deficiency is needed and the lower the ferritin or transferrin saturation the more appropriate the iron treatment (Allen et al., 2018). It is actually admitted that iron supplementation should be considered when serum ferritin $<100\,\mu g/L$ (Allen et al., 2018). In any case, iron supplementation should be prohibited with ferritin $>300\,\mu g/L$ or transferrin saturation $>45\%$.

5.2.1 Oral iron

There are two double-blinded, placebo-controlled studies with conflicting results regarding the improvement in RLS symptoms' severity under oral iron therapy in patients with low to normal ferritin (Davis, Rajput, Rajput, Aul, & Eichhorn, 2000; Wang, O'Reilly, Venkataraman, Mysliwiec, & Mysliwiec, 2009). In the study by Davis et al., patients in the treatment arm of this study had mean serum ferritin levels of 134.8 ng/mL and the primary outcome measure was a dichotomous variable of improvement or no improvement in average quality of sleep as recorded by a visual analog scale with no validated measure of RLS symptoms' severity (Davis et al., 2000). One study showed oral iron to be less effective in substituting iron loss in blood donors compared with intravenous iron (Birgegard, Schneider, & Ulfberg, 2010). Frequent nausea and constipation, and long duration treatment period may also limit patients' compliance to oral iron therapy.

5.2.2 *Intravenous iron*

Data from several open-label and controlled studies of intravenous iron treatment of RLS using different iron formulation such as ferric carboxymaltose (Allen et al., 2011; Cho, Allen, & Earley, 2016; Cho, Allen, & Earley, 2018; Hornyak, Scholz, Kiemen, & Kassubek, 2012; Lieske et al., 2016; Trenkwalder et al., 2017), iron dextran (Cho, Allen, & Earley, 2013; Earley, Heckler, & Allen, 2004; Mehmood, Auerbach, Earley, & Allen, 2014; Ondo, 2010), iron sucrose (Birgegard et al., 2010; Earley et al., 2009; Grote, Leissner, Hedner, & Ulfberg, 2009; Zhang, Chen, & Huang, 2015) and iron gluconate (Earley, Heckler, & Allen, 2005; Lieske et al., 2016) are available and yielded conflicting results likely reflecting variable effects of different iron formulations and dosages, different patient populations and different study design (Trotti, Bhadriraju, & Becker, 2012). Experts' consensus recommends intravenous ferric carboxymaltose for the treatment of RLS in patients with serum ferritin levels $\leq 100\,\mu g/L$ with or without anemia (Allen et al., 2018).

5.3 Closing thoughts

Although compromised iron status is considered as the primary actor in the pathogenetic mechanism of RLS, iron replacement therapies have so far generated unpredictable results and more data are still required to confirm indications, short- and long-term efficacy and tolerance of intravenous iron (Allen et al., 2018).

6. Benzodiazepines

Although successful treatment of RLS and PLMS with clonazepam was reported (Boghen, 1980; Ohanna, Peled, Rubin, Zomer, & Lavie, 1985; Peled & Lavie, 1987; Saletu et al., 2001), data from blinded, controlled studies on the use of anxiolytic agents in patients with RLS are limited, with a small controlled study of clonazepam reporting negative results (Boghen, Lamothe, Elie, Godbout, & Montplaisir, 1986). In a prospective, randomized, open-label study, clonazepam and nortriptyline showed similar efficacy on QoL in women with RLS (Roshi, Tandon, Mahajan, Sharma, & Khajuria, 2018).

6.1 Closing thoughts

Although there is insufficient evidence to support the use of benzodiazepines in RLS, just like $\alpha 2$-δ ligands, clonazepam has been largely used for treating numerous neurological pain conditions including neuropathic pain and RLS. Owing to its central action via the GABA receptors, its anxiolytic effect may improve sleep initiation and maintenance in patients with comorbid anxiety (Limousin et al., 2018). In RLS, and to avoid possible development of tolerance and dependency and sleep apnea, clonazepam could be used on an ad hoc basis in case of symptoms severity exacerbation or in patients with intermittent symptoms (Limousin et al., 2018).

7. Adenosine

Based on the recent evidence of a central hypoadenosinergic state in rodents with brain iron deficiency, a prospective open-label, non-placebo controlled clinical trial showed mitigated efficacy of dipyridamole, a non-selective inhibitor of adenosine transport, as only 6 out of 13 enrolled patients were full responders (Garcia-Borreguero et al., 2018). Data are lacking from controlled clinical studies of dipyridamole treatment for RLS to support the recommendation of this approach.

8. Comparison trials and comparative meta-analysis

8.1 Head to head comparison trials

The comparative long-term effectiveness, cost-effectiveness, and safety of different RLS labeled treatments are important issues, but currently little evidence is available to help resolve uncertainty on these questions.

In RLS, a total of four randomized trials compared the efficacy of iron versus pramipexole (Lee, Lee, Kang, Park, & Yoon, 2014), gabapentin versus ropinirole (Happe et al., 2003) and pregabalin versus pramipexole (Allen, 2014; Garcia-Borreguero et al., 2014).

In one randomized, but not blinded trial to compare the efficacy of oral iron and pramipexole in RLS patients with a serum ferritin between 15 and 50 ng/mL over a 12-week treatment period, no significant difference was observed between the iron and pramipexole groups in terms of treatment efficacy and rate of improvement speed, although one would have expected that the iron group may show delayed response in relation with iron stores restoration (Lee et al., 2014). The impact of these results is seriously limited by the small sample size, lack of placebo control and a high rate of dropout.

One open trial compared ropinirole with gabapentin in terms of efficacy and tolerance and found that both drugs were equally efficient in alleviating RLS symptoms (Happe et al., 2003). In this study, PSG data showed a worsening of sleep parameters with ropinirole, similar reduction of PLMS index in both groups but significant decrease in PLMS-arousal index only with gabapentin (Happe et al., 2003). Total scores of the Pittsburgh Sleep Quality Index improved significantly in the gabapentin group, whereas there were no significant changes in these scores in the ropinirole group (Happe et al., 2003). Again, limitations of this study are the small sample size, the lack of placebo control and the unblinded nature of the trial.

One robust head-to-head comparison trial compared the efficacy of pregabalin with pramipexole and observed a greater reduction in RLS symptoms' severity with pregabalin than with pramipexole over a period of 52 weeks along with a greater subjective improvement in sleep (Allen, 2014). Improvement in objective and subjective measures of sleep maintenance and sleep architecture with pregabalin at 300 mg/day, compared with placebo and pramipexole at 0.5 mg/day, was further confirmed in one randomized, double-blinded, three-way crossover trial (Garcia-Borreguero et al., 2014). In this trial, effects of pregabalin on PLMS-arousal index were however comparable to pramipexole (Garcia-Borreguero et al., 2014).

Polysomnographic comparison of acute effects of pramipexole versus ropinirole was also performed in one prospective double-blind controlled study. Both groups of patients treated with DA showed a significant decrease in PLMS index versus placebo but neither drug significantly improved sleep parameters (Manconi et al., 2011). In this study, direct comparison between the acute effects of pramipexole and ropinirole on PSG parameters was not performed.

In one parallel-group, placebo-controlled, single-blind PSG study that compared the acute effects of gabapentin and ropinirole, the DA showed acute therapeutic efficacy with regard to PLMS measures only, whereas gabapentin was shown to have a less pronounced effect on these measures, but improved objective and subjective sleep and awakening quality as compared with both placebo and ropinirole (Saletu et al., 2010).

8.2 Comparative meta-analysis

Indirect comparison of different drug classes' efficacy and tolerance is also available from very few comparative meta-analysis of randomized controlled trials.

Indirect results from one meta-analysis showed a mildly superior effect of pramipexole over ropinirole on sensitive symptoms of RLS and a lower incidence of DA-related side effects (Quilici et al., 2008), whereas one other treatment comparison meta-analysis confirmed rotigotine to show additional benefit in terms of change in RLS symptoms' severity at week 12 compared to ropinirole, the latter being associated with a higher risk of nausea than the other agents (Sun, van Valkenhoef, & Morel, 2014). More recently, a comparative meta-analysis of the efficacy of DA (pramipexole, ropinirole and rotigotine) and α2-δ ligands (gabapentin enacarbil and pregabalin) concluded to a similar efficacy between the drugs in reducing RLS symptoms severity with however gabapentin enacarbil and rotigotine to be associated with the highest Clinical Global Impression of Improvement responders' rates, compared to placebo, but with those of gabapentin enacarbil to be significantly better than those of ropinirole (Iftikhar, Alghothani, & Trotti, 2017). In this study, nausea was most common with DA, with ropinirole having the highest incidence, followed by rotigotine and pramipexole, compared with placebo, but no significant inter-treatment differences existed across all drug classes for nausea, headache or somnolence. Significant inter-treatment differences were only detected for dizziness between pregabalin and all DA (Iftikhar et al., 2017).

8.3 Closing thoughts

Overall, current evidence from a very limited number of head-to-head trials in adult patients with idiopathic RLS is insufficient to guide the selection of RLS active treatments for short-term or long-term therapy. More research on this topic is needed.

9. Conclusion

Current guidelines state that ropinirole, pramipexole, rotigotine, gabapentin enacarbil (when available), gabapentin, pregabalin and opioids/prolonged release oxycodone–naloxone (when available) are all considered to be effective for short-term RLS treatment (Winkelmann et al., 2018). Guidelines for iron replacement therapy in RLS were also recently established favoring the use of ferric carboxymaltose (Allen et al., 2018). Despite the optimistic conclusions of most clinical trials in RLS, adherence to ropinirole, pramipexole, and gabapentin were shown to be low in newly diagnosed patients with RLS as after 1 year of follow-up, the proportion of persistent users was 25.0%, 25.8%, and 20.6%, respectively (Kim & Hartzema, 2018a). Recently, a decline in DA prescription and an increase in α2-δ ligands prescription in RLS was reported although, despite regularly update experts' recommendations, overall 36% of physician visits in ambulatory care settings were still associated with a prescription of a DA, while only 14% of the visits were associated with a prescription of the α2-δ ligands meaning that DA are still considered as a first line therapy for RLS (Kim & Hartzema, 2018b). In this study, RLS exacerbating drugs were listed in 28% of the physician visits and, among the visits associated with RLS exacerbating drugs, 83% were associated with antidepressants, meaning that communication efforts should be increased towards physicians prescribing major RLS drugs. Concern over tolerance, augmentation and impulse control disorder associated with DA may account for the overall decrease in the percentages of visits associated with DA.

This clearly questions the long-term treatment strategies in RLS and underlies the need for complementary, alternative and novel therapies, be it adenosinergic or other (Garcia-Borreguero et al., 2018; Megelin & Ghorayeb, 2017). This would be better achieved when the pathophysiology of RLS is deciphered.

Conflict of interest

No conflict of interest to declare.

References

Akpinar, S. (1982). Treatment of restless legs syndrome with levodopa plus benserazide. *Archives of Neurology*, *39*(11), 739.

Allen, R. P. (2014). Pregabalin versus pramipexole for restless legs syndrome. *The New England Journal of Medicine*, *370*(21), 2050–2051. https://doi.org/10.1056/NEJMc1402987.

Allen, R. P., Adler, C. H., Du, W., Butcher, A., Bregman, D. B., & Earley, C. J. (2011). Clinical efficacy and safety of IV ferric carboxymaltose (FCM) treatment of RLS: A multi-centred, placebo-controlled preliminary clinical trial. *Sleep Medicine*, *12*(9), 906–913. https://doi.org/10.1016/j.sleep.2011.06.009.

Allen, R. P., Barker, P. B., Wehrl, F., Song, H. K., & Earley, C. J. (2001). MRI measurement of brain iron in patients with restless legs syndrome. *Neurology*, *56*(2), 263–265.

Allen, R., Becker, P. M., Bogan, R., Schmidt, M., Kushida, C. A., Fry, J. M., et al. (2004). Ropinirole decreases periodic leg movements and improves sleep parameters in patients with restless legs syndrome. *Sleep*, *27*(5), 907–914.

Allen, R., Chen, C., Soaita, A., Wohlberg, C., Knapp, L., Peterson, B. T., et al. (2010). A randomized, double-blind, 6-week, dose-ranging study of pregabalin in patients with restless legs syndrome. *Sleep Medicine*, *11*(6), 512–519. https://doi.org/10.1016/j.sleep.2010.03.003.

Allen, R. P., Connor, J. R., Hyland, K., & Earley, C. J. (2009). Abnormally increased CSF 3-Ortho-methyldopa (3-OMD) in untreated restless legs syndrome (RLS) patients indicates more severe disease and possibly abnormally increased dopamine synthesis. *Sleep Medicine*, *10*(1), 123–128. https://doi.org/10.1016/j.sleep.2007.11.012.

Allen, R. P., Picchietti, D. L., Auerbach, M., Cho, Y. W., Connor, J. R., Earley, C. J., et al. (2018). Evidence-based and consensus clinical practice guidelines for the iron treatment of restless legs syndrome/Willis-Ekbom disease in adults and children: An IRLSSG task force report. *Sleep Medicine*, *41*, 27–44. https://doi.org/10.1016/j.sleep.2017.11.1126.

Ashkenazi, R., Ben-Shachar, D., & Youdim, M. B. (1982). Nutritional iron and dopamine binding sites in the rat brain. *Pharmacology, Biochemistry, and Behavior*, *17*(Suppl. 1), 43–47.

Astrakas, L. G., Konitsiotis, S., Margariti, P., Tsouli, S., Tzarouhi, L., & Argyropoulou, M. I. (2008). T2 relaxometry and fMRI of the brain in late-onset restless legs syndrome. *Neurology*, *71*(12), 911–916. https://doi.org/10.1212/01.wnl.0000325914.50764.a2.

Aul, E. A., Davis, B. J., & Rodnitzky, R. L. (1998). The importance of formal serum iron studies in the assessment of restless legs syndrome. *Neurology*, *51*(3), 912.

Bauer, A., Cassel, W., Benes, H., Kesper, K., Rye, D., Sica, D., et al. (2016). Rotigotine's effect on PLM-associated blood pressure elevations in restless legs syndrome: An RCT. *Neurology*, *86*(19), 1785–1793. https://doi.org/10.1212/WNL.0000000000002649.

Beard, J. L., Chen, Q., Connor, J., & Jones, B. C. (1994). Altered monamine metabolism in caudate-putamen of iron-deficient rats. *Pharmacology, Biochemistry, and Behavior*, *48*(3), 621–624.

Benes, H., Mattern, W., Peglau, I., Dreykluft, T., Bergmann, L., Hansen, C., et al. (2011). Ropinirole improves depressive symptoms and restless legs syndrome severity in RLS patients: A multicentre, randomized, placebo-controlled study. *Journal of Neurology*, *258*(6), 1046–1054. https://doi.org/10.1007/s00415-010-5879-7.

Ben-Shachar, D., Finberg, J. P., & Youdim, M. B. (1985). Effect of iron chelators on dopamine D2 receptors. *Journal of Neurochemistry*, *45*(4), 999–1005.

Berger, K., von Eckardstein, A., Trenkwalder, C., Rothdach, A., Junker, R., & Weiland, S. K. (2002). Iron metabolism and the risk of restless legs syndrome in an elderly general population—The MEMO-Study. *Journal of Neurology*, *249*(9), 1195–1199. https://doi.org/10.1007/s00415-002-0805-2.

Bianco, L. E., Wiesinger, J., Earley, C. J., Jones, B. C., & Beard, J. L. (2008). Iron deficiency alters dopamine uptake and response to L-DOPA injection in Sprague-Dawley rats. *Journal of Neurochemistry*, *106*(1), 205–215. https://doi.org/10.1111/j.1471-4159.2008.05358.x.

Birgegard, G., Schneider, K., & Ulfberg, J. (2010). High incidence of iron depletion and restless leg syndrome (RLS) in regular blood donors: Intravenous iron sucrose substitution more effective than oral iron. *Vox Sanguinis*, *99*(4), 354–361. https://doi.org/10.1111/j.1423-0410.2010.01368.x.

Bliwise, D. L., Freeman, A., Ingram, C. D., Rye, D. B., Chakravorty, S., & Watts, R. L. (2005). Randomized, double-blind, placebo-controlled, short-term trial of ropinirole in restless legs syndrome. *Sleep Medicine*, *6*(2), 141–147. https://doi.org/10.1016/j.sleep.2004.12.002.

Bogan, R. K., Bornemann, M. A., Kushida, C. A., Tran, P. V., Barrett, R. W., & XP060 Study Group. (2010). Long-term maintenance treatment of restless legs syndrome with gabapentin enacarbil: A randomized controlled study. *Mayo Clinic Proceedings*, *85*(6), 512–521. https://doi.org/10.4065/mcp.2009.0700.

Bogan, R. K., Fry, J. M., Schmidt, M. H., Carson, S. W., Ritchie, S. Y., & TREAT RLS US Study Group. (2006). Ropinirole in the treatment of patients with restless legs syndrome: A US-based randomized, double-blind, placebo-controlled clinical trial. *Mayo Clinic Proceedings*, *81*(1), 17–27.

Boghen, D. (1980). Successful treatment of restless legs with clonazepam. *Annals of Neurology*, *8*(3), 341. https://doi.org/10.1002/ana.410080322.

Boghen, D., Lamothe, L., Elie, R., Godbout, R., & Montplaisir, J. (1986). The treatment of the restless legs syndrome with clonazepam: A prospective controlled study. *The Canadian Journal of Neurological Sciences*, *13*(3), 245–247.

Cho, Y. W., Allen, R. P., & Earley, C. J. (2013). Lower molecular weight intravenous iron dextran for restless legs syndrome. *Sleep Medicine*, *14*(3), 274–277. https://doi.org/10.1016/j.sleep.2012.11.001.

Cho, Y. W., Allen, R. P., & Earley, C. J. (2016). Clinical efficacy of ferric carboxymaltose treatment in patients with restless legs syndrome. *Sleep Medicine*, *25*, 16–23. https://doi.org/10.1016/j.sleep.2016.06.021.

Cho, Y. W., Allen, R. P., & Earley, C. J. (2018). Efficacy of ferric carboxymaltose (FCM) 500 mg dose for the treatment of Restless Legs Syndrome. *Sleep Medicine*, *42*, 7–12. https://doi.org/10.1016/j.sleep.2017.11.1134.

Cho, Y. W., Hong, S. B., Kim do, H., Lee, H. W., Joo, E. Y., Kim, J. H., et al. (2013). The effect of ropinirole on the quality of life in patients with restless legs syndrome in Korea: An 8-week, multicenter, prospective study. *Journal of Clinical Neurology*, *9*(1), 51–56. https://doi.org/10.3988/jcn.2013.9.1.51.

Chokroverty, S. (2015). Opioid-induced hyperalgesia and dopamine-induced augmentation in an intractable and refractory case of RLS. *Sleep Medicine*, *16*(10), 1304. https://doi.org/10.1016/j.sleep.2015.08.005.

Clemens, S., Rye, D., & Hochman, S. (2006). Restless legs syndrome: Revisiting the dopamine hypothesis from the spinal cord perspective. *Neurology*, *67*(1), 125–130. https://doi.org/10.1212/01.wnl.0000223316.53428.c9.

Connor, J. R., Boyer, P. J., Menzies, S. L., Dellinger, B., Allen, R. P., Ondo, W. G., et al. (2003). Neuropathological examination suggests impaired brain iron acquisition in restless legs syndrome. *Neurology*, *61*(3), 304–309.

Connor, J. R., Ponnuru, P., Wang, X. S., Patton, S. M., Allen, R. P., & Earley, C. J. (2011). Profile of altered brain iron acquisition in restless legs syndrome. *Brain*, *134*(Pt 4), 959–968. https://doi.org/10.1093/brain/awr012.

Connor, J. R., Wang, X. S., Allen, R. P., Beard, J. L., Wiesinger, J. A., Felt, B. T., et al. (2009). Altered dopaminergic profile in the putamen and substantia nigra in restless leg syndrome. *Brain*, *132*(Pt 9), 2403–2412. https://doi.org/10.1093/brain/awp125.

Connor, J. R., Wang, X. S., Patton, S. M., Menzies, S. L., Troncoso, J. C., Earley, C. J., et al. (2004). Decreased transferrin receptor expression by neuromelanin cells in restless legs syndrome. *Neurology*, *62*(9), 1563–1567.

Cundy, K. C., Branch, R., Chernov-Rogan, T., Dias, T., Estrada, T., Hold, K., et al. (2004). XP13512 [(+/−)-1-([(alpha-isobutanoyloxyethoxy)carbonyl] aminomethyl)-1-cyclohexane acetic acid], a novel gabapentin prodrug: I. Design, synthesis, enzymatic conversion to gabapentin, and transport by intestinal solute transporters. *The Journal of Pharmacology and Experimental Therapeutics*, *311*(1), 315–323. https://doi.org/10.1124/jpet.104.067934.

Davis, B. J., Rajput, A., Rajput, M. L., Aul, E. A., & Eichhorn, G. R. (2000). A randomized, double-blind placebo-controlled trial of iron in restless legs syndrome. *European Neurology*, *43*(2), 70–75. https://doi.org/10.1159/000008138.

de Oliveira, C. O., Carvalho, L. B., Carlos, K., Conti, C., de Oliveira, M. M., Prado, L. B., et al. (2016). Opioids for restless legs syndrome. *Cochrane Database Syst Rev*, *6*, CD006941. https://doi.org/10.1002/14651858.CD006941.pub2.

Didriksen, M., Rigas, A. S., Allen, R. P., Burchell, B. J., Di Angelantonio, E., Nielsen, M. H., et al. (2017). Prevalence of restless legs syndrome and associated factors in an otherwise healthy population: Results from the Danish Blood Donor Study. *Sleep Medicine*, *36*, 55–61. https://doi.org/10.1016/j.sleep.2017.04.014.

Dohin, E., Hogl, B., Ferini-Strambi, L., Schollmayer, E., Fichtner, A., Bauer, L., et al. (2013). Safety and efficacy of rotigotine transdermal patch in patients with restless legs syndrome: A post-hoc analysis of patients taking 1–3 mg/24 h for up to 5 years. *Expert Opinion on Pharmacotherapy*, *14*(1), 15–25. https://doi.org/10.1517/14656566.2013.758251.

Dorfman, B. J., & Nirenberg, M. J. (2013). Dopamine agonist withdrawal syndrome in a patient with restless legs syndrome. *Parkinsonism & Related Disorders*, *19*(2), 269–270. https://doi.org/10.1016/j.parkreldis.2012.06.006.

Earley, C. J., & Allen, R. P. (2006). Restless legs syndrome augmentation associated with tramadol. *Sleep Medicine*, 7(7), 592–593. https://doi.org/10.1016/j.sleep.2006.05.011.

Earley, C. J., B Barker, P., Horska, A., & Allen, R. P. (2006). MRI-determined regional brain iron concentrations in early- and late-onset restless legs syndrome. *Sleep Medicine*, 7(5), 458–461. https://doi.org/10.1016/j.sleep.2005.11.009.

Earley, C. J., Connor, J. R., Beard, J. L., Malecki, E. A., Epstein, D. K., & Allen, R. P. (2000). Abnormalities in CSF concentrations of ferritin and transferrin in restless legs syndrome. *Neurology*, *54*(8), 1698–1700.

Earley, C. J., Connor, J., Garcia-Borreguero, D., Jenner, P., Winkelman, J., Zee, P. C., et al. (2014). Altered brain iron homeostasis and dopaminergic function in Restless Legs Syndrome (Willis-Ekbom Disease). *Sleep Medicine*, *15*(11), 1288–1301. https://doi.org/10.1016/j.sleep.2014.05.009.

Earley, C. J., Heckler, D., & Allen, R. P. (2004). The treatment of restless legs syndrome with intravenous iron dextran. *Sleep Medicine*, *5*(3), 231–235. https://doi.org/10.1016/j.sleep.2004.03.002.

Earley, C. J., Heckler, D., & Allen, R. P. (2005). Repeated IV doses of iron provides effective supplemental treatment of restless legs syndrome. *Sleep Medicine*, *6*(4), 301–305. https://doi.org/10.1016/j.sleep.2005.01.008.

Earley, C. J., Horska, A., Mohamed, M. A., Barker, P. B., Beard, J. L., & Allen, R. P. (2009). A randomized, double-blind, placebo-controlled trial of intravenous iron sucrose in restless legs syndrome. *Sleep Medicine*, *10*(2), 206–211. https://doi.org/10.1016/j.sleep.2007.12.006.

Earley, C. J., Kuwabara, H., Wong, D. F., Gamaldo, C., Salas, R., Brasic, J., et al. (2011). The dopamine transporter is decreased in the striatum of subjects with restless legs syndrome. *Sleep*, *34*(3), 341–347.

Earley, C. J., Kuwabara, H., Wong, D. F., Gamaldo, C., Salas, R. E., Brasic, J. R., et al. (2013). Increased synaptic dopamine in the putamen in restless legs syndrome. *Sleep*, *36*(1), 51–57. https://doi.org/10.5665/sleep.2300.

Ekbom, K. A. (1960). Restless legs syndrome. *Neurology*, *10*, 868–873.

Ellenbogen, A. L., Thein, S. G., Winslow, D. H., Becker, P. M., Tolson, J. M., Lassauzet, M. L., et al. (2011). A 52-week study of gabapentin enacarbil in restless legs syndrome. *Clinical Neuropharmacology*, *34*(1), 8–16. https://doi.org/10.1097/WNF.0b013e3182087d48.

Erikson, K. M., Jones, B. C., & Beard, J. L. (2000). Iron deficiency alters dopamine transporter functioning in rat striatum. *The Journal of Nutrition*, *130*(11), 2831–2837.

Erikson, K. M., Jones, B. C., Hess, E. J., Zhang, Q., & Beard, J. L. (2001). Iron deficiency decreases dopamine D1 and D2 receptors in rat brain. *Pharmacology, Biochemistry, and Behavior*, *69*(3–4), 409–418.

Evoy, K. E., Morrison, M. D., & Saklad, S. R. (2017). Abuse and Misuse of Pregabalin and Gabapentin. *Drugs*, 77(4), 403–426. https://doi.org/10.1007/s40265-017-0700-x.

Ferini-Strambi, L. (2002). Restless legs syndrome augmentation and pramipexole treatment. *Sleep Medicine*, *3*(3 Suppl), S23–S25. https://doi.org/10.1016/S1389-9457(02)00144-2.

Ferini-Strambi, L., Aarskog, D., Partinen, M., Chaudhuri, K. R., Sohr, M., Verri, D., et al. (2008). Effect of pramipexole on RLS symptoms and sleep: A randomized, double-blind, placebo-controlled trial. *Sleep Medicine*, *9*(8), 874–881. https://doi.org/10.1016/j.sleep.2008.09.001.

Ferre, S., Garcia-Borreguero, D., Allen, R. P., & Earley, C. J. (2018). New insights into the neurobiology of restless legs syndrome. *The Neuroscientist*. 1073858418791763. https://doi.org/10.1177/1073858418791763.

Garcia-Borreguero, D., Allen, R., Hudson, J., Dohin, E., Grieger, F., Moran, K., et al. (2016). Effects of rotigotine on daytime symptoms in patients with primary restless legs syndrome: A randomized, placebo-controlled study. *Current Medical Research and Opinion, 32*(1), 77–85. https://doi.org/10.1185/03007995.2015.1103216.

Garcia-Borreguero, D., Grunstein, R., Sridhar, G., Dreykluft, T., Montagna, P., Dom, R., et al. (2007). A 52-week open-label study of the long-term safety of ropinirole in patients with restless legs syndrome. *Sleep Medicine, 8*(7–8), 742–752. https://doi.org/10.1016/j.sleep.2006.09.009.

Garcia-Borreguero, D., Guitart, X., Garcia Malo, C., Cano-Pumarega, I., Granizo, J. J., & Ferre, S. (2018). Treatment of restless legs syndrome/Willis-Ekbom disease with the non-selective ENT1/ENT2 inhibitor dipyridamole: Testing the adenosine hypothesis. *Sleep Medicine, 45*, 94–97. https://doi.org/10.1016/j.sleep.2018.02.002.

Garcia-Borreguero, D., Hogl, B., Ferini-Strambi, L., Winkelman, J., Hill-Zabala, C., Asgharian, A., et al. (2012). Systematic evaluation of augmentation during treatment with ropinirole in restless legs syndrome (Willis-Ekbom disease): Results from a prospective, multicenter study over 66 weeks. *Movement Disorders, 27*(2), 277–283. https://doi.org/10.1002/mds.24889.

Garcia-Borreguero, D., Larrosa, O., de la Llave, Y., Verger, K., Masramon, X., & Hernandez, G. (2002). Treatment of restless legs syndrome with gabapentin: A double-blind, cross-over study. *Neurology, 59*(10), 1573–1579.

Garcia-Borreguero, D., Larrosa, O., Williams, A. M., Albares, J., Pascual, M., Palacios, J. C., et al. (2010). Treatment of restless legs syndrome with pregabalin: A double-blind, placebo-controlled study. *Neurology, 74*(23), 1897–1904. https://doi.org/10.1212/WNL.0b013e3181e1ce73.

Garcia-Borreguero, D., Patrick, J., DuBrava, S., Becker, P. M., Lankford, A., Chen, C., et al. (2014). Pregabalin versus pramipexole: Effects on sleep disturbance in restless legs syndrome. *Sleep, 37*(4), 635–643. https://doi.org/10.5665/sleep.3558.

Giorgi, L., Asgharian, A., & Hunter, B. (2013). Ropinirole in patients with restless legs syndrome and baseline IRLS total scores $\geq$ 24: Efficacy and tolerability in a 26-week, double-blind, parallel-group, placebo-controlled study followed by a 40-week open-label extension. *Clinical Therapeutics, 35*(9), 1321–1336. https://doi.org/10.1016/j.clinthera.2013.06.016.

Godau, J., Klose, U., Di Santo, A., Schweitzer, K., & Berg, D. (2008). Multiregional brain iron deficiency in restless legs syndrome. *Movement Disorders, 23*(8), 1184–1187. https://doi.org/10.1002/mds.22070.

Grote, L., Leissner, L., Hedner, J., & Ulfberg, J. (2009). A randomized, double-blind, placebo controlled, multi-center study of intravenous iron sucrose and placebo in the treatment of restless legs syndrome. *Movement Disorders, 24*(10), 1445–1452. https://doi.org/10.1002/mds.22562.

Happe, S., Klosch, G., Saletu, B., & Zeitlhofer, J. (2001). Treatment of idiopathic restless legs syndrome (RLS) with gabapentin. *Neurology, 57*(9), 1717–1719.

Happe, S., Sauter, C., Klosch, G., Saletu, B., & Zeitlhofer, J. (2003). Gabapentin versus ropinirole in the treatment of idiopathic restless legs syndrome. *Neuropsychobiology, 48*(2), 82–86. https://doi.org/10.1159/000072882.

Heim, B., Djamshidian, A., Heidbreder, A., Stefani, A., Zamarian, L., Pertl, M. T., et al. (2016). Augmentation and impulsive behaviors in restless legs syndrome: Coexistence or association? *Neurology, 87*(1), 36–40. https://doi.org/10.1212/WNL.0000000000002803.

Hening, W. A., Allen, R. P., Ondo, W. G., Walters, A. S., Winkelman, J. W., Becker, P., et al. (2010). Rotigotine improves restless legs syndrome: A 6-month randomized, double-blind, placebo-controlled trial in the United States. *Movement Disorders, 25*(11), 1675–1683. https://doi.org/10.1002/mds.23157.

Hening, W. A., Walters, A., Kavey, N., Gidro-Frank, S., Cote, L., & Fahn, S. (1986). Dyskinesias while awake and periodic movements in sleep in restless legs syndrome: Treatment with opioids. *Neurology*, *36*(10), 1363–1366.

Hogl, B., Garcia-Borreguero, D., Trenkwalder, C., Ferini-Strambi, L., Hening, W., Poewe, W., et al. (2011). Efficacy and augmentation during 6 months of double-blind pramipexole for restless legs syndrome. *Sleep Medicine*, *12*(4), 351–360. https://doi.org/10.1016/j.sleep.2010.12.007.

Hogl, B., Kiechl, S., Willeit, J., Saletu, M., Frauscher, B., Seppi, K., et al. (2005). Restless legs syndrome: A community-based study of prevalence, severity, and risk factors. *Neurology*, *64*(11), 1920–1924. https://doi.org/10.1212/01.WNL.0000163996.64461.A3.

Hornyak, M., Scholz, H., Kiemen, A., & Kassubek, J. (2012). Investigating the response to intravenous iron in restless legs syndrome: An observational study. *Sleep Medicine*, *13*(6), 732–735. https://doi.org/10.1016/j.sleep.2012.02.011.

Hyacinthe, C., De Deurwaerdere, P., Thiollier, T., Li, Q., Bezard, E., & Ghorayeb, I. (2015). Blood withdrawal affects iron store dynamics in primates with consequences on monoaminergic system function. *Neuroscience*, *290*, 621–635. https://doi.org/10.1016/j.neuroscience.2015.01.057.

Iftikhar, I. H., Alghothani, L., & Trotti, L. M. (2017). Gabapentin enacarbil, pregabalin and rotigotine are equally effective in restless legs syndrome: A comparative meta-analysis. *European Journal of Neurology*, *24*(12), 1446–1456. https://doi.org/10.1111/ene.13449.

Inoue, Y., Hirata, K., Kuroda, K., Fujita, M., Shimizu, T., Emura, N., et al. (2010). Efficacy and safety of pramipexole in Japanese patients with primary restless legs syndrome: A polysomnographic randomized, double-blind, placebo-controlled study. *Sleep Medicine*, *11*(1), 11–16. https://doi.org/10.1016/j.sleep.2009.03.009.

Inoue, Y., Hirata, K., Uchimura, N., Kuroda, K., Hattori, N., & Takeuchi, M. (2013). Gabapentin enacarbil in Japanese patients with restless legs syndrome: A 12-week, randomized, double-blind, placebo-controlled, parallel-group study. *Current Medical Research and Opinion*, *29*(1), 13–21. https://doi.org/10.1185/03007995.2012.746217.

Inoue, Y., Kuroda, K., Hirata, K., Uchimura, N., Kagimura, T., & Shimizu, T. (2010). Long-term open-label study of pramipexole in patients with primary restless legs syndrome. *Journal of the Neurological Sciences*, *294*(1–2), 62–66. https://doi.org/10.1016/j.jns.2010.04.003.

Inoue, Y., Shimizu, T., Hirata, K., Uchimura, N., Ishigooka, J., Oka, Y., et al. (2013). Efficacy and safety of rotigotine in Japanese patients with restless legs syndrome: A phase 3, multicenter, randomized, placebo-controlled, double-blind, parallel-group study. *Sleep Medicine*, *14*(11), 1085–1091. https://doi.org/10.1016/j.sleep.2013.07.007.

Inoue, Y., Uchimura, N., Kuroda, K., Hirata, K., & Hattori, N. (2012). Long-term efficacy and safety of gabapentin enacarbil in Japanese restless legs syndrome patients. *Progress in Neuro-Psychopharmacology & Biological Psychiatry*, *36*(2), 251–257. https://doi.org/10.1016/j.pnpbp.2011.10.009.

Jama, L., Hirvonen, K., Partinen, M., Alakuijala, A., Hublin, C., Tamminen, I., et al. (2009). A dose-ranging study of pramipexole for the symptomatic treatment of restless legs syndrome: Polysomnographic evaluation of periodic leg movements and sleep disturbance. *Sleep Medicine*, *10*(6), 630–636. https://doi.org/10.1016/j.sleep.2008.05.014.

Jost, W. H. (2004). Ropinirole: Current status of the studies. *Journal of Neurology*, *251* (Suppl. 6). VI/13–18.

Kim, J., & Hartzema, A. G. (2018a). Adherence and persistence to ropinirole, pramipexole, and gabapentin in patients with newly diagnosed restless legs syndrome. *Sleep Medicine*, *44*, 45–52. https://doi.org/10.1016/j.sleep.2017.11.1139.

Kim, J., & Hartzema, A. G. (2018b). Decline in dopamine agonists prescribing and characteristics of drugs prescribed during ambulatory office visits for restless legs syndrome: The National Ambulatory Medical Care Survey 2007–2015. *Sleep Medicine*, *54*, 238–243. https://doi.org/10.1016/j.sleep.2018.11.011.

Kim, K. W., Yoon, I. Y., Chung, S., Shin, Y. K., Lee, S. B., Choi, E. A., et al. (2010). Prevalence, comorbidities and risk factors of restless legs syndrome in the Korean elderly population—results from the Korean Longitudinal Study on Health and Aging. *Journal of Sleep Research, 19*(1 Pt. 1), 87–92. https://doi.org/10.1111/j.1365-2869.2009.00739.x.

Knake, S., Heverhagen, J. T., Menzler, K., Keil, B., Oertel, W. H., & Stiasny-Kolster, K. (2010). Normal regional brain iron concentration in restless legs syndrome measured by MRI. *Nature and Science of Sleep, 2*, 19–22.

Kvernmo, T., Hartter, S., & Burger, E. (2006). A review of the receptor-binding and pharmacokinetic properties of dopamine agonists. *Clinical Therapeutics, 28*(8), 1065–1078. https://doi.org/10.1016/j.clinthera.2006.08.004.

Kvernmo, T., Houben, J., & Sylte, I. (2008). Receptor-binding and pharmacokinetic properties of dopaminergic agonists. *Current Topics in Medicinal Chemistry, 8*(12), 1049–1067.

Lal, R., Ellenbogen, A., Chen, D., Zomorodi, K., Atluri, H., Luo, W., et al. (2012). A randomized, double-blind, placebo-controlled, dose-response study to assess the pharmacokinetics, efficacy, and safety of gabapentin enacarbil in subjects with restless legs syndrome. *Clinical Neuropharmacology, 35*(4), 165–173. https://doi.org/10.1097/WNF.0b013e318259eac8.

Lanza, G., Bachmann, C. G., Ghorayeb, I., Wang, Y., Ferri, R., & Paulus, W. (2017). Central and peripheral nervous system excitability in restless legs syndrome. *Sleep Medicine, 31*, 49–60. https://doi.org/10.1016/j.sleep.2016.05.010.

Lee, C. S., Lee, S. D., Kang, S. H., Park, H. Y., & Yoon, I. Y. (2014). Comparison of the efficacies of oral iron and pramipexole for the treatment of restless legs syndrome patients with low serum ferritin. *European Journal of Neurology, 21*(2), 260–266. https://doi.org/10.1111/ene.12286.

Li, X., Allen, R. P., Earley, C. J., Liu, H., Cruz, T. E., Edden, R. A., et al. (2016). Brain iron deficiency in idiopathic restless legs syndrome measured by quantitative magnetic susceptibility at 7 tesla. *Sleep Medicine, 22*, 75–82. https://doi.org/10.1016/j.sleep.2016.05.001.

Lieske, B., Becker, I., Schulz, R. J., Polidori, M. C., Kassubek, J., & Roehrig, G. (2016). Intravenous iron administration in restless legs syndrome: An observational study in geriatric patients. *Zeitschrift für Gerontologie und Geriatrie, 49*(7), 626–631. https://doi.org/10.1007/s00391-015-0984-y.

Limousin, N., Flamand, M., Schroder, C., & Charley Monaca, C. (2018). French consensus: Treatment of newly diagnosed restless legs syndrome. *Revue Neurologique (Paris), 174*(7–8), 515–521. https://doi.org/10.1016/j.neurol.2018.06.002.

Lipford, M. C., & Silber, M. H. (2012). Long-term use of pramipexole in the management of restless legs syndrome. *Sleep Medicine, 13*(10), 1280–1285. https://doi.org/10.1016/j.sleep.2012.08.004.

Ma, J. F., Wan, Q., Hu, X. Y., Sun, S. G., Wang, W. Z., Zhao, Z. X., et al. (2012). Efficacy and safety of pramipexole in chinese patients with restless legs syndrome: Results from a multi-center, randomized, double-blind, placebo-controlled trial. *Sleep Medicine, 13*(1), 58–63. https://doi.org/10.1016/j.sleep.2011.03.021.

Manconi, M., Ferri, R., Zucconi, M., Oldani, A., Fantini, M. L., Castronovo, V., et al. (2007). First night efficacy of pramipexole in restless legs syndrome and periodic leg movements. *Sleep Medicine, 8*(5), 491–497. https://doi.org/10.1016/j.sleep.2006.10.008.

Manconi, M., Ferri, R., Zucconi, M., Oldani, A., Giarolli, L., Bottasini, V., et al. (2011). Pramipexole versus ropinirole: Polysomnographic acute effects in restless legs syndrome. *Movement Disorders, 26*(5), 892–895. https://doi.org/10.1002/mds.23543.

Margariti, P. N., Astrakas, L. G., Tsouli, S. G., Hadjigeorgiou, G. M., Konitsiotis, S., & Argyropoulou, M. I. (2012). Investigation of unmedicated early onset restless legs syndrome by voxel-based morphometry, T2 relaxometry, and functional MR imaging during the night-time hours. *AJNR American Journal of Neuroradiology, 33*(4), 667–672. https://doi.org/10.3174/ajnr.A2829.

Megelin, T., & Ghorayeb, I. (2017). Cannabis for restless legs syndrome: A report of six patients. *Sleep Medicine*, *36*, 182–183. https://doi.org/10.1016/j.sleep.2017.04.019.

Mehmood, T., Auerbach, M., Earley, C. J., & Allen, R. P. (2014). Response to intravenous iron in patients with iron deficiency anemia (IDA) and restless leg syndrome (Willis-Ekbom disease). *Sleep Medicine*, *15*(12), 1473–1476. https://doi.org/10.1016/j.sleep.2014.08.012.

Mellick, G. A., & Mellick, L. B. (1996). Management of restless legs syndrome with gabapentin (Neurontin). *Sleep*, *19*(3), 224–226.

Mizuno, S., Mihara, T., Miyaoka, T., Inagaki, T., & Horiguchi, J. (2005). CSF iron, ferritin and transferrin levels in restless legs syndrome. *Journal of Sleep Research*, *14*(1), 43–47. https://doi.org/10.1111/j.1365-2869.2004.00403.x.

Montagna, P., Hornyak, M., Ulfberg, J., Hong, S. B., Koester, J., Crespi, G., et al. (2011). Randomized trial of pramipexole for patients with restless legs syndrome (RLS) and RLS-related impairment of mood. *Sleep Medicine*, *12*(1), 34–40. https://doi.org/10.1016/j.sleep.2010.08.005.

Montplaisir, J., Denesle, R., & Petit, D. (2000). Pramipexole in the treatment of restless legs syndrome: A follow-up study. *European Journal of Neurology*, 7(Suppl. 1), 27–31.

Montplaisir, J., Fantini, M. L., Desautels, A., Michaud, M., Petit, D., & Filipini, D. (2006). Long-term treatment with pramipexole in restless legs syndrome. *European Journal of Neurology*, *13*(12), 1306–1311. https://doi.org/10.1111/j.1468-1331.2006.01459.x.

Montplaisir, J., Karrasch, J., Haan, J., & Volc, D. (2006). Ropinirole is effective in the long-term management of restless legs syndrome: A randomized controlled trial. *Movement Disorders*, *21*(10), 1627–1635. https://doi.org/10.1002/mds.21050.

Montplaisir, J., Nicolas, A., Denesle, R., & Gomez-Mancilla, B. (1999). Restless legs syndrome improved by pramipexole: A double-blind randomized trial. *Neurology*, *52*(5), 938–943.

Moon, H. J., Chang, Y., Lee, Y. S., Song, H. J., Chang, H. W., Ku, J., et al. (2014). T2 relaxometry using 3.0-tesla magnetic resonance imaging of the brain in early- and late-onset restless legs syndrome. *Journal of Clinical Neurology*, *10*(3), 197–202. https://doi.org/10.3988/jcn.2014.10.3.197.

Nelson, C., Erikson, K., Pinero, D. J., & Beard, J. L. (1997). In vivo dopamine metabolism is altered in iron-deficient anemic rats. *The Journal of Nutrition*, *127*(12), 2282–2288.

Oertel, W. H., Benes, H., Garcia-Borreguero, D., Geisler, P., Hogl, B., Saletu, B., et al. (2008). Efficacy of rotigotine transdermal system in severe restless legs syndrome: A randomized, double-blind, placebo-controlled, six-week dose-finding trial in Europe. *Sleep Medicine*, *9*(3), 228–239. https://doi.org/10.1016/j.sleep.2007.04.010.

Oertel, W. H., Benes, H., Garcia-Borreguero, D., Hogl, B., Poewe, W., Montagna, P., et al. (2010). Rotigotine transdermal patch in moderate to severe idiopathic restless legs syndrome: A randomized, placebo-controlled polysomnographic study. *Sleep Medicine*, *11*(9), 848–856. https://doi.org/10.1016/j.sleep.2010.02.014.

Oertel, W. H., Hallstrom, Y., Saletu-Zyhlarz, G. M., Hopp, M., Bosse, B., Trenkwalder, C., et al. (2016). Sleep and quality of life under prolonged release oxycodone/naloxone for severe restless legs syndrome: An analysis of secondary efficacy variables of a double-blind, randomized, placebo-controlled study with an open-label extension. *CNS Drugs*, *30*(8), 749–760. https://doi.org/10.1007/s40263-016-0372-1.

Oertel, W. H., Stiasny-Kolster, K., Bergtholdt, B., Hallstrom, Y., Albo, J., Leissner, L., et al. (2007). Efficacy of pramipexole in restless legs syndrome: A six-week, multicenter, randomized, double-blind study (effect-RLS study). *Movement Disorders*, *22*(2), 213–219. https://doi.org/10.1002/mds.21261.

Oertel, W., Trenkwalder, C., Benes, H., Ferini-Strambi, L., Hogl, B., Poewe, W., et al. (2011). Long-term safety and efficacy of rotigotine transdermal patch for moderate-to-severe idiopathic restless legs syndrome: A 5-year open-label extension study. *Lancet Neurology*, *10*(8), 710–720. https://doi.org/10.1016/S1474-4422(11)70127-2.

Ohanna, N., Peled, R., Rubin, A. H., Zomer, J., & Lavie, P. (1985). Periodic leg movements in sleep: Effect of clonazepam treatment. *Neurology, 35*(3), 408–411.
O'Keeffe, S. T., Gavin, K., & Lavan, J. N. (1994). Iron status and restless legs syndrome in the elderly. *Age and Ageing, 23*(3), 200–203.
Ondo, W. (1999). Ropinirole for restless legs syndrome. *Movement Disorders, 14*(1), 138–140.
Ondo, W. G. (2005). Methadone for refractory restless legs syndrome. *Movement Disorders, 20*(3), 345–348. https://doi.org/10.1002/mds.20359.
Ondo, W. G. (2010). Intravenous iron dextran for severe refractory restless legs syndrome. *Sleep Medicine, 11*(5), 494–496. https://doi.org/10.1016/j.sleep.2009.12.002.
Partinen, M., Hirvonen, K., Jama, L., Alakuijala, A., Hublin, C., Tamminen, I., et al. (2006). Efficacy and safety of pramipexole in idiopathic restless legs syndrome: A polysomnographic dose-finding study—The PRELUDE study. *Sleep Medicine, 7*(5), 407–417. https://doi.org/10.1016/j.sleep.2006.03.011.
Partinen, M., Hirvonen, K., Jama, L., Alakuijala, A., Hublin, C., Tamminen, I., et al. (2008). Open-label study of the long-term efficacy and safety of pramipexole in patients with Restless Legs Syndrome (extension of the PRELUDE study). *Sleep Medicine, 9*(5), 537–541. https://doi.org/10.1016/j.sleep.2007.12.004.
Peled, R., & Lavie, P. (1987). Double-blind evaluation of clonazepam on periodic leg movements in sleep. *Journal of Neurology, Neurosurgery, and Psychiatry, 50*(12), 1679–1681.
Pittock, S. J., Parrett, T., Adler, C. H., Parisi, J. E., Dickson, D. W., & Ahlskog, J. E. (2004). Neuropathology of primary restless leg syndrome: Absence of specific tau- and alpha-synuclein pathology. *Movement Disorders, 19*(6), 695–699. https://doi.org/10.1002/mds.20042.
Quilici, S., Abrams, K. R., Nicolas, A., Martin, M., Petit, C., Lleu, P. L., et al. (2008). Meta-analysis of the efficacy and tolerability of pramipexole versus ropinirole in the treatment of restless legs syndrome. *Sleep Medicine, 9*(7), 715–726. https://doi.org/10.1016/j.sleep.2007.11.020.
Rizzo, G., Manners, D., Testa, C., Tonon, C., Vetrugno, R., Marconi, S., et al. (2013). Low brain iron content in idiopathic restless legs syndrome patients detected by phase imaging. *Movement Disorders, 28*(13), 1886–1890. https://doi.org/10.1002/mds.25576.
Roshi, Tandon, V. R., Mahajan, A., Sharma, S., & Khajuria, V. (2018). A prospective, randomized, open-label study comparing the efficacy and safety of clonazepam versus nortriptyline on quality of life in 40+ years old women presenting with restless leg syndrome. *Journal of Midlife Health, 9*(3), 135–139. https://doi.org/10.4103/jmh.JMH_25_18.
Saletu, M., Anderer, P., Saletu-Zyhlarz, G., Hauer, C., & Saletu, B. (2002). Acute placebo-controlled sleep laboratory studies and clinical follow-up with pramipexole in restless legs syndrome. *European Archives of Psychiatry and Clinical Neuroscience, 252*(4), 185–194. https://doi.org/10.1007/s00406-002-0380-7.
Saletu, M., Anderer, P., Saletu-Zyhlarz, G. M., Parapatics, S., Gruber, G., Nia, S., et al. (2010). Comparative placebo-controlled polysomnographic and psychometric studies on the acute effects of gabapentin versus ropinirole in restless legs syndrome. *Journal of Neural Transmission, 117*(4), 463–473. https://doi.org/10.1007/s00702-009-0361-3.
Saletu, M., Anderer, P., Saletu-Zyhlarz, G., Prause, W., Semler, B., Zoghlami, A., et al. (2001). Restless legs syndrome (RLS) and periodic limb movement disorder (PLMD): Acute placebo-controlled sleep laboratory studies with clonazepam. *European Neuropsychopharmacology, 11*(2), 153–161.
Saletu, B., Gruber, G., Saletu, M., Brandstatter, N., Hauer, C., Prause, W., et al. (2000). Sleep laboratory studies in restless legs syndrome patients as compared with normals and acute effects of ropinirole. 1. Findings on objective and subjective sleep and awakening quality. *Neuropsychobiology, 41*(4), 181–189. https://doi.org/10.1159/000026658.
Shimo, Y., Nakajima, A., & Hattori, N. (2015). Dopamine agonist withdrawal syndrome in a patient with restless legs syndrome without impulse control disorder or drug abuse. *Neurological Sciences, 36*(6), 1021–1023. https://doi.org/10.1007/s10072-014-1996-x.

Silber, M. H., Girish, M., & Izurieta, R. (2003). Pramipexole in the management of restless legs syndrome: An extended study. *Sleep*, *26*(7), 819–821.

Silber, M. H., & Richardson, J. W. (2003). Multiple blood donations associated with iron deficiency in patients with restless legs syndrome. *Mayo Clinic Proceedings*, *78*(1), 52–54. https://doi.org/10.4065/78.1.52.

Silver, N., Allen, R. P., Senerth, J., & Earley, C. J. (2011). A 10-year, longitudinal assessment of dopamine agonists and methadone in the treatment of restless legs syndrome. *Sleep Medicine*, *12*(5), 440–444. https://doi.org/10.1016/j.sleep.2010.11.002.

Sommer, M., Bachmann, C. G., Liebetanz, K. M., Schindehutte, J., Tings, T., & Paulus, W. (2007). Pregabalin in restless legs syndrome with and without neuropathic pain. *Acta Neurologica Scandinavica*, *115*(5), 347–350. https://doi.org/10.1111/j.1600-0404.2007.00796.x.

Stiasny-Kolster, K., Kohnen, R., Schollmayer, E., Moller, J. C., Oertel, W. H., & Rotigotine Sp 666 Study Group. (2004). Patch application of the dopamine agonist rotigotine to patients with moderate to advanced stages of restless legs syndrome: A double-blind, placebo-controlled pilot study. *Movement Disorders*, *19*(12), 1432–1438. https://doi.org/10.1002/mds.20251.

Sun, E. R., Chen, C. A., Ho, G., Earley, C. J., & Allen, R. P. (1998). Iron and the restless legs syndrome. *Sleep*, *21*(4), 371–377.

Sun, Y., van Valkenhoef, G., & Morel, T. (2014). A mixed treatment comparison of gabapentin enacarbil, pramipexole, ropinirole and rotigotine in moderate-to-severe restless legs syndrome. *Current Medical Research and Opinion*, *30*(11), 2267–2278. https://doi.org/10.1185/03007995.2014.946124.

Takahashi, M., Nishida, S., Nakamura, M., Kobayashi, M., Matsui, K., Ito, E., et al. (2017). Restless legs syndrome augmentation among Japanese patients receiving pramipexole therapy: Rate and risk factors in a retrospective study. *PLoS One*, *12*(3), e0173535. https://doi.org/10.1371/journal.pone.0173535.

Trenkwalder, C., Benes, H., Grote, L., Garcia-Borreguero, D., Hogl, B., Hopp, M., et al. (2013). Prolonged release oxycodone-naloxone for treatment of severe restless legs syndrome after failure of previous treatment: A double-blind, randomised, placebo-controlled trial with an open-label extension. *Lancet Neurology*, *12*(12), 1141–1150. https://doi.org/10.1016/S1474-4422(13)70239-4.

Trenkwalder, C., Benes, H., Poewe, W., Oertel, W. H., Garcia-Borreguero, D., de Weerd, A. W., et al. (2008). Efficacy of rotigotine for treatment of moderate-to-severe restless legs syndrome: A randomised, double-blind, placebo-controlled trial. *Lancet Neurology*, 7(7), 595–604. https://doi.org/10.1016/S1474-4422(08)70112-1.

Trenkwalder, C., Garcia-Borreguero, D., Montagna, P., Lainey, E., de Weerd, A. W., Tidswell, P., et al. (2004). Ropinirole in the treatment of restless legs syndrome: Results from the TREAT RLS 1 study, a 12 week, randomised, placebo controlled study in 10 European countries. *Journal of Neurology, Neurosurgery, and Psychiatry*, *75*(1), 92–97.

Trenkwalder, C., Stiasny-Kolster, K., Kupsch, A., Oertel, W. H., Koester, J., & Reess, J. (2006). Controlled withdrawal of pramipexole after 6 months of open-label treatment in patients with restless legs syndrome. *Movement Disorders*, *21*(9), 1404–1410. https://doi.org/10.1002/mds.20983.

Trenkwalder, C., Winkelmann, J., Oertel, W., Virgin, G., Roubert, B., Mezzacasa, A., et al. (2017). Ferric carboxymaltose in patients with restless legs syndrome and nonanemic iron deficiency: A randomized trial. *Movement Disorders*, *32*(10), 1478–1482. https://doi.org/10.1002/mds.27040.

Trotti, L. M., Bhadriraju, S., & Becker, L. A. (2012). Iron for restless legs syndrome. *Cochrane Database of Systematic Reviews*, *5*, CD007834. https://doi.org/10.1002/14651858.CD007834.pub2.

Vetrugno, R., La Morgia, C., D'Angelo, R., Loi, D., Provini, F., Plazzi, G., et al. (2007). Augmentation of restless legs syndrome with long-term tramadol treatment. *Movement Disorders*, *22*(3), 424–427. https://doi.org/10.1002/mds.21342.

von Spiczak, S., Whone, A. L., Hammers, A., Asselin, M. C., Turkheimer, F., Tings, T., et al. (2005). The role of opioids in restless legs syndrome: An [11C]diprenorphine PET study. *Brain*, *128*(Pt. 4), 906–917. https://doi.org/10.1093/brain/awh441.

Walters, A., Hening, W., Cote, L., & Fahn, S. (1986). Dominantly inherited restless legs with myoclonus and periodic movements of sleep: A syndrome related to the endogenous opiates? *Advances in Neurology*, *43*, 309–319.

Walters, A. S., Ondo, W. G., Dreykluft, T., Grunstein, R., Lee, D., Sethi, K., et al. (2004). Ropinirole is effective in the treatment of restless legs syndrome. TREAT RLS 2: A 12-week, double-blind, randomized, parallel-group, placebo-controlled study. *Movement Disorders*, *19*(12), 1414–1423. https://doi.org/10.1002/mds.20257.

Walters, A. S., Ondo, W. G., Kushida, C. A., Becker, P. M., Ellenbogen, A. L., Canafax, D. M., et al. (2009). Gabapentin enacarbil in restless legs syndrome: A phase 2b, 2-week, randomized, double-blind, placebo-controlled trial. *Clinical Neuropharmacology*, *32*(6), 311–320. https://doi.org/10.1097/WNF.0b013e3181b3ab16.

Walters, A. S., Ondo, W. G., Zhu, W., & Le, W. (2009). Does the endogenous opiate system play a role in the Restless Legs Syndrome? A pilot post-mortem study. *Journal of the Neurological Sciences*, *279*(1–2), 62–65. https://doi.org/10.1016/j.jns.2008.12.022.

Walters, A. S., Wagner, M. L., Hening, W. A., Grasing, K., Mills, R., Chokroverty, S., et al. (1993). Successful treatment of the idiopathic restless legs syndrome in a randomized double-blind trial of oxycodone versus placebo. *Sleep*, *16*(4), 327–332.

Walters, A. S., Winkelmann, J., Trenkwalder, C., Fry, J. M., Kataria, V., Wagner, M., et al. (2001). Long-term follow-up on restless legs syndrome patients treated with opioids. *Movement Disorders*, *16*(6), 1105–1109.

Wang, J., O'Reilly, B., Venkataraman, R., Mysliwiec, V., & Mysliwiec, A. (2009). Efficacy of oral iron in patients with restless legs syndrome and a low-normal ferritin: A randomized, double-blind, placebo-controlled study. *Sleep Medicine*, *10*(9), 973–975. https://doi.org/10.1016/j.sleep.2008.11.003.

Winkelman, J. W., Bogan, R. K., Schmidt, M. H., Hudson, J. D., DeRossett, S. E., & Hill-Zabala, C. E. (2011). Randomized polysomnography study of gabapentin enacarbil in subjects with restless legs syndrome. *Movement Disorders*, *26*(11), 2065–2072. https://doi.org/10.1002/mds.23771.

Winkelman, J. W., & Johnston, L. (2004). Augmentation and tolerance with long-term pramipexole treatment of restless legs syndrome (RLS). *Sleep Medicine*, *5*(1), 9–14.

Winkelman, J. W., Sethi, K. D., Kushida, C. A., Becker, P. M., Koester, J., Cappola, J. J., et al. (2006). Efficacy and safety of pramipexole in restless legs syndrome. *Neurology*, *67*(6), 1034–1039. https://doi.org/10.1212/01.wnl.0000231513.23919.a1.

Winkelmann, J., Allen, R. P., Hogl, B., Inoue, Y., Oertel, W., Salminen, A. V., et al. (2018). Treatment of restless legs syndrome: Evidence-based review and implications for clinical practice (Revised 2017) (section sign). *Movement Disorders*, *33*(7), 1077–1091. https://doi.org/10.1002/mds.27260.

Zhang, X., Chen, W. W., & Huang, W. J. (2015). Efficacy of the low-dose Saccharum iron treatment of idiopathic restless legs syndrome. *Panminerva Medica*, *57*(3), 109–113.

Zhang, J., Liu, B., Zheng, Y., Chu, T., & Yang, Z. (2015). Pramipexole for Chinese people with primary restless legs syndrome: A 12-week multicenter, randomized, double-blind study. *Sleep Medicine*, *16*(1), 181–185. https://doi.org/10.1016/j.sleep.2014.09.015.

CHAPTER ELEVEN

Treatment of pediatric restless legs syndrome

Lourdes DelRosso[a], Oliviero Bruni[b,*]
[a]University of Washington and Seattle Children's Hospital, Seattle, WA, United States
[b]Pediatric Sleep Center, Department of Developmental and Social Psychology, Sapienza University, Rome, Italy
*Corresponding author: e-mail address: oliviero.bruni@uniroma1.it

Contents

Abstract

Restless legs syndrome (RLS) is not uncommon in children with an estimated prevalence of 2%. There is clear evidence that RLS affects quality of life, sleep, cognition and behavior in children and adults. Although the diagnosis of RLS can be challenging in young children, the International Restless Legs Study Group (IRLSSG) has published guidelines for diagnosis which include description of symptoms in the child's own words. Once the diagnosis is made, treatment options must be explored. It is commonly accepted that non-pharmacological interventions be recommended to all affected families. These include maintaining a consistent bedtime routine, establishing healthy eating habits and exercise, avoiding caffeine and other substances that can exacerbate RLS, and stretching before bedtime. Pharmacological interventions in children are challenged by the lack of solid data supporting effectiveness and long-term safety. Historically and based on pathophysiology, iron supplementation is the first line therapy in children. Recently intravenous iron

Advances in Pharmacology, Volume 84
ISSN 1054-3589
https://doi.org/10.1016/bs.apha.2018.11.001
© 2019 Elsevier Inc.
All rights reserved.

supplementation has shown promising results, following studies in adults. Most studies in children on various pharmacological options follow a robust body of data previously published in adult patient with RLS, yet data in children remain scarce. This chapter will discuss both non-pharmacologic and pharmacologic treatment options for children with RLS.

Abbreviations

ADHD attention deficit hyperactivity disorder
CSF cerebrospinal fluid
FDA federal drug administration
IRLSSG international restless legs study group
NREM non-rapid eye movement sleep stage
PLMD periodic leg movement disorder
PLMI periodic leg movement index
PLMS periodic leg movements of sleep
RLS restless legs syndrome
SSRI selective serotonin reuptake inhibitor
TCA tricyclic antidepressant

1. Introduction

The prevalence of RLS in children has been estimated to be 2% (Picchietti et al., 2007). Children with RLS have various degrees of sleep disturbance, neurocognitive deficits, mood disturbances and decreased quality of life (Abetz et al., 2004). In spite of these consequences, RLS continues to be underdiagnosed in children maybe in part to the difficulty assessing symptoms in young ones. Children may have difficulty verbalizing the classic symptoms of RLS. RLS may also present in different ways in children, as RLS symptoms occur during bedtime they are most likely to interfere with sleep onset and these symptoms may be confused with bedtime resistance and limit setting-type behaviors. The presence of RLS may be unrecognized, especially in infants and preschool children that may present clinically with sleep disturbance before the onset of any RLS feelings, months or years later (Picchietti & Stevens, 2008). This is why it is extremely important to evaluate any symptoms in children related to urge to move and discomfort in the legs, and to inquire about family history of RLS: it is not uncommon to discover, while taking the history of the child, that a family member was also affected by RLS and was not aware of it. The International RLS Study Group (IRLSSG) has published guidelines for the diagnosis of RLS, which, in children, include that symptoms must be able to be described in the child's own words (Allen et al., 2014).

The pathophysiology of RLS has been linked to genetic factors, dopaminergic dysfunction and decreased iron storages. RLS has been found in association with homeobox gene MEIS1, BTBD9 and LBXCOR1 on chromosomes 2p, 6p and 15q, respectively. The presence of each variant is associated with 50% risk of RLS (Winkelmann et al., 2007). Ferritin levels were found to be lower in children with the addition of each BTBD9 allele (Picchietti & Picchietti, 2010). This is an important implication when suspecting RLS or when evaluating children of parents with RLS. Studies in adults have shown decreased iron storages in cerebrospinal fluid (CSF). Ferritin measurements in CSF from patients with RLS have shown to be decreased in proportion to the age on onset, with subjects with RLS onset at a younger age (<45 y/o) having lower ferritin levels than subjects with RLS onset at an older age (Earley, Connor, Beard, Clardy, & Allen, 2005). MRI studies on regional iron brain concentrations have confirmed low iron storages in the substantia nigra and to a lesser extent the putamen in adults with RLS (Allen, Barker, Wehrl, Song, & Earley, 2001). Autopsy studies in adults with RLS have shown decreased ferritin levels in RLS patients. Like these, studies in children have found low iron storages in pediatric RLS (Connor et al., 2003). It is postulated that low iron decreases dopamine levels. Iron is a cofactor for tyrosine hydroxylase (the rate limiting enzyme in conversion of tyrosine to dopamine) in the dopamine synthesis pathway. Because of the overwhelming evidence pointing toward iron deficiency, iron supplementation is often the first step in the treatment of RLS. Besides iron supplementation, management of pediatric RLS includes non-pharmacologic interventions and other pharmacologic options. We will start presenting non-pharmacologic recommendations and then we will present the evidence supporting various pharmacologic treatment options in children.

2. Non-pharmacological management of RLS

Treatment of RLS in children should include non-pharmacological management. Since RLS is often associated with symptoms of difficulty with sleep onset, a review of sleep hygiene and bedtime routines should always be included. Establishing healthy sleep habits is an important aspect of a comprehensive treatment plan to ensure adequate sleep duration, regular bed timings and routine adherence to principles of good sleep hygiene. Along this line, there are many activities that can alleviate symptoms of RLS. By definition and criteria of RLS, movement of legs should relieve symptoms, hence walking or stretching late in the afternoon and a few hours prior to bedtime may be helpful. In this section we will review the most common non-pharmacologic recommendations for the treatment of pediatric RLS (Table 1).

Table 1 Non-pharmacological treatment.

Treatment	
Sleep hygiene	– Allow enough opportunity to sleep – Keep consistent bedtime routines – Turn off electronics – Bedroom dark, uncluttered – Bedding clean, soft
Dietary modifications	– Avoid caffeine
Physical activity	– Aerobic training – Leg exercises
Sensory stimulation	– Massage – Heating pad – Cooling – Rubbing
Avoidance of medications	– Antihistamines – Antidepressants

2.1 Sleep hygiene

Insomnia is often the presenting symptom in children with RLS (Picchietti et al., 2007). Assessment of sleep habits, routines and available opportunities to sleep is important in the evaluation of children with both RLS and difficulty with sleep onset. Sleep hygiene in general refers to allowing enough opportunity to sleep and maintaining a consistent sleep schedule. The bedroom must be conductive to sleep allowing for a cool, dark, clean and uncluttered place with comfortable mattress and bedding. It is important to recommend children to turn off electronics at least an hour prior to bedtime. Although evidence of effectiveness of sleep hygiene alone in the management of RLS has not been assessed, it is the author's opinion that these recommendations will aid in the diagnosis of other confounders and help with overall sleep patterns.

2.2 Dietary modifications

A report on four patients with celiac disease and RLS showed improvement on RLS symptoms with gluten free diet (Manchanda, Davies, & Picchietti, 2009). There are no similar reports in children.

Caffeine. Caffeine consumption has been shown to exacerbate symptoms of RLS. Coffee, chocolates or any other substance containing caffeine should be avoided in the afternoon (Amos et al., 2014).

2.3 Physical activity

Stretching exercises prior to bedtime may provide relief enough to fall asleep. However, strenuous exercise within a few hours of bedtime should be avoided. A study in adults showed that aerobic exercise and lower body resistance training three times a week improved symptoms of RLS (Aukerman et al., 2006). There are various mechanisms by which exercise may improve RLS. One postulated mechanism involves improving circulation or by release of endorphins (Bega & Malkani, 2016). Stretching raise leg exercises have shown to decreased symptoms of RLS by 63% (Dinkins & Stevens-Lapsley, 2013).

2.4 Sensory stimulation

Some patients may report relief using rubbing, massaging, cool pads or heating pads but data in children are lacking. Although not directly studied in RLS patients, massage therapy has shown to increase dopamine in urine by 31% (Field, Hernandez-Reif, Diego, Schanberg, & Kuhn, 2005). Increase in dopamine levels may be responsible for improved symptoms of RLS after massaging the legs. Vibration therapy has been studied in adults (Mitchell, Hilton, Hunsaker, & Ulfberg, 2016) but there is no data in children.

2.5 Avoidance of medications

There are some medications known to exacerbate RLS. Selective serotonin reuptake inhibitors (SSRIs), tricyclic antidepressants (TCAs), metoclopramide, diphenhydramine, nicotine and alcohol are notorious for worsening leg movements at night. Antidepressants with dopaminergic activity (bupropion, trazodone) have not shown to affect or worsen RLS.

3. Pharmacological management of RLS

There are currently no FDA approved medications for the management of RLS in children and the data supporting various treatment options are scarce. In children medication should always be combined with non-pharmacological measures to achieve optimal results and should involve: a detailed discussion of risks versus benefits with the family (Garcia-Borreguero et al., 2013; Picchietti & Picchietti, 2010), the elimination of factors or conditions that may worsen or precipitate RLS and the evaluation of iron status. It is generally accepted to start with iron supplementation if iron storage is low. However, the decision to treat is often based on the presenting symptoms. It is the authors experience that based on the main symptoms, RLS could be perceived as a sleep disruptive disorder, a disorder or nocturnal hyper motor activity, or a condition that produces chronic discomfort even pain. The pharmacologic treatment choices should consider this symptomatology when deciding the best drug treatment to optimize patient care. In some cases, the categories could overlap, and a combination of treatment options could be needed. A common example is the use or iron and gabapentin or melatonin and a dopamine agonist (Table 2).

We have learned a lot from adult data driven decision making in treatment choices for RLS. For example, in children RLS has been associated with ADHD and PLMD, however polysomnographic studies in adults have demonstrated that dopaminergic agents are only effective on the periodic component of the sleep related leg movements. For children with sleep disruption due to PLMS, one might raise the consideration that dopaminergics may not be effective due to polysomnographic evidence that points toward lack of periodicity in leg movements in children (Ferri, Bruni, Novelli, Picchietti, & Picchietti, 2013; Ferri et al., 2008). Another example of data driven treatment selection given by the adult literature is illustrated by the fact that a single oral dose of a dopamine agonists improved NREM sleep instability in adults with RLS (Ferri et al., 2010); while clonazepam

Table 2 Pharmacological treatment.

Treatment	Dose
Ferrous sulfate	3–4 mg/kg/day
Melatonin	1–5 mg at bedtime
Gabapentin	50–100 mg at bedtime
Clonidine	50–100 μg at bedtime
Levodopa-carbidopa	25/100 mg at bedtime
Pramipexole	0.25–0.5 mg at bedtime
Ropinirole	0.5–1.5 mg at bedtime
Levetiracetam	10–20 mg/kg/day
Clonazepam	0.3–0.5 mg/day

(Manconi et al., 2012) and gabapentin (Saletu et al., 2010) were able to improve sleep architecture.

In this section we will review the data on the various pharmacologic treatment options for children with RLS.

3.1 Iron supplementation

The IRLSSG has published recent guidelines on use of iron supplementation as treatment for RLS both in children and adults. The guidelines state that there is not enough evidence to recommend iron for RLS in children (Allen et al., 2018). Iron supplementation nevertheless remains the first line therapy of RLS in children.

Iron deficiency (ID) is prevalent in human infants, especially in the late infancy/toddler period and there is mounting evidence that ID affects motor activity (Felt & Lozoff, 1996). Typically, iron stores increase slowly with supplemental iron over weeks to months, and buildup is delayed by physical growth. The level of iron stores in humans is easily measured by serum ferritin that is the best indicator of early iron deficiency, but can be a challenging marker to interpret: cut-off values differ across centers and literature sources, and as an acute-phase reactant, false elevations can occur from infection or inflammation (Panagiotou & Douros, 2004).

A few studies have shown clinical evidence of subjective improvement of symptoms in children with RLS after iron supplementation. Mohri et al. reported that iron supplementation was effective in 27 out of 30 children ages 2–14 with diagnosis of RLS (Mohri et al., 2012). Amos et al. in a retrospective study of 97 children with RLS (ages 5–18 years old) found out that about 80% of children who received iron supplementation (3–4 mg/kg/day) for RLS improved in symptoms. In this study the median ferritin level was 22.7 ng/mL and 71% of children had ferritin levels lower than 30 ng/mL and the time to improve symptoms was about 3.8 months. Children with lower ferritin levels (18.9 ng/mL) improved symptoms while children with higher ferritin levels (27.4 ng/mL) did not (Amos et al., 2014). Dye et al. reported long-term (up to 2 years) iron supplementation in 105 children (39% with RLS and 61% with PLMD). The authors reported subjective symptomatic improvement in 62.86% and objective decrease in polysomnographic PLMI after up to 2 years follow up (Dye, Jain, & Simakajornboon, 2017). Tilma et al. studied 22 children 0–40 months of age with RLS and low ferritin levels (median 21 ng/mL) with improvement in symptoms after iron supplementation. The improvement was correlated with the increase in ferritin levels (Tilma, Tilma, Norregaard, & Ostergaard, 2013).

Furudate et al. studied RLS symptoms and daytime dysfunction in 25 children with RLS and 28 controls (Furudate, Komada, Kobayashi, Nakajima, & Inoue, 2014). 61% of children with ferritin levels less than 40 ng/mL were treated with iron supplementation alone. After 2 months, if symptoms persisted a second drug was added (clonazepam or pramipexole). Children with ferritin levels more than 40 ng/mL were treated with clonazepam or pramipexole. 50% of children responded to iron alone with full remission of symptoms in some children even after iron discontinuation (Furudate et al., 2014).

Side effects must be taken into consideration when considering iron supplementation for the treatment of pediatric RLS. Small children may have difficulty swallowing pills. Liquid iron may stain the teeth. Common side effects include constipation (Picchietti, 2017). The benefit of oral iron supplementation may be tampered by decreased absorption in children with celiac disease or gastroesophageal reflux. When absorption of oral iron is a challenge, intravenous iron may be considered.

Intravenous iron supplementation has been studied in adults with various iron preparations (iron dextran, iron gluconate, iron sucrose, ferumoxytol, iron isomaltoside and ferric carboxymaltose), however there is a single study on IV iron in 16 children ages 2–16 years old. In this study iron sucrose 1.2–6.6 mg/kg was infused over 2 h. Sleep improved in 62.5% of children (Grim, Lee, Sung, & Kotagal, 2013).

Current recommendations for iron supplementation in children with RLS symptoms suggest treatment when the serum ferritin falls below 35 or even 50 ng/mL (Earley, 2003). Achieving a ferritin level of 80–100 ng/mL will allow saturation of peripheral iron stores. Clinical evidence suggests that oral supplementation may take 3 months or more to achieve adequate ferritin elevations and to have relief for symptoms (Mohri et al., 2012). Oral dosing is usually 3–6 mg/kg/day and supplements should be taken on an empty stomach with vitamin C for improved absorption.

Deficits in serum ferritin often go unrecognized, even with testing, since the lower end of the normal reference ranges typically is listed as being well below the 50 ng/mL level, i.e., below the level where RLS and PLMD symptoms may emerge.

3.2 Dopaminergics

Dopaminergic agents are divided into levodopa and non-ergot derived dopamine agonists (pramipexole, ropinirole, rotigotine). In adults, both carbidopa/levodopa and dopamine receptor agonists are approved for the management of RLS and PLMS, which are widely used, and there is extensive data on their effectiveness. There is scarce data supporting their use in children with RLS. Dopaminergic medications have proven successful in case reports and small open-label studies of children with RLS with and without ADHD but very few double-blind, placebo-controlled trials have been carried out (Konofal, Arnulf, Lecendreux, & Mouren, 2005; Kotagal & Silber, 2004; Muhle et al., 2008; Picchietti & Walters, 1999; Starn & Udall, 2008; Walters et al., 2000).

The effect of L-dopa on symptoms of ADHD and RLS in children was investigated in a 2011 small randomized, double-blind study. Twenty-nine children diagnosed with ADHD and RLS, and 29 with ADHD and no RLS, were either treated with L-dopa or a placebo and assessed pre- and post-intervention. Despite a significant impact on RLS and PLMS, there were no effects on objective neuropsychiatric measures of ADHD (England et al., 2011). Although ADHD and RLS share a significant clinical overlap, multiple therapies may be required to control symptoms in this patient population which is beyond the scope of this chapter.

A case series published by Walters et al. showed that monotherapy either with carbidopa/levodopa in five children and pergolide in two children resulted in improvement RLS, PLMS and daytime symptoms of ADHD (Walters et al., 2000). A case report on a 6 year old boy with ADHD and RLS showed significant improvement in both daytime and night time symptoms using ropinirole (Konofal et al., 2005). In another case report, an 11 year old girl with RLS and depression had symptom improvement with ropinirole but without improvement in PLMI (Cortese, Konofal, & Lecendreux, 2009). In a study using rotigotine in adolescents (13–17 y/o) showed effectiveness (Elshoff et al., 2017). In some cases dopaminergics are used in combination with iron supplementation (Dye et al., 2017).

There are some major limitations to the use of dopaminergic medications in adults: augmentation, withdrawal symptoms and side effects. Common side effects of dopaminergics reported in adults include nausea, sleepiness, insomnia, obsessive compulsive behavior, hallucinations and augmentation. There are limited data on side effects in children and no data on augmentation in children.

3.3 Anticonvulsants

Studies using anticonvulsants for treatment of RLS in children are scarce. Although there are rare studies using carbamazepine (Zucconi et al., 1989) and valproic acid (Eisensehr, Ehrenberg, Rogge Solti, & Noachtar, 2004), there is no evidence of their use in children. Therefore, in this section we will discuss the evidence found for the use of alpha-2-delta ligands and levetiracetam in pediatric RLS.

3.3.1 Alpha-2-delta ligand

Gabapentin is an alpha-2-delta-1 ligand used to treat epilepsy and neuropathies. Its use in children for these diagnosis over long-term periods has proven to be safe with minimal side effects which makes it an attractive treatment option for RLS. The most common adverse reactions reported include sleepiness and dizziness. Polysomnography studies in adults taking gabapentin have demonstrated that it affects sleep structure enhancing slow-wave sleep and reducing sleep-onset latency (Foldvary-Schaefer et al., 2002).

Gabapentin enacarbil has FDA approval for moderate to severe symptoms of RSL in adults but not in children. There are isolated cases of children with RLS treated with gabapentin. Amos et al. studied iron and other treatments in children with RLS. In this cohort, two children were treated with gabapentin alone and showed resolution of symptoms (Amos et al., 2014).

A case report of an effective treatment of gabapentin in a 14-month-old girl affected by psychomotor retardation and severe chronic insomnia with extreme difficulty in falling asleep and multiple nocturnal awakenings with inconsolable crying. Falling asleep was characterized by episodes of kicking, hitting, and jerking of the legs, accompanied by screaming and crying, suggesting discomfort or pain, lasting for about 2–4 h and followed by several night awakenings with the reappearance of legs kicking and cycling movements. The clinical presentation and the worsening at bedtime or when falling asleep suggested a diagnosis of RLS. According to the benefit/risk assessment made together with the parents, gabapentin 50 mg was prescribed at bedtime which induced an immediate improvement of the leg movements and of sleep continuity. After a few days, the symptoms relapsed and gabapentin was increased to 100 and then 200 mg, with a complete disappearance of symptoms (Bruni, Angriman, Luchetti, & Ferri, 2015).

3.3.2 Levetiracetam

Levetiracetam is an antiepileptic medication with various mechanisms of action that inhibit neuronal hyper-synchronization. It also activates gamma-aminobutyric acid (GABA) which may be responsible for the somnolence and fatigue associated with the drug (Verrotti et al., 2015). Although usually well tolerated and with minimal side effect, one of the most common side effects is mood changes and depression, anxiety and sometimes psychosis (White et al., 2003). A single study in which seven boys between 5 and 12 years of age with attention deficit hyperactivity disorder and RLS were given levetiracetam 10–20 mg/kg/day followed by increments of 10 mg/kg/day up to 50–60 mg/kg/day given in two doses showed improvement in symptoms and daytime behaviors. The children were followed at 3 and 6 months and reported improvement in the International RLS Rating Scale (IRLS-RS). The parents also reported improved sleep with less nocturnal awakenings. There were no side effects reported (Gagliano et al., 2011).

3.4 Benzodiazepines

3.4.1 Clonazepam

Clonazepam is a long acting benzodiazepine sometimes used to treat frequent, disturbing parasomnias in children. The long half-life can be attractive for children who naturally sleep longer. There are limited data on it use for RLS in children. Polysomnography studies have shown that clonazepam tends to improve sleep and reduce arousals in RLS patients, but it was not effective in reducing the motor and sensory abnormalities associated with RLS (Manconi et al., 2012; Saletu et al., 2010). A study on 51 children who received treatment for PLMD but not RLS showed that 6 were treated with clonazepam as first line treatment and 5 were treated with a combination of dopamine agonist and clonazepam (Gingras, Gaultney, & Picchietti, 2011). The most common side effect to clonazepam was paradoxical alerting reaction (13%). Although the medication was used clinically assessment of polysomnographic evidence of effectiveness is lacking.

3.5 Other treatments

3.5.1 Clonidine

Clonidine is an alpha-2-adrenergic agonist commonly used for insomnia particularly in children with neurodevelopmental disorders especially if associated with hyperactivity. This effect is thought to be mediated by its antiadrenergic effect that decrease the overactivity of the sympathetic nervous system. Clonidine is widely used as pediatric sleep aid drug (not FDA approved) because it is well tolerated by children, soporific, and rapidly effective. In some instances alpha-2-adrenergics have been given in combination with iron supplementation (Dye et al., 2017). In one randomized, double-blind, placebo-controlled trial clonidine has been effective for RLS sensory symptoms in adults without side effects (Prince, Wilens, Biederman, Spencer, & Wozniak, 1996).

3.5.2 Opioids

They are often reserved for refractory RLS in adults. Opioids treat RLS via their action on dopaminergic receptors. There are no data on opioids in children.

3.5.3 Magnesium

Early evidence showed some positive effect of magnesium on RLS and PLMS in adults (Hornyak, Voderholzer, Hohagen, Berger, & Riemann, 1998) and pregnant women (Bartell & Zallek, 2006). There are no data in children.

3.5.4 Vitamin D

Recently published data have proposed an association between vitamin D deficiency and severity of RLS symptoms (Oran et al., 2014). The authors hypothesized that low vitamin D levels may lead to dopaminergic dysfunction. Vitamin D protects dopaminergic neurons against toxicity and can increase the levels to vitamin D or it's metabolites. A study in 12 adults with RLS and vitamin D supplementation showed improvement in RLS symptoms. Studies in children are lacking (Wali, Shukr, Boudal, Alsaiari, & Krayem, 2015).

3.5.5 Melatonin

Symptoms of RLS are worse at night demonstrating a circadian preference. Both the peak of RLS symptoms and melatonin production occur at similar times in the evening. Studies have shown intricate interactions between melatonin and dopamine with evidence that increase in melatonin production blocks dopamine in various brain areas including the striatum (Zisapel, 2001). Whittom et al. studied exogenous melatonin and bright light in eight adults and showed that melatonin increased motor activity while bright light attenuates symptoms (Whittom et al., 2010). Paradoxically, exogenous melatonin has shown to decrease PLMS (Kunz & Bes, 2001). Melatonin is often prescribed to children with delayed circadian disorder or insomnia. Since insomnia is a common presentation of RLS, sleep physicians may be tempted to prescribe melatonin for RLS. There is no current evidence to support the use of melatonin in children with RLS or PLMS.

4. Conclusion

The first step in the management of pediatric RLS must include non-pharmacological approaches. Lifestyle modifications include: diet and exercise, avoidance of drugs that worsen or provoke the sensory-motor symptoms of RLS and adoption of relieving strategies (Table 1). Iron storage status evaluation is recommended in children and iron supplementation is still considered the first line treatment option. In children who are not responding to oral iron, intravenous iron can be an option. If iron deficiency is not present or there are significant co-morbidities (Angriman, Cortese, & Bruni, 2017) other treatment options can be considered. We have discussed the evidence for the various treatment options studied in the literature including use of dopaminergics, benzodiazepine and anticonvulsant among other less commonly used options. Due to lack of robust data it is prudent to begin with the lowest possible dose and slowly titrate with close monitoring for assessment of effectiveness and evaluation of possible adverse effects. Finally, the natural course of pediatric RLS is not completely understood but there is some suggestion that symptoms may improve over time. It is the authors opinion that a treatment course of 6 months could be followed by a period of observation. Regardless of choice of treatment or observation, children with RLS should be followed periodically for assessment of symptom presence and severity.

Conflict of interest statement

The authors do not have any conflict of interest to declare.

References

Abetz, L., Allen, R., Follet, A., Washburn, T., Earley, C., Kirsch, J., et al. (2004). Evaluating the quality of life of patients with restless legs syndrome. *Clinical Therapeutics*, *26*(6), 925–935.

Allen, R. P., Barker, P. B., Wehrl, F. W., Song, H. K., & Earley, C. J. (2001). MRI measurement of brain iron in patients with restless legs syndrome. *Neurology*, *56*(2), 263–265.

Allen, R. P., Picchietti, D. L., Auerbach, M., Cho, Y. W., Connor, J. R., Earley, C. J., et al. (2018). Evidence-based and consensus clinical practice guidelines for the iron treatment of restless legs syndrome/Willis-Ekbom disease in adults and children: An IRLSSG task force report. *Sleep Medicine*, *41*, 27–44. https://doi.org/10.1016/j.sleep.2017.11.1126.

Allen, R. P., Picchietti, D. L., Garcia-Borreguero, D., Ondo, W. G., Walters, A. S., Winkelman, J. W., et al. (2014). Restless legs syndrome/Willis-Ekbom disease diagnostic criteria: Updated international restless legs syndrome study group (IRLSSG) consensus criteria—History, rationale, description, and significance. *Sleep Medicine*, *15*(8), 860–873. https://doi.org/10.1016/j.sleep.2014.03.025.

Amos, L. B., Grekowicz, M. L., Kuhn, E. M., Olstad, J. D., Collins, M. M., Norins, N. A., et al. (2014). Treatment of pediatric restless legs syndrome. *Clinical Pediatrics (Phila)*, *53*(4), 331–336. https://doi.org/10.1177/0009922813507997.

Angriman, M., Cortese, S., & Bruni, O. (2017). Somatic and neuropsychiatric comorbidities in pediatric restless legs syndrome: A systematic review of the literature. *Sleep Medicine Reviews*, *34*, 34–45. https://doi.org/10.1016/j.smrv.2016.06.008.

Aukerman, M. M., Aukerman, D., Bayard, M., Tudiver, F., Thorp, L., & Bailey, B. (2006). Exercise and restless legs syndrome: A randomized controlled trial. *Journal of American Board of Family Medicine*, *19*(5), 487–493.

Bartell, S., & Zallek, S. (2006). Intravenous magnesium sulfate may relieve restless legs syndrome in pregnancy. *Journal of Clinical Sleep Medicine*, *2*(2), 187–188.

Bega, D., & Malkani, R. (2016). Alternative treatment of restless legs syndrome: An overview of the evidence for mind-body interventions, lifestyle interventions, and neutraceuticals. *Sleep Medicine*, *17*, 99–105. https://doi.org/10.1016/j.sleep.2015.09.009.

Bruni, O., Angriman, M., Luchetti, A., & Ferri, R. (2015). Leg kicking and rubbing as a highly suggestive sign of pediatric restless legs syndrome. *Sleep Medicine*, *16*(12), 1576–1577. https://doi.org/10.1016/j.sleep.2015.07.016.

Connor, J. R., Boyer, P. J., Menzies, S. L., Dellinger, B., Allen, R. P., Ondo, W. G., et al. (2003). Neuropathological examination suggests impaired brain iron acquisition in restless legs syndrome. *Neurology*, *61*(3), 304–309.

Cortese, S., Konofal, E., & Lecendreux, M. (2009). Effectiveness of ropinirole for RLS and depressive symptoms in an 11-year-old girl. *Sleep Medicine*, *10*(2), 259–261. https://doi.org/10.1016/j.sleep.2007.10.023.

Dinkins, E. M., & Stevens-Lapsley, J. (2013). Management of symptoms of restless legs syndrome with use of a traction straight leg raise: A preliminary case series. *Manual Therapy*, *18*(4), 299–302. https://doi.org/10.1016/j.math.2012.11.002.

Dye, T. J., Jain, S. V., & Simakajornboon, N. (2017). Outcomes of long-term iron supplementation in pediatric restless legs syndrome/periodic limb movement disorder (RLS/PLMD). *Sleep Medicine*, *32*, 213–219. https://doi.org/10.1016/j.sleep.2016.01.008.

Earley, C. J. (2003). Clinical practice. Restless legs syndrome. *The New England Journal of Medicine*, *348*(21), 2103–2109. https://doi.org/10.1056/NEJMcp021288.

Earley, C. J., Connor, J. R., Beard, J. L., Clardy, S. L., & Allen, R. P. (2005). Ferritin levels in the cerebrospinal fluid and restless legs syndrome: Effects of different clinical phenotypes. *Sleep*, *28*(9), 1069–1075.

Eisensehr, I., Ehrenberg, B. L., Rogge Solti, S., & Noachtar, S. (2004). Treatment of idiopathic restless legs syndrome (RLS) with slow-release valproic acid compared with slow-release levodopa/benserazid. *Journal of Neurology*, *251*(5), 579–583. https://doi.org/10.1007/s00415-004-0367-6.

Elshoff, J. P., Hudson, J., Picchietti, D. L., Ridel, K., Walters, A. S., Doggett, K., et al. (2017). Pharmacokinetics of rotigotine transdermal system in adolescents with idiopathic restless legs syndrome (Willis-Ekbom disease). *Sleep Medicine*, *32*, 48–55. https://doi.org/10.1016/j.sleep.2016.04.012.

England, S. J., Picchietti, D. L., Couvadelli, B. V., Fisher, B. C., Siddiqui, F., Wagner, M. L., et al. (2011). L-Dopa improves restless legs syndrome and periodic limb movements in sleep but not attention-deficit-hyperactivity disorder in a double-blind trial in children. *Sleep Medicine*, *12*(5), 471–477. https://doi.org/10.1016/j.sleep.2011.01.008.

Felt, B. T., & Lozoff, B. (1996). Brain iron and behavior of rats are not normalized by treatment of iron deficiency anemia during early development. *The Journal of Nutrition*, *126*(3), 693–701. https://doi.org/10.1093/jn/126.3.693.

Ferri, R., Bruni, O., Novelli, L., Picchietti, M. A., & Picchietti, D. L. (2013). Time structure of leg movement activity during sleep in attention-deficit/hyperactivity disorder and effects of levodopa. *Sleep Medicine*, *14*(4), 359–366. https://doi.org/10.1016/j.sleep.2012.12.012.

Ferri, R., Manconi, M., Arico, D., Sagrada, C., Zucconi, M., Bruni, O., et al. (2010). Acute dopamine-agonist treatment in restless legs syndrome: Effects on sleep architecture and NREM sleep instability. *Sleep*, *33*(6), 793–800.

Ferri, R., Manconi, M., Lanuzza, B., Cosentino, F. I., Bruni, O., Ferini-Strambi, L., et al. (2008). Age-related changes in periodic leg movements during sleep in patients with restless legs syndrome. *Sleep Medicine*, *9*(7), 790–798. https://doi.org/10.1016/j.sleep.2007.08.020.

Field, T., Hernandez-Reif, M., Diego, M., Schanberg, S., & Kuhn, C. (2005). Cortisol decreases and serotonin and dopamine increase following massage therapy. *The International Journal of Neuroscience*, *115*(10), 1397–1413. https://doi.org/10.1080/00207450590956459.

Foldvary-Schaefer, N., De Leon Sanchez, I., Karafa, M., Mascha, E., Dinner, D., & Morris, H. H. (2002). Gabapentin increases slow-wave sleep in normal adults. *Epilepsia*, *43*(12), 1493–1497.

Furudate, N., Komada, Y., Kobayashi, M., Nakajima, S., & Inoue, Y. (2014). Daytime dysfunction in children with restless legs syndrome. *Journal of the Neurological Sciences*, *336*(1–2), 232–236. https://doi.org/10.1016/j.jns.2013.11.001.

Gagliano, A., Arico, I., Calarese, T., Condurso, R., Germano, E., Cedro, C., et al. (2011). Restless leg syndrome in ADHD children: Levetiracetam as a reasonable therapeutic option. *Brain and Development*, *33*(6), 480–486. https://doi.org/10.1016/j.braindev.2010.09.008.

Garcia-Borreguero, D., Kohnen, R., Silber, M. H., Winkelman, J. W., Earley, C. J., Hogl, B., et al. (2013). The long-term treatment of restless legs syndrome/Willis-Ekbom disease: Evidence-based guidelines and clinical consensus best practice guidance: A report from the international restless legs syndrome study group. *Sleep Medicine*, *14*(7), 675–684. https://doi.org/10.1016/j.sleep.2013.05.016.

Gingras, J. L., Gaultney, J. F., & Picchietti, D. L. (2011). Pediatric periodic limb movement disorder: Sleep symptom and polysomnographic correlates compared to obstructive sleep apnea. *Journal of Clinical Sleep Medicine*, 7(6), 603–609A. https://doi.org/10.5664/jcsm.1460.

Grim, K., Lee, B., Sung, A. Y., & Kotagal, S. (2013). Treatment of childhood-onset restless legs syndrome and periodic limb movement disorder using intravenous iron sucrose. *Sleep Medicine*, *14*(11), 1100–1104. https://doi.org/10.1016/j.sleep.2013.06.006.

Hornyak, M., Voderholzer, U., Hohagen, F., Berger, M., & Riemann, D. (1998). Magnesium therapy for periodic leg movements-related insomnia and restless legs syndrome: An open pilot study. *Sleep*, *21*(5), 501–505.

Konofal, E., Arnulf, I., Lecendreux, M., & Mouren, M. C. (2005). Ropinirole in a child with attention-deficit hyperactivity disorder and restless legs syndrome. *Pediatric Neurology*, *32*(5), 350–351. https://doi.org/10.1016/j.pediatrneurol.2004.11.007.

Kotagal, S., & Silber, M. H. (2004). Childhood-onset restless legs syndrome. *Annals of Neurology*, *56*(6), 803–807. https://doi.org/10.1002/ana.20292.

Kunz, D., & Bes, F. (2001). Exogenous melatonin in periodic limb movement disorder: An open clinical trial and a hypothesis. *Sleep*, *24*(2), 183–187.

Manchanda, S., Davies, C. R., & Picchietti, D. (2009). Celiac disease as a possible cause for low serum ferritin in patients with restless legs syndrome. *Sleep Medicine*, *10*(7), 763–765. https://doi.org/10.1016/j.sleep.2008.07.014.

Manconi, M., Ferri, R., Zucconi, M., Bassetti, C. L., Fulda, S., Arico, D., et al. (2012). Dissociation of periodic leg movements from arousals in restless legs syndrome. *Annals of Neurology*, *71*(6), 834–844. https://doi.org/10.1002/ana.23565.

Mitchell, U. H., Hilton, S. C., Hunsaker, E., & Ulfberg, J. (2016). Decreased symptoms without augmented skin blood flow in subjects with RLS/WED after vibration treatment. *Journal of Clinical Sleep Medicine*, *12*(7), 947–952. https://doi.org/10.5664/jcsm.5920.

Mohri, I., Kato-Nishimura, K., Kagitani-Shimono, K., Kimura-Ohba, S., Ozono, K., Tachibana, N., et al. (2012). Evaluation of oral iron treatment in pediatric restless legs syndrome (RLS). *Sleep Medicine*, *13*(4), 429–432. https://doi.org/10.1016/j.sleep.2011.12.009.

Muhle, H., Neumann, A., Lohmann-Hedrich, K., Lohnau, T., Lu, Y., Winkler, S., et al. (2008). Childhood-onset restless legs syndrome: Clinical and genetic features of 22 families. *Movement Disorders*, *23*(8), 1113–1121. quiz 1203. https://doi.org/10.1002/mds.22016.

Oran, M., Unsal, C., Albayrak, Y., Tulubas, F., Oguz, K., Avci, O., et al. (2014). Possible association between vitamin D deficiency and restless legs syndrome. *Neuropsychiatric Disease and Treatment*, *10*, 953–958. https://doi.org/10.2147/NDT.S63599.

Panagiotou, J. P., & Douros, K. (2004). Clinicolaboratory findings and treatment of iron-deficiency anemia in childhood. *Pediatric Hematology and Oncology*, *21*(6), 521–534.

Picchietti, D. L. (2017). Should oral iron be first-line therapy for pediatric restless legs syndrome and periodic limb movement disorder? *Sleep Medicine*, *32*, 220–221. https://doi.org/10.1016/j.sleep.2016.05.005.

Picchietti, D., Allen, R. P., Walters, A. S., Davidson, J. E., Myers, A., & Ferini-Strambi, L. (2007). Restless legs syndrome: Prevalence and impact in children and adolescents—The Peds REST study. *Pediatrics*, *120*(2), 253–266. https://doi.org/10.1542/peds.2006-2767.

Picchietti, M. A., & Picchietti, D. L. (2010). Advances in pediatric restless legs syndrome: Iron, genetics, diagnosis and treatment. *Sleep Medicine*, *11*(7), 643–651. https://doi.org/10.1016/j.sleep.2009.11.014.

Picchietti, D. L., & Stevens, H. E. (2008). Early manifestations of restless legs syndrome in childhood and adolescence. *Sleep Medicine*, *9*(7), 770–781. https://doi.org/10.1016/j.sleep.2007.08.012.

Picchietti, D. L., & Walters, A. S. (1999). Moderate to severe periodic limb movement disorder in childhood and adolescence. *Sleep*, *22*(3), 297–300.

Prince, J. B., Wilens, T. E., Biederman, J., Spencer, T. J., & Wozniak, J. R. (1996). Clonidine for sleep disturbances associated with attention-deficit hyperactivity disorder: A systematic chart review of 62 cases. *Journal of the American Academy of Child and Adolescent Psychiatry*, *35*(5), 599–605. https://doi.org/10.1097/00004583-199605000-00014.

Saletu, M., Anderer, P., Saletu-Zyhlarz, G. M., Parapatics, S., Gruber, G., Nia, S., et al. (2010). Comparative placebo-controlled polysomnographic and psychometric studies on the acute effects of gabapentin versus ropinirole in restless legs syndrome. *Journal of Neural Transmission (Vienna)*, *117*(4), 463–473. https://doi.org/10.1007/s00702-009-0361-3.

Starn, A. L., & Udall, J. N., Jr. (2008). Iron deficiency anemia, pica, and restless legs syndrome in a teenage girl. *Clinical Pediatrics (Phila)*, *47*(1), 83–85. https://doi.org/10.1177/0009922807303930.

Tilma, J., Tilma, K., Norregaard, O., & Ostergaard, J. R. (2013). Early childhood-onset restless legs syndrome: Symptoms and effect of oral iron treatment. *Acta Paediatrica, 102*(5), e221–e226. https://doi.org/10.1111/apa.12173.

Verrotti, A., Prezioso, G., Di Sabatino, F., Franco, V., Chiarelli, F., & Zaccara, G. (2015). The adverse event profile of levetiracetam: A meta-analysis on children and adults. *Seizure, 31*, 49–55. https://doi.org/10.1016/j.seizure.2015.07.004.

Wali, S., Shukr, A., Boudal, A., Alsaiari, A., & Krayem, A. (2015). The effect of vitamin D supplements on the severity of restless legs syndrome. *Sleep & Breathing, 19*(2), 579–583. https://doi.org/10.1007/s11325-014-1049-y.

Walters, A. S., Mandelbaum, D. E., Lewin, D. S., Kugler, S., England, S. J., & Miller, M. (2000). Dopaminergic therapy in children with restless legs/periodic limb movements in sleep and ADHD. Dopaminergic therapy study group. *Pediatric Neurology, 22*(3), 182–186.

White, J. R., Walczak, T. S., Leppik, I. E., Rarick, J., Tran, T., Beniak, T. E., et al. (2003). Discontinuation of levetiracetam because of behavioral side effects: A case-control study. *Neurology, 61*(9), 1218–1221.

Whittom, S., Dumont, M., Petit, D., Desautels, A., Adam, B., Lavigne, G., et al. (2010). Effects of melatonin and bright light administration on motor and sensory symptoms of RLS. *Sleep Medicine, 11*(4), 351–355. https://doi.org/10.1016/j.sleep.2009.12.008.

Winkelmann, J., Schormair, B., Lichtner, P., Ripke, S., Xiong, L., Jalilzadeh, S., et al. (2007). Genome-wide association study of restless legs syndrome identifies common variants in three genomic regions. *Nature Genetics, 39*(8), 1000–1006. https://doi.org/10.1038/ng2099.

Zisapel, N. (2001). Melatonin-dopamine interactions: From basic neurochemistry to a clinical setting. *Cellular and Molecular Neurobiology, 21*(6), 605–616.

Zucconi, M., Coccagna, G., Petronelli, R., Gerardi, R., Mondini, S., & Cirignotta, F. (1989). Nocturnal myoclonus in restless legs syndrome effect of carbamazepine treatment. *Functional Neurology, 4*(3), 263–271.

CHAPTER TWELVE

Pharmacological treatments of augmentation in restless legs syndrome patients

Claudia Trenkwalder[a,b,*], Walter Paulus[c]
[a]Department of Neurosurgery, University Medical Center, Göttingen, Germany
[b]Paracelsus-Elena Hospital, Center of Parkinsonism and Movement Disorders, Kassel, Germany
[c]Department of Clinical Neurophysiology, University Medical Center Göttingen, Georg August University, Göttingen, Germany
*Corresponding author: e-mail address: claudia.trenkwalder@med.uni-goettingen.de

Contents

Abstract

Augmentation, a treatment-induced paradoxical worsening of the symptoms of restless legs syndrome (RLS) that is caused by long-term dopaminergic therapy, in particular with higher doses, remains the major challenge of RLS treatment. The mainstay of treatment continues to be preventing augmentation, either by starting RLS therapy with alternative drugs or by sensitizing physicians about the absolute necessity of respecting approved dosages of dopaminergic drugs when treating RLS and never exceeding the maximum recommended dosages. In the case of a positive diagnosis of augmentation, treatment consists of reducing or eliminating dopaminergic therapy, ensuring that serum ferritin is clearly higher than the level assumed to be necessary from a hematological point of view and/or switching treatment to alternative drugs such as $\alpha 2\delta$ ligands, opiates, or to combination therapy.

Advances in Pharmacology, Volume 84
ISSN 1054-3589
https://doi.org/10.1016/bs.apha.2019.02.002
© 2019 Elsevier Inc.
All rights reserved.

1. Introduction

Augmentation can be defined as a worsening of restless legs syndrome (RLS) caused by long-term dopaminergic medication (Allen & Earley, 1996). The term augmentation is somewhat misleading. In analogy to medication-overuse headache or opiate-induced hyperalgesia, a denomination like "medication-induced RLS" might describe the problem better. This is, however, the personal opinion of the authors and not agreed upon in the scientific community. A consensus conference identified the following five major diagnostic features of augmentation (Garcia-Borreguero et al., 2007): a shift in the usual time of RLS symptom onset each day, an increase in the number of body parts with RLS symptoms, shorter latency to symptoms at rest, increased severity of symptoms when they occur, and a worsening (paradoxical) effect of dopaminergic medication on symptoms. The quantitative data available concerning the time of RLS onset and the presence of other features indicated an optimal augmentation criterion of either a 4-h advance in the usual starting time of RLS symptoms or a combination of the occurrence of other features.

Two aspects of medication dispose patients to developing augmentation. First, the half-life of the dopaminergic drug, and second, the receptor profile it targets. From clinical observation it seems that the shorter the half-life and the more the pronociceptive receptors D1 and D5 are targeted, as opposed to the antinociceptive receptors D2, D3, and D4, the higher the risk for augmentation (Paulus & Trenkwalder, 2006). Recently, however, attention has focused on D3 and D1 heterometric ensembles (Clemens & Ghorayeb, 2019) explaining why long-term treatment with D3 receptor agonists may also induce augmentation.

Levodopa, which has the shortest half-life and is the only available drug at present targeting D1 and D5 receptors, has the highest risk of all dopaminergic drugs. Present guidelines (Garcia-Borreguero et al., 2016) state "levodopa may be used for intermittent treatment at most two to three times a week, but should not be used for daily treatment, given the high risk of augmentation with this medication." In the personal opinion of the authors the use of levodopa should, at best, be restricted to an initial "levodopa test" checking for responsiveness of RLS symptoms. Also, the dopamine agonist rotigotine targets D1/D5 receptors to a similar extent as dopamine (Wood, Dubois, Scheller, & Gillard, 2015) (cf. Table 1).

The half maximal effective concentration (EC_{50}) is commonly used as a measure of a drug's potency. It refers to the concentration of a drug that induces a response halfway between the baseline and maximum after a

Table 1 Functional profile of dopaminergic agonists at human recombinant dopamine receptor subtypes.

Compound	D1 pEC_{50}	D2 pEC_{50}	D3 pEC_{50}	D4 pEC_{50}	D5 pEC_{50}
Rotigotine	9.6 ± 0.1	10.4 ± 0.1	8.2 ± 0.2	7.7 ± 0.1	7.7 ± 0.2
Pramipexole	<5	9.1 ± 0.2	8.3 ± 0.1	7.4 ± 0.1	<5
Ropinirole	<5	8.5 ± 0.1	8.1 ± 0.1	6.3 ± 0.1	<5
Dopamine	9.0 ± 0.4	8.6 ± 0.3	8.3 ± 0.1	7.5 ± 0.1	8.2 ± 0.3

The pEC_{50} values reflect the functional potency indicative of the half maximal effective concentration between baseline and maximum response.
Taken from Wood, M., Dubois, V., Scheller, D., & Gillard, M. (2015). Rotigotine is a potent agonist at dopamine D1 receptors as well as at dopamine D2 and D3 receptors. *British Journal of Pharmacology, 172*(4), 1124–1135. doi:10.1111/bph.12988.

specified exposure time. The pEC_{50} is defined as the negative logarithm of the EC_{50}. Table 1 lists pEC_{50} values for common dopamine agonists in comparison to dopamine. What can be seen in this table is that rotigotine has a similar potency to bind to D1 receptors as dopamine, and thus should have a higher likelihood of inducing augmentation. However, by its transcutaneous route of application rotigotine provides stable plasma levels and thereby the lowest rate of augmentation for dopaminergic drugs (see below) (Trenkwalder, Benes, et al., 2008; Trenkwalder et al., 2017), although no head-to-head comparisons are available to demonstrate this.

2. Prophylaxis and awareness for the development of augmentation

The best treatment of augmentation is its prophylaxis. This can be accomplished in several ways. Since the risk of augmentation is almost exclusively due to dopaminergic treatment, avoiding dopaminergic agents is one solution. Unfortunately, the alternatives to dopaminergic agents such as $\alpha 2\delta$ ligands and opioids are often less well tolerated at the efficient dosages. The second possibility that is very likely to avoid augmentation is paying close attention to the dosage: sticking to a low dose of any dopaminergic drug is key. Physicians, mainly neurologists who are not familiar with this problem and are otherwise used to treating Parkinson's disease patients, tend to increase the dose of dopaminergic drugs, in particular when RLS patients complain about a loss of efficacy or incomplete suppression of symptoms. The pathophysiological background of both diseases is based on the availability of dopaminergic neurons. However, unlike Parkinson's disease patients, RLS patients do not suffer from a loss of dopaminergic neurons, and therefore can easily generate a sufficient amount of dopamine from substantia nigra dopaminergic neurons. In late Parkinson's disease, when substantia nigra neurons have almost completely stopped their dopamine production, externally added levodopa has to be converted to dopamine by serotonergic or some glial cells (cf. Clemens & Ghorayeb, 2019). In these severely affected Parkinson's patients this process requires a dose approximately 10-fold higher than that required in RLS patients. In practical terms the dose of, for example, the dopamine agonist pramipexole should not increase beyond 0.35 mg (0.5 mg) compared to a maximal dose in Parkinson's patients of 3.15 mg (4.5 mg) (Table 2).

Long-term data on augmentation are scarce, with the exception of rotigotine for which data from a five-year study provide the augmentation

Table 2 Comparison of maximum dosages of dopaminergic drugs in RLS and Parkinson's disease.

	Maximum dosage for dopaminergic drugs approved for treating RLS	**Maximum dosage dopaminergic drugs approved for treating Parkinson's disease**	**Half-life (h)**
Pramipexole Pramipexole-salt (US, MIRAPEX) Pramipexol dihydrochloride monohydrate = base (Sifrol, Europe)	Europe: 0.54 mg (Base) 0·75 mg (salt) in the USA; (no benefit in clinical trials of 0.75 mg over 0.5 mg) recommended 0.5 mg maximum (0·5 and 0·75 mg). Three doses of European formulation reported effective: 0·088, 0·18, and 0·35 mg. Maximum dose 0·54 mg (mean 0·35 mg) in Europe	Europe: 3.3 mg (3 × 1.1 mg) (base) 4.5 mg (salt) US, FDA approved with 3 × 1.5 mg	8–12
Rotigotine	3 mg	16 mg	5–7 after patch removal
Ropinirole	4 mg	24 mg	6
Levodopa	300 mg (Levodopa/ benserazide)		2
	Maximally allowed dosages for opiates in RLS	**Maximally allowed dosages for opiates in pain treatment**	
Oxycodone-naloxone	40/20 mg	100/50 mg	3.2

rate: those who were able to tolerate rotigotine and who did not suffer from skin reactions over time, had, over 5 years, an augmentation rate of 13%, which consisted of 5% of patients receiving a rotigotine dose within the range approved by the European Medicines Agency (EMA; 1–3 mg/24 h) while the other 8% received 4 mg/24 h (Oertel et al., 2011). An even lower rate of 5–6% of augmentation with dopamine agonist therapy was estimated in a meta-analysis (Liu et al., 2016) that depended on available studies (no data for ropinirole), which is the major criticism here. Direct comparative studies are not available. The augmentation rate of rotigotine seems quite low compared to augmentation rates with pramipexole (Hogl et al., 2011), even after 6 months, or in the 1 year comparative study of pregabalin and pramipexole (Allen et al., 2014).

A less pulsatile application of a dopaminergic therapy, therefore, seems to best fit the needs of RLS patients, although no comparative studies are available to confirm this hypothesis. Alternatively, and intensively discussed as an initial strategy, the α2δ ligands gabapentin enacarbil, gabapentin, or pregabalin should be mentioned (Allen, 2014; Garcia-Borreguero et al., 2016; Trenkwalder et al., 2018). The decision to start with an α2δ ligand may be supported by painful comorbidities, in particular painful small fiber polyneuropathy (Trenkwalder, Allen, Hogl, Paulus, & Winkelmann, 2016). Also, since iron deficiency predisposes to augmentation (Trenkwalder, Hogl, Benes, & Kohnen, 2008), iron status should be checked by measuring serum ferritin and transferrin saturation (TSAT) and supplemented at each stage of RLS (see below for recommended levels), in particular during augmentation (Garcia-Borreguero et al., 2016) or when other treatment problems occur when iron storage levels are low (Trenkwalder et al., 2018). The targeted ferritin levels should be clearly higher than those targeted in hematological disorders, and transferrin saturation should be above 20%. In an iron deficient rat and D3 knockout model some preponderance of female liability to develop hyperactivity was seen, although this is at best an indirect model of augmentation (Klinker, Kohnemann, Paulus, & Liebetanz, 2017). Also, dopamine D(3) receptor deficiency sensitizes mice to iron deficiency-related deficits in motor learning (Klinker, Hasan, Dowling, Paulus, & Liebetanz, 2011).

Another important issue is the awareness of the risk of developing augmentation at any time during RLS treatment. Even for experts it is particularly challenging to separate a "natural" increase of severity in RLS from the beginning of augmentation, even in clinical trials (Hogl et al., 2011). One of the most robust criteria is the temporal shift of the occurrence of symptoms from the evening to at least 4-h earlier during the daytime

(Garcia-Borreguero et al., 2007; Trenkwalder et al., 2018). Since the therapeutic strategy is just the opposite, i.e., increasing the dose versus dose reduction, one of the clinically practical approaches may be to just lower the dose and check if symptoms become (paradoxically) better. There are no data that indicate for how many days or weeks it is necessary to lower the dosage. Fast or abrupt reduction of dopaminergic dosages, especially of dopamine agonists, may lead to a withdrawal syndrome with severe psychiatric and possible heart and blood pressure symptoms (Garcia-Borreguero et al., 2016). There is no consensus on how the reduction of dopaminergic agents should be achieved. Earley and colleagues opt for a sudden withdrawal of medication (personal communication with Dr. C. Earley), whereas others tend to slowly withdraw the medication.

3. Treatment of augmentation

Once the diagnosis of augmentation has been established per definition, any dopaminergic medication needs to be reduced or terminated. Ferritin levels should be measured and adjusted if they are too low. The serum ferritin concentration—an indirect measure of brain iron status—should be at least 112.4 pmol/L (50 μg/L) to rule out the possibility that iron deficiency is responsible for RLS, and in our experience it should be closer to 224.7 μmol/L (100 μg/L) (Trenkwalder, Winkelmann, Inoue, & Paulus, 2015). Furthermore, TSAT should be $<20\%$, if a supplementation of iron is scheduled.

4. Treatment of augmentation with drugs approved for RLS therapy

There are some recommendations about drug holidays in augmented patients, but no trials or any study on non-pharmacological treatment of augmentation. In our clinical experience, which comprises more than 200 patients with severe augmentation (Steinke, Trenkwalder, Zimmermann, Sixel-Doring, & Muntean, 2018), drug holidays are a terrible experience for RLS patients and can lead to severe autonomic reactions such as dopamine withdrawal syndrome and are therefore not recommended.

A flow chart has recently been published by the IRLSSG for the treatment of augmentation (Fig. 1).

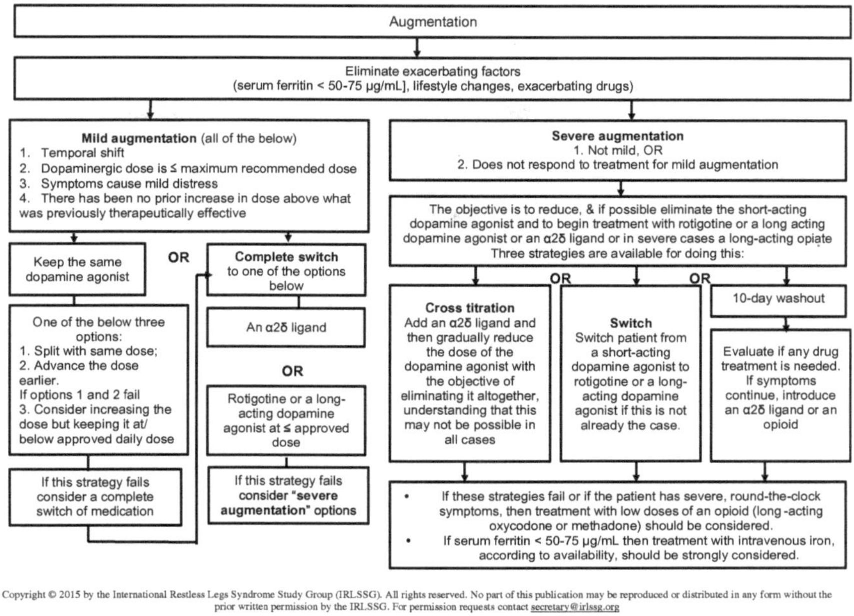

Fig. 1 Augmentation treatment algorithm. Copyright ©2015 by the international Restless Legs Syndrome Study Group (IRLSSG). All rights reserved. No part of this figure may be reproduced or distributed in any form without the prior written permission by the IRLSSG. For permission requests contact secretary@irlssg.org.

With severe augmentation, the reduction of dopaminergic drugs may turn out to be difficult in the first days or weeks due to rebound complaints, which may discourage patients and physicians from further reducing the dosage. In the case of augmentation induced by levodopa a switch to a dopamine agonist at low dose may provide a solution. In case of augmentation induced by a dopamine agonist with a short half-life, e.g., pramipexole, a switch to the rotigotine patch may also provide relief (Trenkwalder, Canelo, et al., 2017), but may not lead to sufficiently treated RLS symptoms when the dosage of a pulsatile dopamine agonist extends the equivalent dosage of for example 2 or 3 mg rotigotine. Switching the patient to one of the α2δ ligands (gabapentin enacarbil, gabapentin, or pregabalin) would be a further option, which has not yet been formally investigated in any RLS augmentation study. The next step would be to switch to opiate therapy, at least during the reduction of the dopaminergic treatment, or when levodopa is stopped (Trenkwalder et al., 2013) and patients cannot tolerate the first days or weeks. During a clinical trial with 1 year of oxycodone/naloxone in severe RLS patients, no cases of augmentation were observed. But even in the case of long-term opioid treatment, a risk of loss of efficacy or augmentation may occur. It is, at present, unclear if an increase in the severity of RLS during long-term opioid therapy is classical RLS augmentation or simply related to opioid-induced hyperalgesia (Ferrini et al., 2013). In case of oxycodone/naloxone in RLS the mean dosages were 10/5–15/7.5 mg slow release oxycodone/naloxone. An interesting question that requires further study is whether such difficult to treat patients would benefit from a low dose of both dopaminergic and opioid receptor stimulation. In almost any area of the brain there is substantial evidence that both systems interact (Li et al., 2016) and that this combination provides more than the sum of its components in terms of RLS symptom release. The latter conclusion reflects the impression of the authors in difficult to treat patients (evidence class IV). A further approach in the latter group consists of a combination of all three drug classes licensed for RLS.

5. Treatment of augmentation with drugs not licensed for RLS (off-label use)

Three strategies of off-label drug use may apply to RLS patients, both with and without augmentation. No systematic review covers the application of any drug in augmentation, but the literature dealing with off-label treatment in RLS may also be of relevance in treating difficult RLS patients once dopaminergic drugs have been removed. One approach pursues the concept of the use of long-half lives of drugs already approved for related diseases**, e.g., slow release pramipexole may be efficient (Maestri et al., 2014). Opiate application therapy with transdermal patch application of fentanyl is quite effective, but not formally studied in RLS to date.

The next approach uses alternative drugs. Drugs that were considered "investigational" ten years ago were dihydroergocriptine, lisuride, methadone, tramadol, clonazepam, zolpidem, amantadine, and topiramate (Trenkwalder, Hening, et al., 2008). At present the situation is as follows: intravenous (IV) ferric carboxymaltose and pneumatic compression devices are considered likely efficacious in idiopathic RLS. Bupropion and clonidine were reviewed, but the lack of data determined a rating of insufficient evidence for efficacy. Iron supplementation with IV iron in particular (Trenkwalder et al., 2017) may be one strategy to avoid augmentation when considered early before dopaminergic treatment starts. According to general treatment recommendations of the IRLSSG in RLS patients, oral iron is non-efficacious in iron-sufficient subjects, "but (65 mg elemental iron) is possibly effective for treating RLS in those with serum ferritin $\leq$75 μg/L (Allen et al., 2018)." This likely also applies for augmented RLS patients, although trials need to confirm this hypothesis.

An ultimate possibility of treatment in difficult to treat patients is the application of intrathecal morphine (Hornyak & Kaube, 2012). Long-term follow up of these rare patients has shown no evidence of the development of tolerance or augmentation, and morphine dosage could even be continuously reduced over time (personal observation).

The advantage of RLS compared to other diseases is that the symptomatic treatment effect becomes clear very soon after treatment initiation, generally within days.

6. Conclusion

Augmentation is per definition induced by too much dopaminergic treatment, over time and/or in dose. The best treatment is prevention, either by starting and ensuring a low dose of dopaminergic treatment and a great deal of awareness of the problem or by starting treatment with a drug from a different class. Following the occurrence of augmentation, dopaminergic treatment must be reduced or eliminated, serum ferritin levels need to be increased substantially above those accepted as normal in hematological diseases and drug treatment should be changed to alternative drugs such as $\alpha 2\delta$ ligands or opiates, or to a combination therapy. As RLS augmentation has been identified as a significant long-term treatment complication for dopamine agonists special monitoring for augmentation is required for all dopaminergic medications as well as for tramadol (Winkelmann et al., 2018).

Conflict of interest statement

C.T. reports personal fees from Paracelsus-Elena-Klinik Kassel, research grants from MJ Fox and EU Horizon 2020 outside the submitted work. C.T. has received honoraries for educational lectures from UCB, Otsouka and Grünenthal.

W.P. reports fees in the area of transcranial electric stimulation and normal pressure hydrocephalus, outside the submitted work.

References

Allen, R. P. (2014). Pregabalin versus pramipexole for restless legs syndrome. *The New England Journal of Medicine*, *370*(21), 2050–2051. https://doi.org/10.1056/NEJMc1402987.

Allen, R. P., Chen, C., Garcia-Borreguero, D., Polo, O., DuBrava, S., Miceli, J., et al. (2014). Comparison of pregabalin with pramipexole for restless legs syndrome. *The New England Journal of Medicine*, *370*(7), 621–631. https://doi.org/10.1056/NEJMoa1303646.

Allen, R. P., & Earley, C. J. (1996). Augmentation of the restless legs syndrome with carbidopa/levodopa. *Sleep*, *19*(3), 205–213.

Allen, R. P., Picchietti, D. L., Auerbach, M., Cho, Y. W., Connor, J. R., Earley, C. J., et al. (2018). Evidence-based and consensus clinical practice guidelines for the iron treatment of restless legs syndrome/Willis-Ekbom disease in adults and children: An IRLSSG task force report. *Sleep Medicine*, *41*, 27–44. https://doi.org/10.1016/j.sleep.2017.11.1126.

Clemens, S., & Ghorayeb, I. (2019). D3 and D1 receptors: The yin and yang in the treatment of restless legs syndrome with dopaminergics. In S. Clemens (Ed.), *Advances in pharmacology, The pharmacology of restless leg syndrome* (Vol. 84). Elsevier, pp. 79–100.

Ferrini, F., Trang, T., Mattioli, T. A., Laffray, S., Del'Guidice, T., Lorenzo, L. E., et al. (2013). Morphine hyperalgesia gated through microglia-mediated disruption of neuronal Cl(−) homeostasis. *Nature Neuroscience*, *16*(2), 183–192. https://doi.org/10.1038/nn.3295.

Garcia-Borreguero, D., Allen, R. P., Kohnen, R., Hogl, B., Trenkwalder, C., Oertel, W., et al. (2007). Diagnostic standards for dopaminergic augmentation of restless legs syndrome: Report from a world association of sleep medicine-International restless legs syndrome study group consensus conference at the Max Planck Institute. *Sleep Medicine*, *8*(5), 520–530. https://doi.org/10.1016/j.sleep.2007.03.022.

Garcia-Borreguero, D., Silber, M. H., Winkelman, J. W., Hogl, B., Bainbridge, J., Buchfuhrer, M., et al. (2016). Guidelines for the first-line treatment of restless legs syndrome/Willis-Ekbom disease, prevention and treatment of dopaminergic augmentation: A combined task force of the IRLSSG, EURLSSG, and the RLS-foundation. *Sleep Medicine*, *21*, 1–11. https://doi.org/10.1016/j.sleep.2016.01.017.

Hogl, B., Garcia-Borreguero, D., Trenkwalder, C., Ferini-Strambi, L., Hening, W., Poewe, W., et al. (2011). Efficacy and augmentation during 6 months of double-blind pramipexole for restless legs syndrome. *Sleep Medicine*, *12*(4), 351–360. https://doi.org/10.1016/j.sleep.2010.12.007.

Hornyak, M., & Kaube, H. (2012). Long-term treatment of a patient with severe restless legs syndrome using intrathecal morphine. *Neurology*, *79*(24), 2361–2362. https://doi.org/10.1212/WNL.0b013e318278b5e7.

Klinker, F., Hasan, K., Dowling, P., Paulus, W., & Liebetanz, D. (2011). Dopamine D(3) receptor deficiency sensitizes mice to iron deficiency-related deficits in motor learning. *Behavioural Brain Research*, *220*(2), 358–361. https://doi.org/10.1016/j.bbr.2011.02.022.

Klinker, F., Kohnemann, K., Paulus, W., & Liebetanz, D. (2017). Dopamine D3 receptor status modulates sexual dimorphism in voluntary wheel running behavior in mice. *Behavioural Brain Research*, *333*, 235–241. https://doi.org/10.1016/j.bbr.2017.06.043.

Li, C., Sugam, J. A., Lowery-Gionta, E. G., McElligott, Z. A., McCall, N. M., Lopez, A. J., et al. (2016). Mu opioid receptor modulation of dopamine neurons in the periaqueductal gray/dorsal raphe: A role in regulation of pain. *Neuropsychopharmacology*, *41*(8), 2122–2132. https://doi.org/10.1038/npp.2016.12.

Liu, G. J., Wu, L., Wang, S. L., Ding, L., Xu, L. L., Wang, Y. F., et al. (2016). Incidence of augmentation in primary restless legs syndrome patients may not be that high: Evidence from a systematic review and meta-analysis. *Medicine (Baltimore)*, *95*(2), e2504. https://doi.org/10.1097/MD.0000000000002504.

Maestri, M., Fulda, S., Ferini-Strambi, L., Zucconi, M., Marelli, S., Staedler, C., et al. (2014). Polysomnographic record and successful management of augmentation in restless legs syndrome/Willis-Ekbom disease. *Sleep Medicine*, *15*(5), 570–575. https://doi.org/10.1016/j.sleep.2014.01.016.

Oertel, W., Trenkwalder, C., Benes, H., Ferini-Strambi, L., Hogl, B., Poewe, W., et al. (2011). Long-term safety and efficacy of rotigotine transdermal patch for moderate-to-severe idiopathic restless legs syndrome: A 5-year open-label extension study. *Lancet Neurology*, *10*(8), 710–720. https://doi.org/10.1016/S1474-4422(11)70127-2.

Paulus, W., & Trenkwalder, C. (2006). Less is more: Pathophysiology of dopaminergic-therapy-related augmentation in restless legs syndrome. *Lancet Neurology*, *5*(10), 878–886. https://doi.org/10.1016/S1474-4422(06)70576-2.

Steinke, S. S., Trenkwalder, C., Zimmermann, J., Sixel-Doring, F., & Muntean, M. L. (2018). Polysomnographic findings in restless legs syndrome (RLS) patients with severe augmentation. *Sleep Medicine*, *48*, 79–85. https://doi.org/10.1016/j.sleep.2018.04.010.

Trenkwalder, C., Allen, R., Hogl, B., Clemens, S., Patton, S., Schormair, B., et al. (2018). Comorbidities, treatment, and pathophysiology in restless legs syndrome. *Lancet Neurology*, *17*(11), 994–1005. https://doi.org/10.1016/S1474-4422(18)30311-9.

Trenkwalder, C., Allen, R., Hogl, B., Paulus, W., & Winkelmann, J. (2016). Restless legs syndrome associated with major diseases: A systematic review and new concept. *Neurology*, *86*(14), 1336–1343. https://doi.org/10.1212/WNL.0000000000002542.

Trenkwalder, C., Benes, H., Grote, L., Garcia-Borreguero, D., Hogl, B., Hopp, M., et al. (2013). Prolonged release oxycodone-naloxone for treatment of severe restless legs syndrome after failure of previous treatment: A double-blind, randomised, placebo-controlled trial with an open-label extension. *Lancet Neurology*, *12*(12), 1141–1150. https://doi.org/10.1016/S1474-4422(13)70239-4.

Trenkwalder, C., Benes, H., Poewe, W., Oertel, W. H., Garcia-Borreguero, D., de Weerd, A. W., et al. (2008). Efficacy of rotigotine for treatment of moderate-to-severe restless legs syndrome: A randomised, double-blind, placebo-controlled trial. *Lancet Neurology*, 7(7), 595–604. https://doi.org/10.1016/S1474-4422(08)70112-1.

Trenkwalder, C., Canelo, M., Lang, M., Schroeder, H., Kelling, D., Berkels, R., et al. (2017). Management of augmentation of restless legs syndrome with rotigotine: A 1-year observational study. *Sleep Medicine*, *30*, 257–265. https://doi.org/10.1016/j.sleep.2015.10.006.

Trenkwalder, C., Hening, W. A., Montagna, P., Oertel, W. H., Allen, R. P., Walters, A. S., et al. (2008). Treatment of restless legs syndrome: An evidence-based review and implications for clinical practice. *Movement Disorders*, *23*(16), 2267–2302. https://doi.org/10.1002/mds.22254.

Trenkwalder, C., Hogl, B., Benes, H., & Kohnen, R. (2008). Augmentation in restless legs syndrome is associated with low ferritin. *Sleep Medicine*, *9*(5), 572–574. https://doi.org/10.1016/j.sleep.2007.07.020.

Trenkwalder, C., Winkelmann, J., Inoue, Y., & Paulus, W. (2015). Restless legs syndrome-current therapies and management of augmentation. *Nature Reviews. Neurology*, *11*(8), 434–445. https://doi.org/10.1038/nrneurol.2015.122.

Trenkwalder, C., Winkelmann, J., Oertel, W., Virgin, G., Roubert, B., & Mezzacasa, A. (2017). Ferric carboxymaltose in patients with restless legs syndrome and nonanemic iron deficiency: A randomized trial. *Movement Disorders*, *32*(10), 1478–1482. https://doi.org/10.1002/mds.27040.

Winkelmann, J., Allen, R. P., Hogl, B., Inoue, Y., Oertel, W., Salminen, A. V., et al. (2018). Treatment of restless legs syndrome: Evidence-based review and implications for clinical practice (Revised 2017)(section sign). *Movement Disorders*, *33*(7), 1077–1091. https://doi.org/10.1002/mds.27260.

Wood, M., Dubois, V., Scheller, D., & Gillard, M. (2015). Rotigotine is a potent agonist at dopamine D1 receptors as well as at dopamine D2 and D3 receptors. *British Journal of Pharmacology*, *172*(4), 1124–1135. https://doi.org/10.1111/bph.12988.

FSC
www.fsc.org
MIX
Papier | Fördert gute Waldnutzung
FSC® C083411

Kolibri 360 GmbH
Ferdinand-Jühlke-Straße 7
99095 Erfurt, Deutschland
produktsicherheit@kolibri360.de